T4-AHH-556

Lungara

Assisting in emergencies

a resource handbook
for UNICEF field staff

Prepared for UNICEF by Ron Ockwell

United Nations Children's Fund
May 1986

© United Nations Children's Fund, 1986

UNICEF House, EMOP
Three United Nations Plaza
New York, NY 10017, USA

UNICEF, EMOP
Palais des Nations
CH-1211 Geneva 10, Switzerland

ISBN : 92-806-3147-0

First printing: 1986
Second printing: 1988
Third printing: 1992
Fourth printing: 1994

This *Handbook* is also being issued in French and, eventually, Spanish.

Parts 2,3 and 5 may be reproduced, translated into other languages or adapted to meet local needs without prior permission from UNICEF, provided (a) that parts used are distributed free or at cost – not for profit, and (b) acknowledgment is given to UNICEF as the original source.

The Emergency Operations Unit (EMOP), UNICEF, New York would be grateful to receive copies of any adaptations or translations into other languages.

Foreword

UNICEF has, since its inception in 1946, played a prominent role in focusing the attention of governments and people around the world on the particular needs of children and extending co-operation to assist a wide variety of programmes benefiting children in all kinds of situations.

In the context of promoting and assisting actions which help to assure the survival and healthy development of children, UNICEF gives particular attention to children in the most deprived communities and the least developed countries. The "silent emergencies" which are the reality of the daily lives of many millions of children around the world and the promotion of cost-effective ways of tackling such situations is necessarily UNICEF's main focus, but the particular needs of children in "loud" emergencies as a result of drought, war, and other disasters which often command the world's headlines also call for appropriate, urgent and sometimes substantial responses from UNICEF.

This *Handbook* has therefore been prepared as a practical tool to help UNICEF field staff—and all those who collaborate with UNICEF and the UN system in general—to meet the needs of children in as appropriate a manner as possible wherever they are affected by such disasters.

This first edition is the result of considerable consultation both within UNICEF and with other collaborating organizations and individuals. It is hoped that it will in future be improved in the light of continuing experience and the contributions of all who seek to assure the well-being of the most vulnerable of all people and the most valuable resource for the future—the young child.

James P. Grant

Acknowledgements

Ron Ockwell, who has prepared and produced this *Handbook*, worked for UNICEF in the emergency relief and rehabilitation operations in Nigeria (1969-71), Bangladesh (1971-75), Kampuchea/Thailand (1979-80) and the Sahel (1984), and in inter-agency liaison in connection with emergencies, in Geneva, (1981-82). He also works as a consultant analyst on information systems in social services in England.

Many other people have contributed suggestions for the content of this *Handbook* and/or reviewed and commented on parts of the drafts. UNICEF is grateful to all who have so given of their time and expertise — many staff of UNICEF and WHO and other individuals including S. Cairncross, P. Diskett, J. Howard, T. Jeggle, M. Lowgren, T. Lusty, N. & S. Morris, A. Moser, E. Ressler, J. Seaman, J. & J. Williamson and others.

The chapters on assessment and programming and the sectoral elements in Parts 3 and 5 have drawn heavily on many of the existing publications which are listed as "further references" in the various annexes, especially those of WHO, FAO, UNHCR, UNDRO, the Ross Institute, OXFAM, the International Disaster Institute and the study on unaccompanied children in emergencies.

UNICEF is also grateful to WHO, FAO, UNHCR, OXFAM, the Ross Institute and Oxford University Press for permission to reproduce certain tables and diagrams in Part 5. The sources are noted in each case.

The credit for whatever may be good about the *Handbook* is therefore widely shared. The responsibility for any errors or omissions rests, however, with the author and UNICEF. Suggestions for corrections and improvements should be sent to:
The Emergency Operations Unit,
UNICEF, 866 UN Plaza,
New York, N.Y.10017, USA.

Preface

Purpose

This *Handbook* has been prepared to help UNICEF field staff to co-operate with governments, local administrations and other organizations in identifying the particular needs of children in various kinds of emergency situations, and in planning and organizing actions to meet those needs in the most appropriate manner.

It is a "resource book" to be turned to when specific guidance or information is required, and to be scanned when you want to be reminded of aspects to consider.

It brings together as much as possible of the information which may be needed to help determine priorities, plan programmes and define what, if any, inputs from UNICEF might be appropriate. The technical guidelines are derived/summarized from many of the existing publications of other competent organizations and incorporate the lessons of UNICEF's experience. A rudimentary understanding of UNICEF procedures and forms is assumed.

Structure

Part 1 provides very brief guidelines/aide-mémoire concerning UNICEF policies and organizational arrangements for emergencies.

Part 2 contains similarly brief guidelines for making assessments, formulating assistance proposals, managing and monitoring implementation, and making final evaluations.

Part 3 suggests the kinds of needs which might arise in different situations and the specific kind of role and interventions which might be appropriate for UNICEF within the larger context of the overall emergency assistance operation.

Part 4 summarizes aspects to which attention may need to be given to assure efficient operations within a UNICEF field office, and provides a brief summary of relevant organizational rules and procedures.

In Part 5, 36 separate "annexes" provide specific guidelines for various kinds of programme interventions which might be appropriate in particular circumstances.

Part 6 contains a number of additional annexes concerning various aspects of organizational procedures, including sample formats for telexes, etc.

Summary notes on "What to do when confronted by an emergency", objectives for UNICEF and a table suggesting the needs which may arise in different types of emergency follow the table of contents. An alphabetical index is included at the back.

Using the *Handbook*

Guidance regarding UNICEF policies, programming processes and requirements, field office operations, etc., should be quickly found in Parts 1, 2 and 4 through reference to the table of contents.

If initial assessment has indicated that needs exist in a particular sector (food supplies, health, etc.), refer to the appropriate chapter in Part 3 for guidelines concerning detailed aspects to be considered and the kind of response interventions which might be appropriate.

When the necessity for action to meet a particular kind of need has been identified, refer to the relevant annex in Part 5 for guidelines as to what may need to be done and defined in planning and organizing such an activity, and the kind of inputs which might be considered.

In Parts 1, 2 and 4 references are given under each sub-heading to the corresponding section/sub-section of the desk manual (Book E of the UNICEF Field Manual) where further details and explanations can be found.

In Part 5, lists are provided at the end of each annex of other publications which may be referred to for additional information, and which will be useful to those who are responsible for the actual management of programmes and the delivery of services in the field. The letters E/F/S/A after each reference indicate the languages—English, French, Spanish, Arabic respectively—in which the publications are available.

Preparedness and recognition

Guidelines for actions to be taken to be prepared to respond effectively when emergencies occur, to alert populations to impending hazards and to recognize the early signs of slow-onset situations (especially droughts) are provided in the desk manual. They are summarized only very briefly in Annex 1.

Abbreviations used in this *Handbook*

Organizations

FAO	Food and Agriculture Organization of the United Nations
ICRC	International Committee of the Red Cross
ILO	International Labour Organisation
LRCS	League of Red Cross and Red Crescent Societies
PAHO	Pan American Health Organization (Regional Office of WHO)
UN	United Nations
UNDP	United Nations Development Programme
UNDRO	Office of the United Nations Disaster Relief Co-ordinator
UNESCO	United Nations Educational, Scientific and Cultural Organization
UNHCR	United Nations High Commissioner for Refugees
UNICEF	United Nations Children's Fund
UNIPAC	UNICEF Supply Division (Procurement and Assembly Centre), Copenhagen
UNRC	United Nations Resident Co-ordinator
WFP	World Food Programme
WHO	World Health Organization

UNICEF in-house abbreviations

AS	Adminstrative services (in NYHQ)
BAL	Basic assistance list
CCF	Cash call-forward
CRC	Contract review committee
DIPA	Division of information and public affairs
DOP	Division of personnel
EOU	Emergency operations unit (in NYHQ)
GEHQ	Geneva office
GS	General service (level of staff appointments)
LPO	Local purchase order
NPO	National professional officer
NYHQ	New York headquarters
PA	Procurement authorization
PAM	Personnel Administration Manual
PFO	Programme funding office
RSDS	Recruitment and staff development section (in NYHQ)
SCF	Supply call-forward
SIMS	Supply input monitoring system
SL(N)	Supply list (non-standard: items not in UNIPAC catalogue)
TA	Travel authorization
TAD	Target arrival date

Other common abbreviations

$	United States dollars
CSM	Corn-soya-milk (blended food)
DPT	Diphtheria-pertussis-tetanus (vaccine)
DSM	Dried skim milk
EPI	Expanded programme of immunization
ETA	Estimated time of arrival
FCM	Full cream milk powder
FFW	Food-for-work
FPC	Fish protein concentrate
HEM	"High energy milk" (feeding mixture)
ICSM	Instant corn-soya-milk
MCH	Mother and child health
MUAC	Mid-upper-arm circumference
NGO	Non-governmental organization
ORS	Oral rehydration salts
PEM	Protein-energy malnutrition
SFP/C	Supplementary feeding programme/centre
TFP/C	Therapeutic feeding programme/centre
WSB	Wheat-soya blend (blended food)

Measures

cm	centimetre
g	gram
ha	hectare
kg	kilogram
m	metre
ml	millilitre
MT	metric ton
m^3 or cu m	cubic metre

Abbreviations for other measures and conversion factors between metric, British and US units are given in Annex 53.

Contents

Part 4 FIELD OFFICE OPERATIONS

Part 5 GUIDELINES FOR PROGRAMME INTERVENTIONS

Food, nutrition and income

Health

Water supplies

Part 6 REFERENCE ANNEXES

Sample formats for:

SUMMARY NOTES

The following pages provide a very brief summary—aide mémoire—of the objectives and probable priorities for UNICEF in different kinds of emergencies, and the essential actions to be taken by a UNICEF Representative/field office.

What to do when confronted by an emergency

Immediate actions

In all cases a UNICEF representative must collaborate with the responsible government departments, the UN Resident Co-ordinator and other concerned agencies (UN and NGOs) to:

• Rapidly, systematically assemble and review all data available on the area and all reports on the current situation.

• Make a rapid initial assessment focusing on the particular situation and needs of young children:

—Participate in and/or organize joint field assessment visits;

—Collect information from all sources;

—Identify and seek to fill any gaps in the information available;

—Build-up an overview of the situation and needs so that priorities can be rationally determined.

• Organize any limited inputs immediately necessary to save lives.

• Ensure that thorough assessments are made of sectors in which significant problems/needs exist or may be anticipated. Mobilize appropriate technical expertise as soon as the need for such is identified.

• Formulate and carefully prioritize specific proposals for any substantial assistance necessary from UNICEF. Maintain a dialogue with HQ during this process to ensure necessary support and resource mobilization, and get final approval from NYHQ.

During programme implementation:

• Monitor and assist programme operations continuously; adjust interventions as necessary; maintain close and continuous co-ordination with all others concerned throughout the entire process.

Priorities

● Ensure that proposed interventions form a coherent, integrated package of practical measures which meet specifically identified priority needs—a "programme" with clear objectives.

● Concentrate on children in the most deprived communities and the most "vulnerable" households. Give particular attention to the needs of destitute and single-parent families, and unaccompanied children.

● Seek ways of increasing the capacity of families to care adequately for their children. Try to ensure that their health, nutritional and other physical needs, and their emotional/psychological needs are met in line with the principles and priorities suggested.

● Advocate to government and others any strengthening or modification of policies or practices which is believed to be desirable for the ultimate well-being of children and their families.

● Promote awareness among media and donor representatives of the situation and needs of children.

● Reinforce government capacity and, if necessary, assist directly to ensure expeditious implementation and efficient utilization of UNICEF resources.

Actions to ensure efficient UNICEF response:

● If there are security risks, take reasonable precautions to ensure the safety of UNICEF personnel and equipment in co-ordination with the UN Resident Co-ordinator. Keep NYHQ informed.

● Clearly define responsibilities within the local UNICEF office(s), establish temporary field outposts and/or an operations room in the country office if necessary.

● Redeploy available staff, mobilize in-country expertise and ask for temporary additional staff if necessary to ensure sufficient capacity and expertise for all aspects and phases of operations.

● Ensure efficient local financial arrangements (and cash flow) to support approved field operations.

● Provide the best possible specifications for all supplies and personnel required.

● Keep HQ continuously informed on the situation, actions taken, proposals being developed, and supplies which might be needed. Telex sitreps regularly.

● Address all reports and major communications to Chief EOU/NYHQ (or other designated focal point) repeated simultaneously to GEHQ and the Regional Director.

Objectives for UNICEF

Major objectives	Activities which might need to be strengthened, intensified or initiated.

Food, nutrition and income

▶ Ensure that sufficient and appropriate food is available and able to be prepared for infants, young children, pregnant and lactating mothers—in both the short and long terms.

▶ Ensure the identification and appropriate treatment of children suffering from severe malnutrition.

(See Chapter 8)

Restoring/adapting/intensifying local agricultural production and market exchange systems—seeds, tools, irrigation, support to co-operatives, etc. (*Annex 2*)

In the mean time, employment (cash-for-work / food-for-work) programmes, food grants and/or general free food distributions where necessary to ensure that all population groups have access to sufficient basic food to maintain reasonable nutritional health. (*Annex 2*)

Weaning foods: assuring mothers are able to obtain and prepare suitable foods—suitable food items, demonstrations, etc. Breast-feeding: providing for infants whose mothers have been lost or cannot lactate. (*Annex 3*)

Nutrition status surveys/screening to determine and monitor the nutritional status of various communities, establish priorities and, where necessary, to select the most malnourished children for admission to special, selective feeding programmes—expertise, funds. (*Annex 4*)

Therapeutic feeding (nutrition rehabilitation) for severely malnourished children—equipment, funds, etc. (*Annex 6*)

Supplementary" feeding for selected vulnerable groups *may*, in some situations, also be appropriate to ensure the health of new-born infants and prevent deterioration of the nutritional condition of young children and other particularly vulnerable individuals. (*Annex 5*)

Health

▶ Ensure that measures are taken to tackle any immediate health problems affecting children and their mothers, and to protect them against foreseeable health risks.

Reinforcing personnel to ensure the efficient organization and delivery of essential health care at community level (in the context of sustainable long-term services)—funding posts, training. (*Annex 8*)

▶Ensure that essential health care services for children and their mothers are provided/restored as quickly as possible and in a way to encourage and facilitate further development and improvement through subsequent long-term programmes.

(See Chapter 9)

Restoration/provision of facilities and equipment essential for the delivery of basic health care services at community level—repair materials, funds, equipment (sets), transport. *(Annex 9)*

Drugs and essential supplies for community level health services focusing on the illnesses most affecting children—e.g. intestinal parasites, respiratory infections, skin diseases, specific vitamin deficiencies (also taking account of appropriate distribution policies and any local production possibilities). *(Annexes 10, 11)*

Immunization to protect children against measles and other particular, preventable diseases which are (or could become) prevalent in the locality—cold chain, vaccines, etc. *(Annex 12)*

Epidemiological surveillance to detect signs of any particular health problems and enable early action to be taken to contain any outbreak of communicable disease. *(Annex 13)*

Public health and treatment measures to contain any actual outbreaks of communicable disease. *(Annex 14)*

Prevention and treatment of diarrhoeal diseases in children—oral rehydration therapy. *(Annex 15)*

Water supply

▶Ensure the availability of sufficient safe water for hygiene and domestic use at household level and for institutions and services benefiting children.

▶Ensure the availability and efficient use of water for household or community-level food production.

(See Chapter 10)

Distribution and storage of water to conserve and protect available supplies, and make reasonably safe water accessible to community services and all population groups—tanks, pipes, transport, competent technicians, etc. *(Annex 16)*

Rehabilitation and/or new exploitation of water sources—materials, funds, technicians, etc. *(Annex 17)*

Improvement of water quality—by storage, filtration and/or chemical treatment. *(Annex 18)*

Objectives for UNICEF (continued)

Major objectives	Activities which might need to be strengthened, intensified or initiated.

Hygiene and sanitation

▶Prevent the spread of disease and promote the establishment of a safe environment.

▶Provide the means for reasonable personal and domestic hygiene.

(See Chapter 11)

Latrines or other arrangements for the safe disposal of human excreta which minimize risks of contamination of the environment, especially water supplies, or the proliferation of vectors—materials, funds, sanitarians. (Annexes 20, 21)

Facilities for the best possible personal and domestic hygiene—liberal use of soap and water. (Annex 22)

Removal/reduction of other health hazards in the environment; especially control of vectors—chemicals, funds, sanitarians. (Annex 23)

Shelter and household functioning

▶ Safeguard the lives of young children by ensuring the availability of necessary shelter, clothing and household items essential to their survival and the satisfactory functioning of the family units to which they belong.

(See Chapter 12)

Materials to improvise emergency shelter materials (where necessary)—plastic sheeting, tarpaulins, etc. (Annex 24)

Clothing and blankets for young children—where the climate requires; basic household utensils where they cannot be salvaged. (Annex 25)

Child care and psycho-social needs

▶Preserve/restore stable family environments for children and normal community life and services for their benefit.

▶Ensure appropriate care and protection for children who are unaccompanied, and rehabilitation training and services for those who are disabled.

▶Ensure that other children with special needs—physical, psychological or emotional—are provided the particular help and assistance they need.

Community-based social services to: help people to meet their own needs—resolve personal problems and inter-personal conflicts (where necessary)—prevent family separations (where possible)—rehabilitate disabled children. (Annex 27)

Special programmes for unaccompanied children, where necessary, to: arrange care which meets their emotional and developmental as well as physical needs—assure any necessary protection—reunite them with their families (wherever possible and not harmful to their individual emotional, social and psychological needs). (Annex 28)

▶(Re-)Establish any special support services necessary to help parents—especially single parents and those who are destitute—to care for their children.

(See Chapter 13)

Logistics and overall management

▶Ensure the timely delivery to the target communities/institutions of supplies for programmes assisted by UNICEF or otherwise of importance for children.

▶Ensure efficient management of overall operations so that programmes benefiting children are able to be implemented efficiently.

(See Chapter 14)

Additional for displaced populations

▶Avoid the congregation of people in temporary camps, if possible.

▶When displacement is inevitable, ensure basic needs are met.

▶Help displaced families and communities to return to their homes or resettle elsewhere (if necessary) as soon as possible.

(See Chapter 12 and Annex 26)

Restore and develop education in the community, especially for young children and women—materials, funds, training. (Annex 29)

Manpower and expertise to establish and manage the necessary logistic operations expeditiously and efficiently. (Annex 30)

Measures to restore/increase (where necessary) the capacity of ports and airports to receive and on-forward supplies—repairs, generators, other equipment. (Annexes 31, 32, 35)

Measures to deliver supplies to locations within the affected area as and when needed—engaging contractors, using existing trucks, boats, etc., mobilizing additional means of transport. (Annex 33)

Adequate warehousing, equipment and record systems for the storage and handling of materials provided by UNICEF—or provided by others for programmes of concern to UNICEF—at all locations where temporary storage and/or stock-piling is necessary. (Annexes 34, 35, 36)

Measures to minimize health hazards, provide essential services, and make life tolerable for displaced children and families until they can return home or be permanently resettled. (Annex 26)

Practical assistance to "returnees"—tools, seeds, other raw materials, (re-)establishment of services, etc.

Needs which may arise in different types of emergency

Sectors in which UNICEF assistance might be considered

- ■ Needs frequently experienced
- □ Needs sometimes experienced
- C Depending on climate; may be needed if weather is cold and/or wet.
- .. Needs rarely arise (or usually of low priority).

Where disasters occur in combination—e.g. floods following a tropical storm—the combined effects/needs must be considered.

Sector in which needs may arise	Sudden, cataclysmic disasters			Long-term, continuing emergencies		
	Earthquakes	Storms	Floods	Droughts, famines[8]	Conflicts	Displaced populations
Food, nutrition and income						
Short-term general ration distribution	■[1]	■	□	■	■	■
Agricultural production	..[C]	■	■[R]	■	□	■
Long-term selective provision of employment and/or food	□[C]	..	■	■	■	■
Nutrition surveillance[2]	..	□	□	■	□	■
Special feeding[2]	..	..	□	■	□	□
Health services						
Reinforcement of management and personnel	■[3]	□	□	□	■	■
Reconstruction, transport and equipment	■	■	□	..	■	■
Drugs and other supplies	■[3]	..	□	■	■	■
Surveillance for communicable diseases	..	■	□	■	■	■
Immunization	..	..	■	■	□	■
Diarrhoea control	..	..	□	■	□	■
Water supplies						
Distribution, storage, treatment	■[C]	..	■[C]	■	□	■
Rehabilitation/development of sources	■[4]	□[5]	□[5]	■	□[5]	■
Sanitation						
Excreta disposal	■[C]	..	□[C]	..	■	■
Garbage/refuse disposal	■	□	□[C]	..	■	■
Personal hygiene	■[C]	..	□[C]	..	■	■
Vector control	□	..	..	..	■	■

Shelter and household functioning

	Fires, landslides, local floods, tsunamis	Floods, landslides, storm surge	Displaced populations	Displaced populations
Emergency shelter	C[6]	C		C
Reconstruction	■[6]	■		■
Blankets	C	C	□[7]	C
Household utensils etc.	■	□	C[7]	■

Child care and social services

	Fires, landslides, local floods, tsunamis	Floods, landslides, storm surge	Displaced populations	Displaced populations
Community social services	■□□	■□□	■□	■■■
Unaccompanied children	■□■	■□□		■■■
Schools/education				■■■

Overall management and logistics

	Fires, landslides, local floods, tsunamis	Floods, landslides, storm surge	Displaced populations	Displaced populations
Reinforcement of management capacity and systems	■□□	■□□	■□□	■■■
Transport, vehicles, fuel, spares, maintenance				
Storage facilities				

Possible secondary effects/disasters				■ □

U Primarily in urban areas.
R Primarily in rural areas.
1 Only if major irrigation works damaged.
2 Assuring appropriate weaning foods and food for vulnerable groups (possible supplementary feeding); therapeutic feeding for severely malnourished children; combating Vitamin-A or other specific deficiencies.
3 For casualty treatment in first few days only.
4 Only if ground-water flows changed.
5 If wells or usual surface sources contaminated or inaccessible.
6 Depending on the type of construction.
7 Only in cases of destructive "flash" floods (in valleys).
8 "Food emergencies" without displacement.

Volcanic eruptions: Possible needs (and secondary effects) are similar to those for earthquakes within the area directly affected by the eruption. There may be population displacements.

Tsunamis (tidal waves caused by earthquakes): Possible needs are similar to those of tropical storms plus floods, with the added complication of contamination of wells and agricultural land by salt water.

Epidemics: Needs usually include specific drugs, transport, surveillance, improvement of water supplies, personal hygiene and sanitation. Reinforcement of health service management may also been required.

Emergency programming response process

Steps	Questions/decisions for UNICEF	Possible follow-up
1. Initial investigations and immediate response		
Rapidly assemble and analyse all available relevant information	Is immediate UNICEF assistance necessary to assure survival of children and families?	Limited inputs to assure survival: possible diversions, local purchases and, exceptionally, airfreighting if necessary.
Identify any immediate survival needs.	Is UNICEF intervention necessary to assure proper assessment of children's needs?	Advise EOU and UNIPAC of the type and quantities of supplies which *might* be required.
Determine what arrangements being made for thorough assessment.		
Visit field site unless already clear that no UNICEF intervention will be needed	Are additional UNICEF staff needed to help make a thorough assessment?	Request EOU-DOP/NYHQ for extra temporary staff.
2. Thorough assessment		
Co-operate with government, UNDP Res. Rep. and others in assessing for:	Is UNICEF assistance necessary?	Ensure that needs of children are fully considered by government and others.
–Continued survival;	What are the priorities for UNICEF?	
–Recovery and rehabilitation. Focus on particular needs of children.	What kinds of interventions/inputs: –For continued survival? –For recovery and rehabilitation?	Mobilize any necessary specialist personnel available locally.
Identify desirable interventions including possible alternative strategies, their implications and any constraints.	What extra staff and/or specialists are needed to investigate further and develop specific programme proposals?	Request EOU-DOP/NYHQ to seek and assign any extra personnel needed from outside.

Determine local capacity and the assistance plans of others.

Define priorities.

What level of funding might be feasible?

Advise EOU and UNIPAC of the types and quantities of supplies and personnel which could be needed.

Seek indication of feasible funding level.

Regular programme considerations

Assess the impact of events on planned regular programme activities.

Are planned activities still relevant and priority in the new situation?

Should plans be modified?

Review with government; agree any appropriate reprogramming to meet the new situation and priorities.

Inform NYHQ and get approval.

3. Programme formulation

Define for each proposed intervention:
- Specific objectives;
- Target groups, locations, numbers;
- What exactly will be done;
- Mechanisms for implementation;
- Personnel and facilities necessary;
- Material and cash inputs required;
- Logistic support arrangements;
- Implementation schedule;
- Budget.

Prepare concise Plan of Action.

Will resources be needed additional to the existing BAL?

What extra staff/specialists will be required for implementation? (Prepare job descriptions.)

What are the best mechanisms for implementation/distribution

What supplies can be obtained locally? What must be imported?

Inform NYHQ as early as possible of the kind of interventions being envisaged and level of funding which might be needed.

Send details of specific proposals as soon as possible.

Determine whether suitable personnel are available in-country and how their services might be obtained.

Inform UNIPAC and EOU of likely needs for offshore and local procurement.

Continued on next page...

Steps	Questions/decisions for UNICEF	Possible follow-up
4. Approval and agreements		
Obtain NYHQ approval of proposals and authorization to commit funds.		Amend existing BAL and/or raise new one for any extra resources provided.
		Establish agreements/understandings with government and any other involved parties.
		Recommend any local candidates for recruitment to professional posts; request HQ to seek/assign personnel needed from outside.
5. Implementation		
Assist government in setting-up and implementing planned operations.	Are any changes necessary in: –Planned inputs or schedule? –Personnel requirements? –Budget.	Seek HQ approval for specific increases in local purchase authority, petty cash and other financial arrangements believed appropriate and justified.
Monitor operations continously.		Advise NYHQ of any changes in plans.
6. Phase out and evaluation		
Carefully phase out emergency activities into long-term programmes.	What was achieved? What lessons to be learned?	Final report.
Evaluate the emergency programme.		

Part 1 POLICIES AND ORGANIZATION

This Part provides a brief summary of the general policies of UNICEF for responding to emergency situations and responsibilities for deciding and organizing UNICEF co-operation in such situations.

The resources which can be called on are described together with reporting requirements.

Specific guidelines for defining appropriate UNICEF responses within the framework of these policies and arrangements are provided in Parts 2 and 3; guidelines for assuring efficient internal UNICEF operations in Part 4.

Chapter 1

UNICEF POLICIES

What is an emergency?

(Manual 1.1)

... A situation of hardship and human suffering arising from events which cause physical loss or damage, social and/or economic disruption with which the country or community concerned is unable to fully cope alone.

It may result from a "natural disaster"—either high impact (e.g. earthquake) or slow-onset (e.g. drought)—or be of "man-made" causes (e.g. war, civil unrest).

- **The relevance for UNICEF is a particular deterioration in the situation of children and/or a disruption of services on their behalf.**

- **The same policies and principles apply regardless of the causes of the situation or whether the government has declared an "emergency".**

Table 1

Likely effects on young children

The following are some of the most frequent and serious effects:

—Lack of shelter and warmth (leading to respiratory diseases and death in harsh climates);

—Lack of clean water (leading to diarrheoal diseases and dehydration);

—Lack of suitable foods and/or the means to prepare food (leading to malnutrition);

—Loss of or separation from parents and family care;

—Lack of health and social care due to interruption of services;

—Increased exposure to endemic diseases due to disruption of preventive/control programmes and poor sanitation;

—Increased prevalance of measles and other diseases of squalor in crowded camps/settlements.

Children in poor and underpriviledged communities are the most vulnerable: their resistance to hardship and disease is already weak on account of poor nutrition and a precarious state of general health.

A loss or reduction in household income and/or purchasing power can itself precipitate the privations listed above.

In conflict situations, children are sometimes also abducted, conscripted, imprisoned, tortured, abused and even deliberately killed—all in contravention of the Geneva Conventions. They may also be traumatized by the sight of parents and others being killed.

What is the role of UNICEF?

(*Manual 1.2*)

... To try to ensure that the particular needs of children are appropriately met. (This does not, however, mean that UNICEF necessarily has to meet them itself.)

In all cases:

- **Ensure that an adequate assessment is made of the situation and needs of children;** *and*

- **Advocate (to government and others) policies and specific measures which will most appropriately assure the well-being of young children.**

Where found necessary:

- **Assist the government and others in making the assessment and organizing necessary responses;** *and*

- **Provide, within the limits of resources able to be mobilized, material and other inputs required.**

To intervene or not?

If needs are being adequately met by others:
— Do not divert effort and resources from long-term programmes.

If there are important needs of children and mothers which are *not* being covered in time by assistance from other sources, and UNICEF *is* able to deliver and assure timely distribution:
— Help to provide the assistance necessary to ensure the survival of children and the restoration of family life and community services.

UNICEF decisions and response must in all cases be based on a thorough *assessment* which determines not only the apparent needs but also the intentions and capacities of the community concerned, the government, and other agencies (UN, Red Cross and NGOs).

Carefully examine and evaluate all requests for specific assistance: don't just accept and act on them, or refer them to HQ.

Obligations

The fundamental principles of UNICEF assistance also apply in emergencies:

(a) Actions are taken in consultation with and with the consent of the government concerned; *and*

(b) UNICEF shares with the government the responsibility of ensuring that:
— Assistance is dispensed/distributed efficiently, equitably and without discrimination; *and*
— Proper utilization and accountability for the assistance is reasonably assured.

5

What kind of response?

(Manual 1.2)

The type and magnitude of any UNICEF response must necessarily be determined by the:
—Priority needs of children in the actual situation;
—Policies of the government;
—Capabilities, actions and intentions of others;
—Level of resources able to be mobilized; and
—Absorption/implementation capacity.

Within this context, assistance proposed should also be generally in line with the overall policies and priorities of UNICEF—particularly:
—Community participation;
—Preservation of a stable family environment;
—Goals of child survival and development;
and also take account of any special competences (and limitations!) UNICEF may have in the country/area concerned.

Assistance interventions should form a coherent, integrated package designed to meet specifically identified needs—i.e. a "programme" with clear objectives, not disjointed *ad hoc* actions.

Consider implementation capacity as well as "needs". There is little point in expending money and effort in rushing supplies to a country if the capacity does not then exist to deliver them to the communities in need.

Priorities in emergency assistance

Keep any purely "relief" inputs to the minimum necessary and ensure that they are specifically targeted for the most vulnerable.

Once survival is assured, focus effort and resources on the restoration and improvement of community and family life, household production, and the rehabilitation and development of services for children and their mothers.

6 Seize any opportunities for initiating new approaches to meeting these needs.

If other priority needs can be met by other organizations, focus UNICEF efforts on actions which:

— Constitute an *expansion, acceleration and/or adaptation* of ongoing or already planned programme activities where these are relevant to the current situation;

— Help communities and individual households to care adequately for their own children; *and*

— Have the potential to contribute towards the overall goals of UNICEF and the long-term development of the communities concerned (including reducing their vulnerability to future disasters).

Special responsibilities

UNICEF has an interest and responsibility for all aspects affecting the well-being of children. It does not have a specific responsibility for any particular sector.

If requested to "co-ordinate" efforts and assistance in any sector (e.g. child feeding or water supply):

— Consider the implications carefully and ensure that the role is clearly defined; *and*

— Ensure that UNICEF has on the spot—or can rapidly make available—the necessary management and technical capacity.

What resources are available?

(*Manual 2.2*)

Diversions

Up to $25,000 worth (supplies and/or cash) from regular programmes on agreement between the Representative and the government.

Reprogramming

Unlimited reallocation of existing commitments (of general resources) subject to government agreement and NYHQ's approval.

Emergency reserve

Additional funds subject to Executive Director's approval through EOU.

Specific purpose contributions

Funds received in response to a special appeal issued by the Executive Director, or jointly by UN.

Noted projects or Special Board allocations

Additional UNICEF funds approved by NYHQ and Executive Board.

Except for diversions, convey (telex) proposals to EOU/NYHQ with sufficient detail and explanation for them to be evaluated, approved and funded: see p. 42

Diversions and reprogramming remain charged to existing BAL and call-forward ceiling. Other sources are additional to the existing BAL and ceiling.

Noted project funds can be reprogrammed only with the prior approval of the donor(s) concerned.

In some situations, in-kind donations may also be appropriate and available: see p. 154

Co-ordinating within the UN and with others

(Manual 1.3)

Ensure close informal as well as formal collaboration and co-ordination with other UN agencies, bilateral assistance organizations, the Red Cross/Crescent and non-governmental organizations (NGOs). Co-operate fully with co-ordinating groups/mechanisms established by the government, the UNDP Resident Representative and others.

Within the UN

- **Co-operate fully with UNDP Resident Representative who co-ordinates UN response at country level and is the representative of UNDRO.**

- **Maintain close and continuous direct contacts also with representatives of WFP, WHO, FAO, UNHCR and any UNDRO personnel present.**

- **Help to ensure good liaison and co-ordination between the UN Team and NGOs.**

- **Ensure that the UN Team is at all times fully informed of UNICEF's assessment of the situation and needs of children, the actual and planned inputs of UNICEF, and any requirement for additional funds.**

Within the UN, agencies are responsible to take actions in response to emergencies in accordance with their own areas of competence, their respective mandates and the resources available to them, within an overall, co-ordinated "team" approach. The specific roles of UNDRO, UNDP and others are briefly summarized in Annex 46.

For major/complex emergencies a UN "lead entity" or special representative of the Secretary General may be appointed and then be responsible for co-ordination. Executive Board approval is necessary before UNICEF could accept a "lead entity" role.

Co-operation is often informal to assure a complementarity between agencies' actions. Formal agreements should normally be established for any jointly financed projects.

With bilateral and other aid organizations

- **Establish and maintain close contact with local representatives of the EEC, major bilateral donors and other organizations providing emergency and development assistance.**

This is in addition to ensuring co-ordination with their assistance operations through established government and UN mechanisms.

Try to ensure the complementary use/allocation of resources, including any directly at the disposal of the local missions. Promote joint field visits and meetings with government where appropriate.

With Red Cross/Crescent and NGOs

- **Co-ordinate closely with the Red Cross/Cresent and NGOs in all aspects and phases of response.**

- **Co-operate with any co-ordinating mechanisms which exist between NGOs. Promote the establishment of co-ordinating mechanisms if they do not already exist.**

- **Consider joint projects where appropriate and the government approves. See Chapter 5, p. 40.**

The Red Cross/Crescent and NGOs are often able to act very quickly at community level, especially where they were already established with long-term programmes in the area before the emergency.

CHAPTER 2.

RESPONSIBILITIES AND ORGANIZATION

Responsibilities for UNICEF response

(Manual 3.1, 3.2)

The UNICEF Representative* is responsible for ensuring that the situation and needs of children are adequately assessed, for determining what—if anything—might be an appropriate response from UNICEF, and co-operating with the responsible national authorities in organizing any such programmes. See Table 2.

The Executive Director remains ultimately responsible for UNICEF actions and performance and he, or specifically delegated senior staff, is finally responsible for overall policy aspects and approving any proposed, significant UNICEF response.

---

* In some situations, another staff member may be specifically assigned by the Executive Director to plan and manage UNICEF's response in the particular situation.

The case of a sub-office

If an emergency occurs in a country where there is only a UNICEF sub-office, the Representative either delegates responsibility—with corresponding authority—to staff resident on the spot, or immediately proceeds to the country to fulfill his/her responsibilities directly.

If communications are cut between the afflicted country and that where the Representative is located, resident staff should—until contact is re-established with the Representative, HQ or the Regional Director—assume the responsibilities and follow, to the best of their abilities, the guidelines provided in this *Handbook* and the *UNICEF Field Manual,* Book E.

A Representative may also request the UNDP Resident Representative to propose any appropriate UNICEF interventions or, in instances of broken communications, the regional office or HQ may establish contact directly with UNDP.

Table 2

Specific responsibilities of Representatives

All aspects outlined in Parts 2 and 4 of this *Handbook*! In particular, assuring:

—Understandings with government and co-operation with other agencies;

—Thorough and expeditious assessments which identify the real needs of children and the most appropriate and practical ways of meeting them;

—Appropriate formulation of proposals for UNICEF co-operation;

—Effective and efficient implementation with close monitoring, carefully planned phasing out and appropriate evaluation;

—Efficient operations within the country office with attention to any security aspects as well as normal "support" functions;

—Appropriate handling of relations with the media and donor representatives at the country level; *and*

—Regular and comprehensive reporting to NYHQ repeated simultaneously to GEHQ and the regional director.

An important element is redeploying available *staff* and recognizing when specific additional staff support and/or expertise is needed, requesting such assistance promptly, and mobilizing personnel who as are available in-country.

HQ and regional office organization

(*Manual 3.3*)

The Emergency Operations Unit (EOU), NYHQ

The Chief/EOU, working closely with the relevant programme desks, is responsible (*inter alia*) for:
— Ensuring the co-ordination of actions of all HQ divisions in responding to the needs of field offices co-operating in emergency situations;
— Providing policy and technical guidance to field offices on the planning and general management of emergency assistance operations;
— Administering the emergency reserve and endorsing to the Executive Director any proposals for releases and/or appeals for specific purpose contributions; *and*
— Co-ordinating at the international level with the U.N. and other concerned agencies in respect of emergency assistance operations.

In the case of a major emergency requiring a substantial response from UNICEF, a "*task force*" is established within NYHQ bringing together designated representatives of all concerned divisions to ensure maximum co-ordination and effective response to field needs.

In all instances, a "*focal point*" will be designated in NYHQ. This will usually be the Chief/EOU.

The Emergency Desk, GEHQ

The Emergency Officer/GEHQ works in close collaboration with the Chief/EOU and is responsible for:
— Liaison and co-ordination with UNDRO and the other humanitarian organizations/agencies based in Geneva and elsewhere in Europe; *and*
— Supporting the vital public information and fund raising functions of GEHQ (particularly through the National Committees for UNICEF and the EEC).

The desk also helps, when appropriate, to facilitate communications between field offices, NYHQ and UNIPAC.

Regional offices

The Regional Director and the regional advisors are available to provide advice and guidance. Staff of the regional office may be among the first to be mobilized to provide temporary, additional assistance to offices within the region which need such support.

The regional supply officer may, depending on local and regional markets and transport possibilities, have a major role in arranging delivery of urgently needed supplies. The regional information officer will provide guidance and support in media relations.

Supply Division/UNIPAC

UNIPAC maintains a stockpile of items frequently required in emergencies (see catalogue pink pages) and assures rapid dispatch of any items in stock in the warehouse. Procurement and shipment of other supplies is undertaken on an accelerated basis—subject to adequate specifications and full call-forward details being provided.

What help is available?

(*Manual 3.3*)

Help available within UNICEF

Additional, temporary personnel:
    HQ; regional office; staff roster; recruitments (see Chapter 15).

General policy and programme advice and guidance:
    EOU (NYHQ and GEHQ); regional office.

Guidance on dealing with donors and media:
    EOU; PFO; DIPA; regional office (see Chapter 19).

Specifications for supplies:
    UNIPAC; regional supply officer.

Preparation of documentation:
    Area/regional office; EOU/NYHQ.

Where to look for help elsewhere

Technical advice for programmes:
- WHO Co-ordinator and experts; FAO Representative and experts; ILO and other agency experts.
- National training and research institutes.
- Regional training and research bodies.
- Bilateral and other technical assistance personnel—e.g. EEC, USAID, Ford Foundation, etc.
- Non-governmental organizations (NGOs) already working in the field.

Guidance and practical assistance in logistics:
- WFP; ILO; bilateral aid organizations; major NGOs.
- Reputable clearing and forwarding agencies.
- National transport and storage organizations.

Additional, temporary personnel:
- National research and training institutes.
- NGOs.

Reporting

(*Manual 3.4*)

Send all communications and reports concerning emergencies to Chief EOU/NYHQ (unless another focal point has been specifically designated) and repeat them simultaneously to GEHQ (for the emergency officer) and the Regional Director.

When preparing reports, remember that up-to-date information is essential to HQ for: internal management—public information—appeals and reports to donors—co-ordination with other agencies at the international level; etc.

Recognition-surveillance data

For slow-onset situations:
- Send regular summary reports of data concerning selected "indicators" with comments and interpretation.
- Send Sitrep 01 when it is decided that some action is to be taken.

Emergency alert

As soon as a sudden emergency strikes, send an alert telex. Follow up with Sitrep 01.

"Sitreps"

- Telex/cable Sitrep 01 within the first few days after an emergency strikes (or is recognized): include as much detail as is available of the nature of the situation, any action taken and any recommendations for further action by UNICEF.

- Send further details, as they become available, in subsequent sitreps.

For Sitrep 01, use the format provided in Annex 37. For subsequent sitreps, use the format provided in Annex 38.

Agree an appropriate frequency of reporting with EOU/NYHQ. In major emergencies, sitreps might be sent *daily* during the first phase of operations: otherwise as agreed—but not less than *weekly*.

Other Reports

Prepare written, narrative reports at fixed intervals. Agree the frequency—every one to three months—with EOU/NYHQ.

Pouch to EOU/NYHQ, GEHQ and the regional office copies of field visit reports by UNICEF personnel and others, and minutes of significant meetings.

For large-scale operations—and any taking place in particularly difficult and sensitive circumstances—keep a simple chronological record (a diary) of all significant events and decisions; also a complete chrono file. Start these at the very beginning.

Important considerations

- If any of the information contained in a sitrep should *not* be used for public information purposes, say so explicitly in the sitrep itself.

- Be precise; choose your words carefully.

- **To the extent possible, agree terminology and figures with the representatives of other major agencies involved.**

Do not simply refer to "affected populations" and people "at risk". Specify the *way* in which the population (or specific groups within it) have been "affected" and the nature and circumstances of the "risk" faced.

Part 2 ASSESSMENT AND PROGRAMMES

This second part of the *Handbook* provides guidelines for the various stages of programming operations from initial assessment through to post-facto evaluation of programmes.

Complementary actions must be taken simultaneously to assure the necessary capacity and efficient functioning of the UNICEF office itself: see Part 4.

CHAPTER 3
PROCESS AND PRINCIPLES OF PROGRAMMING

Sequence of programming operations

(*Manual 5.1*)

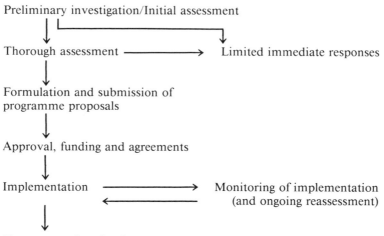

Preliminary investigation/Initial assessment

Thorough assessment ⟶ Limited immediate responses

Formulation and submission of programme proposals

Approval, funding and agreements

Implementation ⟶ Monitoring of implementation (and ongoing reassessment)

Phase out and evaluation

Essential characteristics of the process are:

—*Intensive* assessment efforts at the start of any emergency operation. *Ongoing* process of monitoring and surveillance thereafter, throughout the implementation period.

—*Limited* actions to meet urgent survival needs on the basis of the rapid initial assessment while the more complete assessment is continuing.

—Major interventions on the basis of *thorough assessments*—but a willingness to take calculated risks and support initiatives which, on the basis of the best available information and advice appear to be worthwhile.

Activities within any particular sector should follow the above sequence. Activities in different sectors may, however, commence at different times and proceed at different rates. The table on p. xxiv provides a summary overview of the process and the actions and decisions involved.

Dialogue with HQ while developing proposals:

- **Keep EOU/NYHQ and GEHQ continually informed of the information available and of ideas being developed for possible UNICEF assistance. If certain information or reports are unconfirmed or may be untypical, say so.**

Advise EOU and UNIPAC as early as possible of the types and quantities of supplies which *might* be needed from UNICEF; *and*

Suggest to EOU and PFO any supplies which might be welcome as in-kind contributions (although possibly not being a high priority for the allocation of UNICEF funds directly).

HQ and UNIPAC can then:

—Offer appropriate guidance and support;

—Indicate whether the proposals are likely to be able to be approved and funded;

—Alert potential donors if special funds will be required for the programmes being prepared;

—Respond more quickly if and when you issue specific supply call-forwards for such items; *and*

—Suggest useful actions to any potential contributors of in-kind donations.

(See also p. 154 regarding in-kind contributions.)

Principles

(*Manual 5.2*)

- **Observe the principles of development-oriented humanitarian assistance summarized in Table 3 (next page).** *

- **Plan interventions on the basis of thorough assessment, careful analysis and the best possible advice;** *and*

- **Preserve a strictly impartial, humanitarian focus.**

Don't assume that programmes which were apparently successful in response to an emergency elsewhere will automatically be appropriate in a different situation.

Don't rush into major actions and expenditures on the basis of inadequate information and understanding.

Remember that assistance agencies (you) carry the responsibility for the long-term effects of their (your) decisions and actions as well as being accountable for resources expended.

Be aware of and sensitive to the political context of the situation. Endeavour to be dispassionate in the provision of assistance related to children's needs wherever it is needed. Avoid UNICEF involvement or supplies being used for political—or primarily religious—purposes. Avoid being associated with any particular vested interests locally or internationally.

---

* For practical suggestions on how to promote and achieve real community participation see:

> *Achieving success in community water supply and sanitation projects*—SEARO/WHO, New Delhi (1985)

> *Ask a silly question* (community participation, entry points and the demystification of planning), D. Drucker—unpublished paper available from, *inter alia,* Institute of Child Health, London

> *Towards a programmer's guide,* report of regional water and sanitation workshop, Thailand, 1981—UNICEF (EAPRO), Bangkok

Table 3

Principles of development-oriented humanitarian assistance

Self-help and community participation

- Promote the maximum community participation, initiatives and self-help in all phases of operations.

- Use and reinforce existing structures and processes where possible rather than create new ones.

Recognize and respect the abilities of the affected people to cope with and tackle many of their own problems. Work in partnership with the community from the beginning in establishing priorities, planning and implementing programmes.

Seek ways in which local expertise, labour, materials and facilities can be mobilized. Focus assistance inputs on elements not otherwise available. Select and train project personnel to establish stable relationships of confidence and mutual respect with those being helped.

Work with decentralized levels of government where possible. Consider working with local councils, committees, co-operatives, womens groups, youth groups, traditional leaders, etc. where these are viable/credible.

Preserve community and family environment

- Do everything reasonably possible to preserve family unity and to enable household units to continue functioning or resume operating as soon as possible.

Avoid evacuations and the setting up of camps if at all possible, and promote the earliest possible return to their homes of people who have been evacuated or displaced.

Priorities and long-term considerations

- Allocate resources to the maximum extent possible to activities which will be of lasting benefit: keep any "relief" phase as short as possible.

- Safeguard the interests of the most vulnerable and under-priviledged.

Ensure that social/organizational structures and any materials remaining at the end of emergency operations will contribute positively to long-term social and economic development and the reduction of vulnerability to future similar events.

Be cautious about initiating new services which may not be able to be continued in the long term—when fewer resources might be available.

Innovate with care

- **Identify and be ready to capitalize on any positive aspects inherent in the situation *but* promote innovations only on the basis of good technical advice and relevant previous experience.**

Don't experiment with untested ideas. Understand and be prepared also to respect and accomodate traditional taboos. Get advice from social anthropologists as well as engineers, agronomists, etc.

Allocation and distribution

- **Ensure that assistance is fairly distributed on the basis of need, and in a manner to avoid undermining existing self-reliance systems or accentuating social divisions.**

Consider the social as well as organizational, logistic and economic implications of possible alternative arrangements, and whether supplies should be distributed as free hand-outs, by sale (possibly subsidized), as loans to be repaid in cash or kind, or as some combination.

Work through existing structures and services where feasible: adapt or reinforce them if necessary.

Establish strict criteria for any selective distributions. Where possible, representative community bodies should be responsible for deciding and supervising actual allocations.

Appropriate and standardized provisions

- **Ensure that standards of provision and service are reasonably uniform/equitable between different areas and communities, and equipment appropriate to the general situation locally.**

Ensure the maximum possible co-ordination and agreement on standards between all involved organizations.

Avoid providing unduly sophisticated equipment which cannot be properly maintained and used by the personnel normally available.

Provision for displaced populations should generally be similar to that enjoyed by the neighbouring, indigenous communities amongst which they are (temporarily) settled. Where possible, efforts may be made to increase the level of service for both groups simultaneously.

CHAPTER 4

MAKING ASSESSMENTS

Questions to be answered by assessments

(Manual 5.3)

The questions to be answered by the rapid, initial assessment are listed in Table 4. A more detailed check-list is suggested on pp. 31-36.

Other important needs, such as the restoration of communications, power supplies, etc. may exist and be vital for the communities and authorities concerned, but these are areas in which UNICEF could not normally assist.

Table 5 lists the basic questions for the ongoing, thorough assessment. These should be answered for each of the main sectors (water, food, etc.) where a need appears to exist, and separately for each distinct area or population group.

Detailed check-lists for each of the main sectors of direct concern to UNICEF are suggested in Part 3.

Table 4

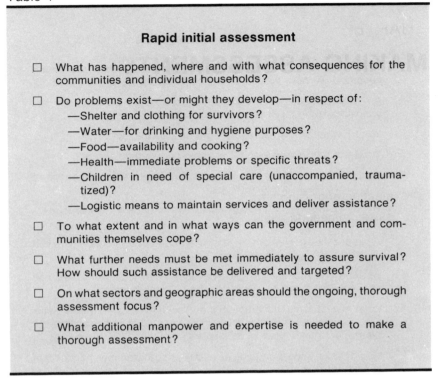

Rapid initial assessment

☐ What has happened, where and with what consequences for the communities and individual households?

☐ Do problems exist—or might they develop—in respect of:
—Shelter and clothing for survivors?
—Water—for drinking and hygiene purposes?
—Food—availability and cooking?
—Health—immediate problems or specific threats?
—Children in need of special care (unaccompanied, traumatized)?
—Logistic means to maintain services and deliver assistance?

☐ To what extent and in what ways can the government and communities themselves cope?

☐ What further needs must be met immediately to assure survival? How should such assistance be delivered and targeted?

☐ On what sectors and geographic areas should the ongoing, thorough assessment focus?

☐ What additional manpower and expertise is needed to make a thorough assessment?

UNICEF role in assessments

(Manual 5.3)

Collaborate with government, the UN team and other concerned organizations from the outset to:
—Define the particular areas to be focused on and information to be sought—both qualitative and quantitative: differentiate that to be obtained immediately from that which may be sought later;
—Divide responsibilities by sector and/or geographic area, and establish arrangements for "pooling" available information: try to agree a common framework for recording and reporting information;
—Co-ordinate arrangements for field visits/surveys and the use of available transport; *and*

Table 5

Ongoing thorough assessment

☐ What are people doing to help themselves? What resources are on hand and en route from all sources? What unmet needs exist?

☐ Are basic services able to continue functioning? Do available personnel have the facilities to live and work effectively?

☐ What further problems/needs might be anticipated?

☐ What are the priorities of the affected people themselves?

☐ How might the priority needs be met? What are the implications of alternative feasible interventions?

☐ Which are the priority target groups? What criteria should be used for allocations and distributions?

☐ What are the policies of the government and others concerned with regard to emergency assistance?

☐ What organizational and logistic capacity exists to deliver assistance to and within the area? How could it be strengthened?

☐ What mechanisms (governmental and/or NGO) exist to utilize/distribute assistance at the local level? How could they be reinforced? What more might need to be created?

☐ How (if at all) should ongoing development programmes be modified to help meet the new situation and any changed priorities? What opportunities exist for beginning new development processes?

—Ensure that the initial assessment covers *all* communities within the affected area as quickly as possible.

Ensure that all relevant base-line information available in UNICEF and other offices is assembled and used to best advantage.

Mobilize personnel and participate in survey/fact-finding missions:
  —Mobilize relevant expertise from all sources (institutes and other agencies) and, if necessary, take the initiative to organize field visits.
  —Redeploy UNICEF staff and request NYHQ and/or the Regional Office for temporary additional staff to help in the assessment process, if necessary.

A check-list for organizing field visits and a sample format for a field visit report are provided in Annex 42.

Focus on the situation and needs of children, especially among the most deprived population groups:

—Make a deliberate effort to observe the condition of children, to identify their real needs and priorities;

—Look for signs of sick, malnourished or unaccompanied children;

—Check to what extent services are functioning to meet the needs of children in general; *and*

—Encourage others to do the same and ensure that, within the overall context, the particular needs of children are properly considered by the government and others involved so that appropriate actions are taken.

For the overall assessment, a multidisciplinary approach is essential. Teams should normally include agriculturalists, epidemiologists, sanitarians, engineers, logisticians and social scientists.

How and where to get information

(*Manual 5.3*)

Systematically gather information on the current situation from all available sources:

—Get reports (formal and informal) from local administrations and existing service delivery networks—health, rural development, agriculture, water resources, public works, etc.;

—Talk with community leaders, extension workers, NGO staff, journalists and other experienced observers coming from the area;

—Make on-the-spot observations and enquiries, including spot-checks of individual dwellings to observe conditions, household resources and talk to the people themselves; *and*

—Arrange sample surveys if necessary to gather specific data. (Keep such surveys simple, but try to arrange that proper sampling techniques are used—see Table 4/1, p. 191.)

Use established communication/reporting channels to the extent that they are still functioning. Use telephone, police radio, etc. to communicate and get information if necessary and possible.

Direct observations and spot-checks are essential to determine the actual impact on households, the perceptions and priorities of the people themselves. They are particularly important in communities where sick children tend to be kept out-of-sight. (Spot checks should, if possible, be made on a proper random sample basis.) Do not attempt complete house-to-house surveys, nor to address questionnaires to survivors and other respondents in the early stages.

Low level reconnaissance flights *may* be able to provide valuable indications of the extent and general nature of physical damage and the response of the communities themselves *if* undertaken by persons who know the area well.

Evaluating and using information

(*Manual 5.3*)

Record all relevant information received, noting the source/origin and the date.

Evaluate all information:
- Is information consistent? Cross-check and compare reports from different sources.
- Are the reports/figures plausible? Check against available base-line data and experience.
- What biases may be influencing the reports?

Responses from people whose livelihoods and/or families are directly affected *may* be emotional and exaggerated. Technical specialists often, albeit unconsciously, display a bias towards their own field of specialization in suggesting priorities.

Update information on a continuous basis.
- Initial information and impressions can be misleading. Needs evolve and priorities change as days pass after a disaster. Some health, social and other effects/needs may not be apparent at all in the first few days, but only emerge—or be detected—later.

Don't generalize from data relating to only a small area. The actual situation and needs may vary considerably over short distances within the affected area.
- While information is lacking on certain affected areas, use the available base-line data—and the experience of local personnel—to estimate what differences might be expected between those areas and others already visited or for which reliable information is available.

Table 6 lists aspects to be kept always in mind when making assessments.

Possible immediate needs

Assistance necessary to ensure immediate survival of children should be arranged without delay, but using a minimum of resources pending thorough assessment.

Table 6

What to aim for (and avoid) in assessments

- **Determine the "impact" on the lives of the communities and people affected, and the delivery of services: don't just accumulate figures for material losses.**

Differentiate "needs" from "wants". Distinguish needs which are a direct consequence of the event/disaster from "chronic" needs which existed previously.

- **Understand the population's own perceptions, priorities and capacities. Find out what they need to be able to further help themselves.**

Don't underestimate their ability to improvise and adapt. Don't assume that those who speak the language of outside assistance agencies/personnel necessarily represent their communities!

- **Make specific, quantitative estimates of needs, but avoid making elaborate calculations with figures of doubtful validity!**

Try to get reasonable estimates of *rates*—e.g. the percentage of families in need of temporary shelter—and then impute totals, rather than seeking absolute numbers directly.

It *may* be better, initially, to make theoretical estimates based on census data and knowledge of typical effects of similar previous events, rather than rely on the early, subjective estimates of people in the area (which often turn out to be grossly inaccurate).

- **Be thorough: avoid hasty actions. Resist the inevitable pressures to "do something" quickly.**

Avoid assumptions and preconceptions of what needs might exist and what kind of interventions be appropriate—unless they are based on very thorough understanding and analysis of the effects of previous similar disasters in the same area.

Table 7 lists some of the possible immediate survival needs. See Part 5 for detailed considerations relating to each of these sectors of possible need and assistance.

UNICEF action to meet immediate needs might include diversion of in-country supplies, local procurement and/or airfreight from UNIPAC. Actions may be financed by diversions, releases from the emergency reserve and/or reprogramming: see p. 7.

29

Table 7

Possible immediate survival needs

Shelter

Materials to arrange safe, temporary shelter: e.g. plastic sheeting, tarpaulins and rope, tools.

Personal protection

Blankets and/or clothing, especially for children.

Water

Protection of wells; immediate or temporary repairs to piped systems; establishment of storage tanks, truck deliveries and/or treatment for at least minimum quantities of water (if no short-term alternative).

Food

Protection of available stocks against contamination; assurance of at least survival rations (energy) for families and suitable items for young children (weaning); provision of supplies for hospitals and other institutions.

Special feeding

Suitable food items, utensils and other needs of any existing special feeding programmes (supplementary or therapeutic).

Household functioning

Utensils for food preparation, water collection; fuel for cooking, etc.

Health care

Personnel, equipment and supplies to attend to any major, immediate health problems and provide at least minimum maternity and post-natal care.

Sanitation

Temporary sanitation measures: digging latrines; disposing of garbage; instructions to population on personal hygiene and protection against any prevalent vector-borne diseases; soap, disinfectant, tools.

Child care

Arrangements for the emergency and interim care of any unaccompanied children.

Logistics

Necessary transport and handling arrangements to deliver needed immediate assistance.

Initial assessment

Nature of event

☐ What was/is the nature and cause of the emergency situation?

☐ When and where did it strike? What is the extent of the affected area?

☐ What was/is the severity in different locales?

Baseline data

☐ What was the population of the affected area before the disaster—the size and location of communities?

☐ What are the ethnic and cultural characteristics of different groups: language—average family size—typical household living arrangements?

☐ What are the ecological and economic characteristics of the area—degree of self sufficiency—normal sources of supplies?

☐ What traditional community coping/response mechanisms exist?

☐ What political and administrative structures exist in the areas affected?

☐ What type of services and development programmes were operating?

Impact of events

☐ On population numbers and distribution:
  - Have people evacuated or migrated?
  - Have families become divided?
  - What are the reported numbers of casualties—dead, injured and missing?

☐ On food and agriculture
  - Food stocks and/or distribution mechanisms?
  - Crops, irrigation systems, etc.?

☐ On health
  - Health service facilities and supply systems?
  - Health workers and control programmes?

☐ On shelter and personal protection
  - Family dwellings rendered inhabitable?
  - Essential household property lost?

☐ On water and sanitation
  —Water supplies?
  —Sewerage systems or other sanitation arrangements disrupted?

☐ Child care and other social services; schools?

☐ On communications and Logistics
  —Telecommunications within the area and to outside locations?
  —Transport routes and capacity?

☐ On economy activity—employment and income generating opportunities?

Present situation

☐ What weather conditions at present?

Community response

☐ What are the people/survivors already doing to help themselves?

☐ Are traditional coping mechanisms operating?

☐ If not, what are the reasons?

☐ Have any self-help groups/arrangements been established?

Food, nutrition and income

☐ Are any particular groups without adequate food? If so, is it due to lack of supplies or lack of purchasing power?

☐ Are households able to prepare food?

☐ Are children malnourished?

Health

☐ Are there any immediate health problems?

☐ Are there adequate medical personnel? Do they have the facilities and supplies to live and work?

Shelter and personal protection

☐ Is survival threatened by lack of shelter, clothing, etc.?

Water and sanitation

☐ Are at least minimum quantities of safe water available to all communities?

☐ Is lack of adequate sanitation posing immediate health risks?

Child care

☐ Are there children in need of special care: unaccompanied—traumatized—disabled?

☐ Are traditional care arrangements/social services functioning?

Logistics

☐ Can supplies be brought into the area? What specific constraints?

Administration

☐ Are there any problems of law and order?

☐ Is the local administration functioning effectively?

Assistance

☐ What is the government already doing/planning? Has there been an official request for aid?

☐ What other organizations are present? What are they doing/planning?

Probable evolution

☐ What weather conditions are forecast for the immediate future? What are the implications for: survival—communications—logistics?

☐ Are any secondary disasters likely to ensue?

☐ What health risks arise from changes in the environment in which people are living?

☐ How are the people expected to respond: what further actions will they be taking for themselves?

☐ Are disruptions to market mechanisms, supply systems and employment opportunities likely to be short- or long-term effects?

☐ What policies and actions are the government and others expected to pursue?

Conclusions for action

The following immediate actions [specify actions, target beneficiaries and locations] are required to meet *immediate* needs for:

☐ Access to food supplies . . .

- ☐ Household functioning . . .
- ☐ Health care . . .
- ☐ Shelter and personal protection . . .
- ☐ Water supplies . . .
- ☐ Sanitation . . .
- ☐ Special care for children . . .

Further actions [specify sectors and general nature] are needed to meet *short-, medium-* and *long-term* needs for:

- ☐ Food production and marketing/distribution . . .
- ☐ Employment/income opportunities . . .
- ☐ Household functioning . . .
- ☐ Health care . . .
- ☐ Shelter and personal protection . . .
- ☐ Water supplies . . .
- ☐ Sanitation . . .
- ☐ Special care for children . . .

Priorities

- ☐ The overall priorities of the various communities are . . .
- ☐ The most severely affected areas and population groups are . . .
  [Specify what must to be done to ensure that their needs receive priority.]
- ☐ Special considerations arising from the nature of the area/location are . . .
- ☐ More detailed surveys and investigations should be undertaken to determine needs and identify appropriate responses in respect of: . . .

Capacity and organization

- ☐ Local capacity to handle the required relief and rehabilitation operations should be strenthened by: . . .
- ☐ Other in-country capacity which should be mobilized includes: . . .
- ☐ To ensure effective co-ordination and control at local and national levels, action should be taken to . . .
- ☐ The following needed supplies are available within the country: . . .

Additional considerations for displaced populations

Reasons/motivation for movement

☐ Where are the people now—concentrated in large groups or scattered?

☐ Why have they moved? Is displacement expected to be temporary or permanent?

☐ Are they still moving? If so, at what rate? Are further movements likely?

☐ Are there political implications—international or local? Is UNHCR or the ICRC involved in assuring any necessary protection?

Characterstics of the population

☐ What is the ethnic and cultural background of the people? What are their traditions and normal life style?

☐ What are the precentages of men, women, children (0-5 and 5-10 years) and old people in the population?

☐ What resources, if any, have they brought with them? Are they able to survive and support themselves, at least in the short-term?

☐ How are they received by the indigenous population of the area?

☐ Is the condition of new arrivals better or worse than those who came earlier? What differences? Why?

Location and social organization

☐ What particular difficulties/hazards are faced in the present location? What can be done to improve the situation? Is a better site available?

☐ How is the camp organized? Are different groups concentrated in separate sections?

☐ What social and other structures exist? Who are the apparent leaders? What is the basis of their influence? To what extent do they have the confidence and support of different population groups?

☐ What tensions/rivalries exist within the population?

Resources and services

☐ Are the new arrivals placing strain on the area's resources (including water and cooking fuel) and services? Is the local population being adversely affected?

☐ What services are available/being provided? What other assistance is already being provided or planned?

35

Conclusions for action

☐ ... 000 people are likely to be displaced until ...

☐ The organization of the population and the implementation of programmes should be promoted through the following community structures: ...

☐ Practical actions to improve the site, layout and facilities include: ...

☐ To ensure service delivery:
  —Existing delivery and distribution systems should be strengthened by ...
  —New systems must be created to ...

Additional considerations in conflict situations

☐ What particular risks are faced by:
  —The civilian population in general?
  —Children in particular?

☐ Is there evidence of children being abducted, conscripted, imprisoned, tortured, abused or deliberately killed? Have children been severely traumatized by their experiences?

☐ What is being done to protect and help children within their family and community environment?

Conclusions for action

☐ Further actions necessary to protect and help children are: ...

CHAPTER 5

FORMULATING SPECIFIC PROPOSALS

Planning for action

(Manual 5.4)

- **For each proposed UNICEF intervention, define all the aspects listed in Table 8 on the basis of a thorough assessment, good technical advice and close collaboration with:**
  - a. **The government, local authorities, reliable local organizations and the communities themselves;** *and*
  - b. **Other concerned UN agencies (notably UNDP, WFP, WHO and FAO) and other involved organizations.**

Take account of established policies and principles, and maintain a dialogue with HQ throughout the assessment and planning process: see Chapter 3.

As an example, Annex 5 provides particularly detailed guidelines for aspects to be determined in planning a supplementary feeding programme.

Documenting proposals

Explicitly record all the elements listed in Table 8, a summary of the assessment findings and conclusions, and the particular assumptions on which the proposals are based.

In the case of a substantial programme, prepare a formal (but concise) Plan of Action for signature with the government. More detailed guidelines of aspects to consider and what to include in a Plan of Action are provided in Annex 43.

Table 8

Aspects to be defined
(Elements of a Plan of Action)

☐ The specific objectives;

☐ The target groups, locations and the estimated number of beneficiaries;

☐ The specific nature of the proposed activities; the particular inputs; the manner in which inputs are intended to be used and the processes by which they are to be transported, allocated and distributed;

☐ Mechanisms and responsibilities for implementation, including criteria and arrangements for distribution, accounting, supervision, etc.;

☐ The technical expertise and other personnel required, and from where they will be provided;

☐ Responsibilities and arrangements for monitoring implementation and evaluating outcomes;

☐ The planned phasing and specific time schedule of operations (and consequent schedule for delivery of inputs);

☐ The planned budget, including requirements for each phase;

☐ The extent—and limits—of UNICEF's commitments; and

☐ The complementary inputs required from government or other organizations (materials, finance, personnel, logistics and other facilities).

National policies

Understand the policies of the government with respect to:
— Meeting the needs of children in particular;
— The distribution of assistance (food and other items);
— The role of local institutions and NGOs (both national and international).

Advocate any strengthening or modification of policies or practices which is believed to be desireable for the ultimate well-being of children and their families.

Evaluating proposals

☐   Do all concerned at national and local levels understand and agree the policies, objectives and practical strategies?

☐   Are the proposed interventions in line with the principles outlined in Table 3 (p. 22-23)? Do they form a coherent programme?

☐   Are they in fact feasible technically, organizationally and politically?

☐   Will the proposed actions complement those of other organizations (and not duplicate)?

(What is the estimated cost per beneficiary?)

Defining priorities and objectives

(*Manual 5.4*)

● **Define short-term objectives precisely and in operational terms. Specify the:**
— **Target areas/populations;**
— **Outcomes hoped for; *and***
— **Period during which objectives should be achieved.**

In addition, specify the long-term objectives towards which the emergency intervention is expected to contribute, and include training and capacity development objectives wherever possible.

Focus on the most fundamental needs of children and families, including social and psychological as well as material needs.

39

Determine priorities jointly with the communities and local authorities taking account of: national policies—the capabilities and intentions of others—the possibility of contributing to long-term development—the relationship to on-going and planned UNICEF programmes. See Chapter 1, p. 6.

It may be best to leave activities in which UNICEF has no relevant local experience to others, *if* others are ready and able to take them on.

Determining practical strategies

(*Manual 5.4*)

Decide the means by which the objectives can best be achieved: what exactly should be done—what inputs and services be provided—how to target them.

If there are alternative ways of meeting needs and achieving the objectives, evaluate each of them:

☐ What are their implications in terms of both short-term efficiency and long-term effects?

☐ How will they help to develop local capacity and reduce the vulnerability of the communities to future, similar events as well as meeting immediate needs?

Responsibility for implementation

Organize programmes and deliver assistance through established channels to the extent possible. The government or indigenous organizations designated by it should normally be responsible for implementation:

☐ Does government capacity need strengthening? How?

☐ Will co-operation with NGOs be beneficial and feasible? Does the government agree?

If there is no reasonable alternative, UNICEF may itself undertake certain operational responsibilities:

—Define the role carefully in agreement with the government; and

—Assure the necessary staff as well as budget.

In a joint project with an NGO the NGO might, for instance, be responsible for field implementation and/or supervision while UNICEF provides some or all of the necessary funds and/or logistics support.

Phasing of large-scale projects:

Plan as a series of self-contained phases able to be implemented in succession as and when funds and general progress in implementation permit.

Consider rapid, small-scale pilot projects in selected areas or institutions in advance or as a first phase of the envisaged large-scale programme.

Each phase should result in specific, practical benefits independent of whether the planned subsequent phases are able to be implemented or not. (This is particularly important in respect of proposed long-term interventions and rehabilitation projects for which total funding is often not able to be guaranteed at the outset.)

Plan carefully the eventual phasing out "emergency" assistance into appropriate long-term programmes. These must be sustainable with the resources which can be expected to be available in the future: see Chapter 7, p. 51.

Rehabilitation of institutions

If local organizational and technical capacity and physical facilities are limited (disrupted and/or over-stretched):
— Focus initially on selected, individual institutions and communities;
— Deliver inputs specifically designed and packaged for their particular needs.

Deliver bulk materials and supplies (to be stocked and then allocated against assessed needs) only when capacity is assured to handle and administer such an operation.

Delivery of inputs

Schedule the delivery of inputs according to carefully determined priorities taking account of practical/logistic considerations and the possible value of flexibility to manage and adjust deliveries in response to evolving needs and actual operational progress:
— Provide the most basic and essential items first: leave until later any refinements—inputs which though useful are not immediately necessary.
— Would small, initial deliveries and a subsequent steady flow be preferable to a single, large delivery?
— Define whether, in case it proves to be impossible to deliver the desired quantities in the initial weeks/months, the undelivered quantities will still be required in the subsequent months or not.

"Better late than never" does not always apply. Supplies, particularly foodstuffs, which arrive later than planned and when they are no longer needed may be a positive embarrassment and detrimental to the process of recovery, acting as a disincentive to local production.

Some losses and waste will be inevitable, the amount depending in the items and the situation. Make an appropriate allowance for this when planning quantities to be ordered. Five per cent may be the minimum which should be added in most instances.

Getting HQ approval and funding

(*Manual 5.4*)

Once specific proposals are finalized:
— Convey/confirm details as in Table 8 to EOU/NYHQ by telex, repeated to GEHQ and regional director;
— Propose how the interventions should be funded; *and*
— Ensure that sufficient background information as indicated for Sitrep 01 (Annex 37) has also been provided.

Inform EOU-PFO/NYHQ and GEHQ immediately of any subsequent changes in objectives, activities, phasing, location etc. so that up-to-date information is always available for submission to potential donors.

A list of supply requirements is *not* a sufficient basis either for a release from the emergency reserve or for an approach to be made to potential donors for any specific purpose contributions which might be needed.

EOU/NYHQ will react as quickly as possible with approval in principle of the proposals, or to request reconsideration of them, and advice whether, how and when funds may be approved/obtained.

Agreements with government

(*Manual 5.4*)

Ensure that government officers, personnel of other organizations and community leaders all understand:
— The policies and responsibilities of UNICEF, particularly the strictly humanitarian focus and the requirement of non-discriminatory use/distribution of UNICEF assistance;

—That UNICEF's resources and capabilities are limited, and that assistance is dependent on mobilizing resources and can only be provided for selected, defined purposes; *and*

—That the type and quantity of assistance which UNICEF *may* be able to provide in response to a major emergency is exceptional, and will not be able to be continued on the same basis in the long-term when the organization will not be able to mobilize the same level of resources.

Foresee—jointly—from the beginning:

—How the emergency interventions will be phased out and what kind of long-term programmes might be appropriate and feasible as a follow-on; *and/or*

—How any special UNICEF operations will be taken over by the local authorities.

See Chapter 7, p. 51.

For minor "relief" inputs and "diversions"

Exchange letters describing the essentials of the proposed action. Specify the nature and quantity of the UNICEF inputs, how and where they are intended to be used.

Such letters should be adequate for early "relief" inputs—and limited "diversions" of regular programme supplies or funds—whose use and value does not depend on significant complementary commitments from either the government or the community itself. It must be clear that UNICEF's commitment is not open-ended.

For more significant interventions

● **Prepare and sign a concise — but specific — Plan of Action with the responsible government authority. Give copies to all concerned.**

For substantial emergency assistance and rehabilitation funded by programme amendments, releases from the emergency reserve or special contributions, a formal Plan of Action should ensure that strategies are agreed and the means of implementation assured. (Complementary technical, financial and administrative inputs are usually required from the government.)

Include specific provision for review and possible revision during implementation.

Collaboration with NGOs

(*Manual 5.4*)

If, in agreement with the government, it is found appropriate to collaborate with an NGO in a particular project:

- **Verify the capacity and ability of the NGO to implement the intended programme;**

- **Define responsibilities clearly and draw up a specific agreement with the NGO concerned, especially if any UNICEF funds or supplies are to be entrusted or any equipment (e.g. vehicles) to be loaned;** *and*

- **Arrange for appropriate reports to be provided by the organization concerned to both UNICEF and the government.**

A sample format for an agreement with an NGO is included as Annex 43.

NGOs which were already established in the area before the emergency with long-term programmes of their own may be particularly competent and able to profit from their knowledge of the area and their established relationships.

Especially in politically sensitive situations, check the bona fides and motivations of the NGO and its personnel. Ask HQ if necessary. Ensure that they do not engage in any inappropriate political or proselytizing activities.

To the extent necessary and possible, provide technical guidance, including copies of any relevant publications.

CHAPTER 6

MANAGING IMPLEMENTATION

Organizing for implementation

(*Manual 7.2*)

Once HQ approval has been obtained and funding been confirmed, co-operate with government to ensure that:

— Sufficient and appropriate personnel are rapidly mobilized to set in motion all aspects of operations; *and*

— Systems, criteria and controls are established at the outset, and enforced as soon as ever possible.

Table 9 lists the main elements of initiating a field operation. Note that:

— The start-up phase requires a greater concentration of experience and expertise than maintaining operations once established; *and*

— If inappropriate practices become established, they will be difficult to change, and records never catch up.

Specific role of UNICEF

The responsibility of UNICEF Representatives and field staff does not end with the preparation of plans, agreements and the delivery of UNICEF inputs. It extends to helping to assure (a) the achievement of objectives through expeditious implementation of the programmes and (b) the efficient utilization of UNICEF resources.

In emergencies more than in normal operations, it *may* be necessary for staff to support and assist government counterparts and others by participating actively in the organization, monitoring and supervision of operations.

If, exceptionally, UNICEF assumes direct responsibility for certain operations, provide information and reports regularly to the government on the status of operations under UNICEF control.

Table 9

Setting up an operation

Mobilize personnel
- —Get sufficient, competent personnel on the job quickly to set in motion all aspects of operations. Identify and mobilize appropriate in-country resources.
- —Prepare, reproduce and distribute clear, concise operational guidelines—in an appropriate language—for all categories of workers. Provide necessary orientation/training quickly.

Organize logistic capacity
- —Borrow, rent, requisition or purchase all necessary means of transport, warehouses and cargo handling equipment. Ensure security of materials.
- —Organize fuel supplies and maintenance arrangements for all transport units.
- —Arrange for the receipt, clearance, handling, temporary storage and onforwarding of consignments arriving at ports, airports, and any in-country transshipment points.
- —Arrange for ordering and receiving supplies from local suppliers.

Line-up supplies and funds
- —Establish mechanisms for co-ordinating deliveries of inputs from all sources.
- —Schedule and control the ordering and shipment of inputs. Ensure proper specifications. Carefully monitor the "pipeline".
- —Obtain and schedule the release/transfer of funds from government and other contributors.

Establish communications
- —Assure fast, reliable communications between all important operational bases and co-ordinating offices. Get radios if necessary.

Operational procedures

—Produce guidelines—in an appropriate language—describing the programme objectives and strategies, the criteria for allocations and arrangements for implementation/distributions. Give copies to *all* interested parties.

—Establish procedures (responsibilities, communication channels and forms) by which supplies can be requisitioned. Specify procedures and responsibilities for stock control and record keeping in all stores. Provide personnel with clear instructions, and training.

—Designate persons authorized and responsible to disburse funds for procurements, wages and other operating costs. Arrange for funds to be available to them (probably imprest accounts).

—Specify the amounts which may be spent for particular purposes, accounting requirements and arrangements for replenishments.

Operational reporting

—Establish arrangements by which central and regional focal points receive regular, up-to-date reports from all operating units on:

—The progress, achievements and obstacles encountered in implementation;

—Supplies actually used/distributed, stocks received and balances remaining on hand;

—Expenditures incurred; cash transfers received and balances on hand;

—The movements and work of field personnel; *and*

—Any recommendations for changes in inputs, procedures or other actions to overcome difficulties and enhance the effectiveness of the programme.

—Provide operational units at all levels with adequate stocks of forms for recording and reporting, and guidelines on how to use the forms.

Supervision

—Schedule regular supervision of field level operations by personnel competent in all aspects of the operation—the relevant technical specialism (e.g. nutrition), logistics, administration and accounting.

Monitoring and adapting

(*Manual 7.2*)

• Carefully and continuously monitor the execution of planned actions and their outcomes, see Table 10;

- Ensure that all concerned understand and remember the specific objectives of the programme;

- Adjust inputs and/or mechanisms and procedures if found necessary as more information and experience is acquired and the situation itself changes; *but*

- Ensure that any departures from the processes and procedures defined in the Plan of Action are the result of deliberate and agreed decisions, and communicated to all concerned.

Select specific, quantifiable indicators by which the outcome of the programme can be assessed. Collect and analyse data on these from regular reports, spot-check obervations and surveys.

Outcome indicators may be related to the objectives either directly or indirectly. Some examples: number of installations completed—number of people using them— number of seriously malnourished children rehabilitated—changes in the percentage of children malnourished—changes in the quantity and/or quality of water available to and used by the target population; etc.

In the case of major distribution programmes in difficult situations, it may be necessary to establish special arrangements—including staff capacity—to monitor the movement and end-use of supplies on a continuous and systematic basis.

In such cases, obtain the services of personnel fluent in both the local language and that of the overall programme administration. Persons with experience in designing and organizing sociological surveys, including the application of sampling techniques, should plan and supervise the monitoring efforts.

Table 10

Monitoring programme implementation

Carefully analyse reports from all operational units in respect of:
- —Movements, stock levels and rates of utilization of supplies;
- —Rates of expenditures against different budget headings;
- —Reported accomplishments.

Make regular observations and spot checks of:
- —Actual movements, stocks and end-use of supplies; and
- —Processes of training, contracting, storage, distribution and supervision.

Organize occasional sample surveys to determine:
- —The adequacy of targeting;
- —Actual end-use of inputs and the final result/outcome.

Questions for implementation monitoring

Answers to these questions will help to determine what is actually happening, and what can and should be done to improve the effectiveness and efficiency of operations.

Delivery of inputs

☐ Is the receipt and handling of supplies at ports smooth and efficient? Have deliveries been on schedule? What quantities have been received? What percentage losses/damage?

☐ Are local purchase operations proceeding smoothly and on schedule?

☐ Is the movement of supplies to the area of need being effected quickly and efficiently? Are all storage facilities and recording systems adequate?

☐ Have funds been available for approved disbursements when and where necessary? Have any requirements been overlooked?

Organization and supervision

☐ Is the general organization and management of the programme proceeding smoothly? Do all concerned understand the arrangements and procedures, and their own responsibilities?

☐ Is necessary technical expertise available and being used?

Distribution

☐ Is the actual distribution of supplies and disbursement of funds proceeding as intended (in accordance with the Plan of Action)? If not, why not?

☐ What quantities have actually been distributed? What quantities should have been distributed according to the Plan?

Targeting

☐ Who is in fact receiving and benefiting from the inputs?

☐ What percentage of the planned target population is actually receiving and benefiting as intended (percentage "coverage")? If this is low—why?

☐ What precentage of those receiving/benefiting in fact belong to the planned target population (percentage "focussing")? If this is low—why?

Use of inputs

☐ Are the inputs being used as anticipated? If not, why not? Are the inputs in fact appropriate? What needs to be changed?

☐ Are there significant problems of loss, misuse or resale of any items? If so, which and why?

Costs

☐ Are costs in line with the estimates in the Plan? If not, what are the implications for the programme budget?

☐ What is the actual cost per activity? What cost per beneficiary?

Outcome

☐ What outcomes can be measured and/or observed? To what extent are the objectives being achieved?

☐ Is this an adequate/acceptable level of performance?

Continuation/adaptation

☐ Has the situation changed in such a way as to make a change of plan necessary? How is the situation now expected to evolve?

☐ What specific actions should be taken *now* to increase the efficiency and maximise the impact of the programme and the achievement of the objectives?

☐ Should the programme in fact be continued with the original objectives? Should operations be expanded—or restricted?

CHAPTER 7

PHASING OUT AND EVALUATING

Phasing out

(*Manual 7.3*)

Try to phase in appropriate long-term follow-up programmes as the emergency assistance is ending. In general:

—Reduce material inputs;

—Continue training and surveillance activities;

—Consolidate self-sustaining activities (e.g. food production) and any maintenance facilities for equipment; *and*

—Reduce the role of any outside personnel.

Ideally, the emergency assistance (except for very short-term "relief" measures) should have been conceived as the first, intensive phase of a long-term development programme, and the phasing out of extraordinary "emergency" inputs have been foreseen and planned for from the beginning with the community and local administration.

Evaluating

(Manual 7.3)

Evaluation is intended to determine the extent to which the programme was implemented as planned and the objectives met, and what results were actually achieved. This is important for:

— Accountability to both donors and the intended beneficiaries;

— Deciding whether an intervention should be continued, or what form a longer-term follow-up programme should take; *and*

— Drawing "lessons" for future programmes in the same area, and for the organization of responses to similar emergency situations.

Planning evaluations

- **Establish at the outset: the specific purpose(s) of the evaluation — to whom the findings are addressed — who will be responsible for organizing it.**

- **Decide whether it should be an "internal" or "external" evaluation.**

- **Fix the time schedule: ensure that results will be produced quickly enough to be useful!**

Include both "process" aspects (concerning the actual organization of operations) and "gross outcome" (changes detected in the situation): see below.

Questions for evaluations

Warning and preparedness arrangements

☐ Was the disaster/emergency predictable?

☐ Was there an early warning system? Did it operate properly? If not, why not? What errors were made?

☐ Were the government and assistance agencies properly prepared? Was necessary baseline data on the area to hand?

☐ What improvements need to be made for the future?

Effectiveness of the general assessment

☐ Was the initial assessment conducted in a co-ordinated, systematic and expeditious manner?

☐ Was the extent of the disaster correctly understood/determined?

☐ Were any areas/communities neglected, initially?

☐ Were the most severely affected communities correctly identified? Were the numbers of people "affected" is particular ways accurately estimated?

☐ Were the major problem areas/sectors correctly identified in the initial assessment?

☐ What improvements need to be made for the future?

Sectoral needs and programmes

[The following general questions should normally be addressed for each sector and major assistance programme:]

Planning

☐ Were the needs and priorities properly assessed? If not, what was the extent and cause of the error?

☐ Were the wishes of the communities themselves properly understood? Did they contribute to and participate in the planning and implementation?

Implementation Process

☐ Was the delivery of inputs satisfactory? *

☐ Was the distribution of supplies satisfactory? *

☐ Was targeting satisfactory? Were distribution/allocation criteria and processes appropriate? *

☐ Were inputs well used? Were there significant problems of loss, misuse or resale of any items? *

☐ Were actual costs reasonable? Were funds available when and where needed?*

---

* See "Implementation monitoring" pp. 49-50 for elaboration of these questions.   **53**

☐ Was overall management satisfactory? Were responsibilities for implementation adequately and appropriately defined?

☐ Was necessary expertise available when and where needed? Was it properly used?

☐ Did personnel perform adequately?

Outcome

☐ What outcomes have been measured? To what extent have objectives been achieved? Who has benefited, and in what ways?

☐ Was suffering and hardship allieviated?

☐ Has the vulnerability of the communities concerned to future similar events been reduced?

☐ Has local capacity for coping with such situations in the future—and for accelerating general development—been increased?

☐ Did the programme contribute to shortening the time otherwise necessary for recovery? Has it contributed to broad development goals?

☐ Did local purchases disturb the local market? Did they serve to stimulate the local economy?

☐ Were imports really necessary? What effect did they have on the local market and economy?

☐ What lessons should be learned?

Internal UNICEF operations

☐ Was the UNICEF office aware of any early warnings?

☐ Was the UNICEF office itself "prepared"?

☐ Was collaboration with other UN agencies smooth and effective?

☐ Were UNICEF's policies clear? Were there good communications and full understanding between HQ and the field?

☐ Were funds able to be mobilized when needed?

☐ Was supply performance satisfactory? Were the materials delivered appropriate?

☐ Were suitable, additional personnel able to be mobilized when needed?

54 ☐ What lessons need to be learned?

Part 3 POSSIBLE NEEDS AND RESPONSES

This Part provides guidelines concerning the kinds of needs which *might* arise in different situations, the general priorities and the kinds of programme responses which might be appropriate.

In each major sector (food and nutrition—health—water supplies—hygiene and sanitation—shelter and household functioning—child care and psycho-social needs—logistics) a summary is given of the kind of *overall* needs and priorities which might arise. This provides the context within which any UNICEF intervention has to be considered. What might be an appropriate role for UNICEF is then outlined with indications of the kinds of inputs which might be considered.

It does *not* follow that UNICEF should necessarily be involved in any or all of the sectors and possible interventions mentioned! Others not mentioned may be appropriate in some situations. Responsibility for providing assistance to striken populations rests with the government. UNICEF offers co-operation within the limits of its policies and resources.

In all cases, decisions must be based on thorough assessment which takes account not only of "needs" but also the capacities and intentions of the communities themselves, the government and other assistance organizations: see Chapter 1.

A detailed check-list is provided for each sector. Answers may not be quickly available to all of the questions but these represent aspects which it is relevant

to consider in formulating any major assistance programme proposals.

Within the framework of the principles described in
Chapter 3, focus on practical measures to enhance
local efforts and initiatives. Mobilize appropriate
technical expertise in the various fields as soon as the
need for such is identified.

CHAPTER 8

FOOD, NUTRITION AND INCOME

Possible problems/needs

- Actual and/or foreseeable lack of access to adequate food for either the entire population of a particular area or certain subgroups within it.

- Lack of means to prepare and cook food.

- Actual or foreseeable serious levels of malnutrition — especially among children.

Immediate and short-term problems may arise from:
- Damage/loss of public and/or private food stocks (floods, storms, conflicts);
- Disruption of the transport and marketing system which brings food into the area (earthquakes, floods, storms, conflicts);
- Loss of food processing equipment (grinders, etc.), cooking utensils; lack of cooking fuel (earthquakes, floods, storms, conflicts);

57

— Loss of employment/earning opportunities and/or rises in food prices, hence reduced purchasing power of labourers and artisans (droughts, earthquakes, floods, storms, conflicts).

Medium-term (up to 18 months) supply problems from:
— Loss of purchasing power (as above);
— Major reduction of yield or total loss of standing crops/plantations (droughts, floods, storms, crop infestations);
— Prevention of timely planting (droughts, floods, storms, conflicts — including forced consumption of seed stocks or non-availability of seeds, draught animals, fuel, etc.).

Long-term problems from:
— Loss or reduced fertility of cultivable land (tsunamis, storm surges, landslides, erosion or general degradation due to prolonged drought);

Table 11

Malnutrition

Severe malnutrition is often found when droughts or major social/economic disruptions have occured/been developing over some time and no adequate action been taken early enough.

It would not normally be expected in the immediate aftermath of a sudden disaster (unless already chronic in the area), but could develop progressively as a result unless adequate action is taken in time.

The existence of malnutrition (among children) does not necessarily mean that there is an absolute shortage of food in the area and a need to bring food in. It can also be the result of:

—Lack of purchasing power.
—A maldistribution of available supplies/resources between different communities and households, or between individuals within households.
—Disease—infections causing reduced absorption of nutrients, loss of appetite or increase of requirements.
—Ignorance and/or taboos preventing children (and mothers) from eating certain available foods.

Young children are nearly always the worst-affected by a general food shortage as well as any particular shortage of those items most valuable and suitable for weaning. See Annex 4, p. 238, on how to recognize different forms of malnutrition.

Displaced populations may be or rapidly become destitute, lacking any food stocks, land (and therefore future crops) and purchasing power. They may also lack the means—utensils and cooking fuel—to prepare food.

Increases in levels of malnutrition may occur, but are not automatic or immediate results of sudden disasters. See Table 11.

General aims and priorities

- To ensure availability of necessary basic food to all;

- To treat those already suffering from severe malnutrition;

- To expedite the re-establishment of local food production, processing and distribution systems.

After floods, droughts and other events which have interrupted normal agricultural activity:
- The restoration of local production is normally the highest priority. (Timely availability of appropriate seeds may be the most important requirement of farmers.)
- Large-scale employment and/or food supply/distribution programmes may be necessary until the next main harvest or the re-establishment of earning opportunities and food markets.

After earthquakes, floods and some other sudden, cataclysmic events:
- The provision of cooked food may be necessary for a few days.
- Food stocks must be inspected and contaminated food be disposed of.
- The re-establishment of normal distribution and marketing systems, income earning opportunities and arrangements for food preparation are then the priorities.

In all cases:
- Organize treatment for those already suffering severe malnutrition.
- Act to prevent the condition of other "vulnerable groups" from deteriorating before other measures to restore food availability produce results.
- Ensure efficient storage (protection), preservation and processing of all available supplies, and of the next crop when harvested.

Table 12

Types of feeding programme

Feeding programmes aim to provide individuals with free food to make up the difference between (a) what they need to re-establish and maintain reasonable nutritional health and (b) what they are able to obtain/earn for themselves from stocks, current production, cash and/or food-for-work employment.

Where feeding (free food) is considered necessary for particular population groups, it may be provided in the form of cooked meals (daily) or "dry" rations (at weekly or longer intervals) to be prepared and cooked at home.

Three types of feeding are usually distinguished:

"General" feeding

Basic foods/meals are provided for all members of all households within particular population groups, e.g. the entire population of a disaster-affected area, all registered refugees/displaced persons, selected socio-economic groups within a population. Rations may be intended to cover total nutritional needs for a certain period (where the population is totally dependent), or only a part of their needs (when the people have some other sources). Standard, fixed rations are provided either for each family or each individual.

"Supplementary" feeding

Additional food is given to selected, nutritionally vulnerable individuals to compensate for specific deficiencies—in energy, protein, vitamins and minerals—in the food otherwise available to them. It is intended to be in addition to their normal share of household food, including any general emergency distributions. Target "vulnerable groups" usually include young and moderately malnourished children, pregnant and lactating women, see Table 5/3, p. 208. The size of rations depends on the assessed deficiencies in other food expected to be available to the selected beneficiaries.

"Therapeutic" feeding (nutritional rehabilitation)

Special, intensive feeding provided under close medical supervision for severely malnourished children.

In practice, if "feeding" is necessary at all, an integrated package of measures should be envisaged which is appropriate to the local socio-economic situation as well as observed nutritional needs. The very clear separation which has often been made between general and supplementary feeding may not always be appropriate.

General principles

All actions related to ensuring access to food supplies and restoring/increasing local food production should be planned as an integrated "package." The implementation of all separate interventions must be closely co-ordinated.

While trying to ensure the preservation of life and nutritional health, emphasize the restoration of self-reliance:

— Always try to help people where they are; avoid the creation of relief camps. Strengthen appropriate community and government structures as necessary.

— Free distributions of basic foodstuffs are not necessary in all situations. Assuring sufficient availability at fair prices—and the opportunities for people to work and earn money (or food itself)—may be possible and more appropriate.

— Phase out as quickly as possible any general food distributions which might be necessary initially but which, if prolonged, may retard the regeneration of local production, distribution and marketing systems, and create dependency.

Where food distribution and/or special feeding programmes are necessary:

— The community itself must be involved as much as possible in planning and organizing operations. Distributions should generally be selective, ensuring that commodities reach those who need them most. Cultural considerations must be taken into account.

— Distribution sites and feeding centres must be located as close as possible to the communities concerned. (This makes take-up easier and forestalls migrations towards areas where food is believed to be more readily available.)

— Similar practices and criteria should be followed in all places and by all organizations involved in food/feeding programmes.

— All feeding operations and food distributions must be organized and scheduled in close co-ordination with each other and with the delivery of health and other services within the community.

— Food items which are familiar locally should be used, to the extent possible, in all feeding programmes. But pragmatism is also needed: in many situations whatever can be obtained quickly will have to be used!

— All concerned must be aware of the length of time for which the programme inputs are expected to be provided.

In all cases:

— Ensure mobilization—and co-ordination—of available nutritional expertise. (A central food and nutrition committee may be formed to establish specific guidelines and to monitor both needs and programmes.)

— Ensure public health measures to protect food supplies and reduce infection.

—Provide relevant health and nutrition education—for women and community leaders—focusing on a few specific behaviour modifications relevant to the local situation and possibilities.

—Ensure any complementary inputs needed to enable women to take appropriate actions within the resources available to them. Include demonstrations on how to best use the food items available.

Take account of what is available locally at different seasons to the various population groups. Don't underestimate the ability of people to adapt and exploit local sources not normally used.

Role of UNICEF

Specific objectives

- **To ensure that sufficient and appropriate food is available and able to be prepared for infants, young children, pregnant and lactating mothers — in both the short and long terms.**

- **To ensure the identification and appropriate treatment of children suffering from severe malnutrition.**

Possible programme interventions

If local food production has been disrupted:

—Complement the inputs of FAO and others by timely assistance to household and community-level food production, processing and storage.

If adequate supplies of basic foods are not available in the area:

—Promote and assist arrangements to ensure the supply in all locations of sufficient food for sale at affordable prices, and the provision of income-earning opportunities if necessary; *and/or*

—Complement, where necessary, the inputs of WFP and others for any food-for-work operations or general emergency feeding by assistance to: organizing deliveries and distributions—providing tools—ensuring necessary utensils and cooking fuel—demonstrating to women the best use of available items (especially any unfamiliar ones); *and*

—Ensure monitoring of nutritional status and, where necessary, promote and assist appropriate measures to ensure that young children, pregnant and lactating women receive adequate and suitable food. This might include supplementary feeding until their access to sufficient suitable food from other sources is assured.

If availability of basic foodstuffs from local sources *plus* any relief rations remains inadequate in total energy and/or deficient in other nutrients, seek improvements in rations while also promoting local production of nutritious items.

If communities/households lack the means to prepare and cook food:
— Assist the organization and operation of communal kitchens where these are necessary initially.
— Ensure the availability of necessary utensils, water and cooking fuel to households as and when feasible.

If items suitable for infant feeding are not available (to all or to particular sub-groups):
— Encourage WFP and other food donors to provide appropriate items.
— Promote the local production of suitable foods and demonstrations to show women what can be done with what is available.
— If necessary, arrange the provision and distribution of suitable items until local production or other organizations can take over.
— Promote and assist the preparation of weaning food by mothers on a communal basis where this is suitable.

If adequate quantities of basic foods are available in the area but certain population sub-groups do not have access to them:
— Promote income-earning opportunities for those groups, especially their women.
— Promote improved food production, processing and storage by those groups in particular.
— Provide complementary inputs for food-for-work programmes or any general emergency feeding considered necessary in the mean time.
— Ensure monitoring of their nutritional status and, where necessary, promote and assist appropriate measures to ensure that young children, pregnant and lactating women receive adequate and suitable food.

If serious levels of malnutrition already exist:
— Ensure—by systematic nutritional status screening—the identification of priority communities and the individual children in need of special feeding.
— Determine the underlying causes and assist the expansion/establishment and operation of appropriate therapeutic feeding programmes and, where considered necessary and appropriate, supplementary feeding and necessary public health measures.
— Ensure ongoing monitoring of nutritional status of children.

63

In the case of displaced populations:

—Complement the inputs of WFP and others for employment and/or basic feeding, if necessary.

—Promote any possible production of nutritious foods by the displaced people themselves.

—Ensure initial screening and ongoing monitoring of nutritional status of children.

—Assure the availability/preparation of suitable weaning foods and, where necessary, assist the establishment of special feeding programmes.

In all cases:

—Encourage mothers to breast-feed their infants for as long as possible and promote the best possible weaning practices in the circumstances.

—Ensure the availability/provision of substitutes (wet nurses and/or special feeding) for infants whose mothers have died/disappeared or cannot lactate.

—Promote appropriate health and nutrition education, and public health measures to protect children against infection.

Complementing FAO and WFP

The UN organizations should, jointly as a team, assist the government in defining and then implementing an appropriate emergency food and nutrition policy. WFP is then, within the UN, responsible for the mobilization of bulk foodstuffs and FAO for mobilizing resources for the restoration of (large scale) agricultural production.

By providing complementary inputs at the level of local communities, UNICEF can have a vital role in stimulating small-scale/household food production and also ensuring that communities are able to take full advantage and benefit from the inputs of the other organizations. Such inputs may include: tools—vegetable seeds—materials for small-scale irrigation, fishing, animal husbandry, etc.

Only in the most exceptional circumstances should UNICEF be directly involved in providing basic food supplies (general feeding) for entire population groups, or the restoration of staple crop production.

(If the situation is critical and neither government nor any other agency is able to make basic commodities available quickly enough UNICEF might, in close co-ordination with WFP, undertake local purchase and distribution of limited quantities of basic foods to ensure survival in the days until others are able to deliver—if rapid delivery and appropriate distribution of such UNICEF inputs can be reasonably assured.)

Ensuring appropriate food for "vulnerable groups"

In an effort to meet the particular needs of young children (including the moderately malnourished), pregnant and lactating women, "supplementary feeding centres" are often set up and operated by outside organizations. This has been the case especially for displaced and drought-affected populations. In many situations other approaches may, however, be possible—and preferable—to ensure that families have sufficient basic food/rations and are able to prepare foods suitable for young children.

Supplementary feeding programmes (SFPs) which provide on-the-spot feeding (prepared meals) over an extended period for selected vulnerable groups require the commitment of considerable human and financial resources for planning, initiation, ongoing operation and supervision. They have been important in saving the lives of malnourished children in some situations, especially in the early phases of assistance to populations who were already malnourished and weak.

However, some experience and recent research suggests that, in many instances, apart from being expensive:

—The benefits of such "supplementary" feeding to the intended recipients are much less than hoped for as many of the children are then given less than their normal share of the family food at home;

—The most needy and vulnerable individuals are not always included—or do not actually attend regularly; *and*

—The crowding together of large numbers of children in feeding centres greatly increases the risks of spreading communicable diseases.

A greater nutritional impact may, in some situations, be possible by providing families with sufficient food, advice and help in preparing appropriate food for young children, where necessary, and assuring follow-up home visits by basic PHC-type workers. Resources are thus focused on helping families directly rather than on the establishment and management of SFP operations as such.

The necessary food might be provided as supplementary "dry rations" through an appropriate SFP. In some circumstances it might be possible to completely integrate such rations with any "general" feeding programme serving the same population either by ensuring an adequate, basic family ration or by arrangements which provide each family with rations tailored to its particular needs.

(Dry rations of "supplementary" food are also likely to be shared with other members of the family, but responsibility for the allocation of available food resources is not removed from the family and evidence suggests that the impact on the intended beneficiaries may sometimes be better than that achieved through on-the-spot feeding.)

Decide on a strategy to help mothers—and communities in general—to care for their children on the basis of a thorough assessment of the local situation, including social and cultural factors. (See also Annex 5, p. 202.) **65**

Nutritional status

Baseline data

☐ What nutrition status data has been gathered in the area in the recent past?

☐ What levels of malnutrition have been observed in "normal" times in the area?

☐ What specific deficiencies are common/endemic?

Present situation

☐ Do clinics, nutrition rehabilitation units, hospitals report any change in numbers of new cases of malnutrition seen/admitted?

☐ Are any systematic surveys being undertaken now?

   —If so: By whom? What coverage? Are samples representative? What results?

   —If not: What proportion of children are markedly thin? Are there obvious physical signs of oedema, hair colour changes? (See p. 237)

☐ Are levels of moderate and/or severe malnutrition significantly different from the seasonal norm?

☐ Are there signicant differences between different areas and communities? Which are the worst affected?

☐ What therapeutic and/or supplementary feeding programmes are in operation? Where? By whom? With what criteria, commodities, supervision? How many beneficiaries?

Probable evolution

☐ What are the underlying causes of the observed malnutrition: absolute lack of food in the area—lack of purchasing power—infections—poor feeding practices?

☐ Is access to food—basic items and foods suitable for weaning—likely to get better or worse? When?

☐ How are weaning and young children likely to be affected?

Conclusions for action

☐ Abnormal levels of malnutrition exist—or can be anticipated—in the following areas/communities . . .

☐ The most important present/expected nutritional deficiences are . . .

☐ The numbers of severely malnourished children in need of intensive, therapeutic feeding are . . .
[Estimate numbers in each distinct area/community.]

☐ The nutritional health of infants, young children (including those moderately malnourished), pregnant and lactating women in those areas can best be assured by . . .

☐ More thorough nutrition status surveys (if needed) and ongoing surveillance should be organized by . . .
[Specify the mechanisms to be used and resources required.]

If special therapeutic feeding programme (TFP) operations are necessary:

☐ Resources already available to expand or establish an appropriate TFP include . . .

☐ Additional resources required are . . .

☐ Mobilization, training and supervision of field personnel/auxilliaries will be organized by . . .

If supplementary feeding (SFP) operations are considered necessary:

☐ The numbers to be provided for are . . .
[Estimate ˆnumbers of each proposed target group in particular locations/population groups.]

☐ Resources already available to expand or establish an appropriate SFP include . . .

☐ Additional resources required are . . .

☐ Mobilization, training and supervision of field personnel/auxiliaries will be organized by . . .

Sources of information: health workers and field-based agricultural/rural development workers (government and others)—nutrition institutes/units—community leaders—womens groups—WHO and other agencies' personnel.

Data from clinics and administrative centres alone is not sufficient: get out into the more isolated communities to investigate conditions. If reliable nutrition status data are not available, consider organizing a small survey on-the-spot. Ensure that any sample is "representative". See Table 4/1, p. 191.

Food: production and access to supplies

Baseline data

☐ Local food habits: what items are usually consumed and how are they prepared:
  —For the family in general?
  —For weaning and young children?

☐ On what sources and systems of supply do different communities normally depend for their food: Own production?—Cash employment and market purchases?

☐ What crops are grown or gathered? By whom? What are the crop cycles? What inputs are normally required? How are they obtained/provided?

☐ What animals are raised? How many? Who owns them?

☐ What does hunting and fishing normally contribute to the diets of different population groups?

☐ What other local sources exist which are used only when times are hard?

☐ What are the main sources of cash income?

☐ What are normal market prices at different seasons?

☐ Do government rationing/subsidy mechanisms normally operate for any items?

☐ Do any traditional taboos affect the feeding of children, pregnant and lactating women?

Impact of events

☐ Have household food stocks been destroyed?

☐ Have government and market traders' stocks been lost, or supply lines disrupted?

☐ What is the stage of the agricultural cycle? To what extent have standing crops been affected?

☐ Has there been any loss/damage to farm animals, tools, machinery, seed stocks?

☐ To what extent have herds been affected? What effects on the potential for hunting and fishing?

☐ What effects on cash employment and other income-earning opportunities?

Present situation

☐ What are people eating now? From where are they getting the food?

☐ Are basic items—staples, beans, fish, meat, salt, edible oil, etc.—available in the market? At what prices? Are these different from the seasonal norm?

☐ What usable stocks are on hand: In household stocks?—With traders?—In government stocks? (Estimate quantities available per head of population.)

☐ Are any groups unable to obtain/buy what is available in local stocks?

☐ What cattle, goats, etc. are available?

☐ What food surpluses are available elsewhere in the country?—Where?— What prices?

☐ If food relief is already being distributed, is it reaching those most in need? Are there any special arrangements for "vulnerable groups"?

☐ What is the quality of present diets?

☐ Are utensils, water and fuel for cooking available in all communities? What fuel is used? How long will supplies last?

Probable evolution

☐ Is an absolute food shortage in the area likely:
   —In the immediate future?
   —In the medium term?

☐ What harvests (crops and yields) are now anticipated in the near future?

☐ What additional or alternative crops and household vegetables could be planted now or in the near future?

☐ When must seeds be planted? Can land be prepared in time (is sufficient tilling capacity available)? Are sufficient and the right varieties of seed and other inputs on hand? What yields might then be harvested, when?

☐ When might normal cash employment opportunities be restored? What other income-earning opportunities could be available? When?

☐ What normally unused foods might be exploited (roots, small animals, leaves, etc.)? How much might they contribute towards daily requirements during particular periods?

☐ What potential will there be for hunting, catching fish? Is the necessary equipment—boats, nets, etc.—available?

☐ What are the policies and intentions of the government and other agencies concerning access to food supplies?

☐ Could government and/or other (private) marketing systems deliver sufficient supplies if people had the necessary purchasing power?

☐ What possibilities exist for providing cash-for-work opportunities and/or food-for-work? What particular projects would be feasible? Where? During what periods?

☐ What relief and other food deliveries are expected? When will they arrive?

☐ What are the logistics considerations—any present and foreseeable constraints on deliveries?

Conclusions for action

☐ Access to basic food supplies is/will be adequate/inadequate for . . .
[Specify for each distinct area/community the number of people concerned and the amounts of food which they will be able to provide/obtain themselves during particular periods.]

☐ Exploitation of available, little-used sources of food can be immediately increased by . . .

☐ To restore/increase local food production, the measures and inputs required are:
—For large scale production . . .
—For household operations . . .

☐ Inputs must be delivered by (date) . . .

☐ They can be obtained from . . .

☐ Distribution/implementation should be organized by/through . . .

☐ Employment (income) can be provided for the destitute by . . .
[Specify: types of project, cash-for-work and/or food-for-work—when, how and by whom they could be organized—the inputs required.]

☐ Complementary measures required to ensure the availability of food supplies for purchase by the population at fair prices are . . .

☐ Special, selective provisions are required for particularly vulnerable households and individuals as follows: . . .
[Specify target groups, numbers, locations, quantities of food they require and for how long.]

70

☐ The kinds of foods needed—and acceptable—are: . . .

☐ The quantities required month-by-month are: . . .

☐ Distribution should be organized by/through . . .

☐ Further surveys/investigations should be undertaken by . . . to define more specifically:
   —Food needs and production potential . . .
   —Employment and food supply (marketing/distribution) possibilities . . .

Sources of information: ministry of agriculture — agricultural extension workers (government and others) — community/rural development workers — local authorities—community leaders—farmers' groups/co-operatives—FAO, ILO and other agencies' personnel.

CHAPTER 9

HEALTH

Possible problems/needs

- **Inadequacy of basic service delivery capacity due to loss of personnel, facilities, transport, etc. and/or previous deficiencies.**

- **Inadequate availability of drugs and other essential supplies.**

- **Outbreaks of specific communicable diseases.**

- **Casualties (the majority usually minor) requiring treatment.**

Previous preventive and/or long-term treatment or control programmes may also have been interrupted.

Normal seasonal patterns of disease incidence can be expected to continue, and should be anticipated: e.g. increases in diarrhoea during a wet season and in malaria thereafter.

Service capacity may be disrupted on account of:
- Damage to premises and/or loss or damage to equipment;
- Loss/departure of staff, temporarily or permanently; and/or
- Loss of means of transport and/or shortage of fuel (earthquakes, storms, floods, conflicts).

Supplies may be short on account of:
- Destruction of stocks locally and/or centrally;
- Logistic problems hampering restocking/resupply arrangements; and/or
- Disruption of local production (earthquakes, storms, floods, conflicts).
- Unusual demand (displaced populations, epidemics).
- Inadequate resources/foreign exchange to continue normal purchases/importations.

Pre-existing immunization and other long-term preventive, treatment and control programmes may be disrupted for any or all of the above reasons.

Epidemics:
- Measles outbreaks are common in crowded camps and settlements.
- Outbreaks of other, already endemic communicable diseases are possible in particular circumstances — if people are debilitated and/or overcrowded (see Table 13).
- An epidemic outbreak may occur unconnected with any other disastrous event and itself constitute an emergency situation.

N.B. Increased concern and medical attention in the aftermath of a disaster frequently results in higher reporting of existing problems than was previously the case, although the actual prevalence may not have increased.

If any increase in the transmission of an endemic, communicable disease is generated, the outbreak will typically occur 4-6 weeks after the disaster itself. This should allow sufficient time for epidemiological surveillance to be (re-)established so that any outbreak can be detected early.

General aims and priorities

- To save lives by providing, in the immediate aftermath of the disaster/event, necessary medical treatment and care for casualties and the sick.

- To preserve the health of the surviving population by restoring/providing appropriate health services, anticipating and — to the extent possible — preventing/mitigating any foreseeable outbreaks of disease.

Table 13

Possibility of outbreaks of disease

Disasters do not generate "new" diseases but, by altering the environment, *may* increase transmission of diseases which *already* exist in the region through:
— Faecal contamination of water (or the food chain) due to the disruption of any pre-existing utilities, especially sewerage systems.
— Disruption of private ways of life and consequent disruption of personal hygiene.
— Increases in population density (overcrowding) with poor hygiene and sanitation—a major risk in already densely populated areas and in temporary camp settlements.
— Population movements—migrants bringing new diseases into an area or themselves being exposed to diseases to which they have no natural resistance.
— The disruption of pre-existing vector control programmes (especially for malaria and dengue).
— The creation of environments unusually favourable for vector propagation (especially after heavy rains or floods).

Corpses rarely present a direct health hazard unless they are directly contaminating water supplies or are victims of cholera, but removal and disposal in a culturally appropriate manner will normally be a high social priority. (Ritual burial may however be a risk in a few instances; e.g. cholera, African haemorrhagic fevers.)

Outbreaks of **diarrhoea, dysentries, measles** and **pertussis** are likely in the early months of camp settlements. All are diseases of squalor which particularly affect and may be fatal for children.

Scabies is likely wherever there are problems of water availability. Neonatal tetanus is also possible.

Respiratory diseases are common among displaced populations. TB increases in crowded camps.

Malaria, where endemic, may become a major problem especially among non-immune populations who have been displaced into malarial zones.

Anaemias and other specific nutritional deficiencies—especially of vitamins A, B1 and C—are possible wherever food supplies are limited. (See Table 7/1, p. 239.)

There is no danger of **typhus** or **cholera** unless the infections were already present in the area before the event, or are brought in subsequently. Salt water inundations (storm surges/tsunamis) may actually inhibit cholera.

Where there are specific health/medical problems affecting large numbers of people, act within the first few days to:
— Treat casualties (earthquakes, conflicts).
— Organize the specific treatment for any widespread communicable disease (displaced populations, epidemics).
— Determine the causes and intensify vector control and other public health measures to remove them.

Where there are obvious health risks:
— (Re-)Establish appropriate vector control and other public health measures.

In all cases:
— Emphasize preventive and control measures, with high priority to ensuring necessary food and water supplies, reasonable personal hygiene and environmental sanitation.
— Re-establish and reinforce pre-existing services in line with the principles of primary health care: ensure necessary supplies, mobility and supervision at community level—keep to a minimum the involvement of and dependence on outside medical teams.
— Rapidly (re-)institute epidemiological surveillance to detect any outbreaks of communicable disease which might occur in the weeks following a sudden disaster, or within any camp/settlement of displaced persons.

Attention may be needed to strengthening the national and local health administrations as well as action to provide community-level care.

In the case of displaced populations:
— Expand and reinforce existing services in the area to cope with the increased demand and/or create new service delivery arrangements if necessary.
— Involve the people themselves as much as possible in organizing services.
— Train paramedical workers within the community as quickly as possible.

Where they meet a real, popular need, can complement other services but lack the means to re-establish themselves spontaneously, it may be appropriate to promote the re-establishment of traditional medecine services in close co-ordination with ("modern") PHC services.

N.B. Medical needs are often exaggerated following sudden disasters. Large numbers of doctors and massive inputs of drugs are *not* always needed.

General principles

The assurance of appropriate food and water supplies, shelter and environmental sanitation are all vital components of total health care and, in most situations, must have the highest priority.

Resources should *not* be invested in mass vaccination campaigns—except of children against measles. (In some areas other vaccinations may, exceptionally, also be indicated by local epidemiology: e.g. meningitis, yellow fever, Japanese encephalitis.)

Any reports of epidemics should be quickly investigated to check the validity of the diagnoses and determine the actual prevalence of cases.

Emergency health services/operations should be subject to clear overall direction—ensuring effective use and control of all available resources and supplies—and appropriate guidelines be provided to all engaged in health-related activities. This might include standardization of services and treatment schedules when a variety of organizations are involved in service delivery.

Arrangements for health care must be also co-ordinated with those for food distribution and other community services.

Local health personnel in the area should be given maximum support, and the use of outside teams—especially expatriates—be kept to a minimum.

Local health personnel in the area should be given maximum support, and the use of outside teams—especially expatriates—be kept to a minimum.

Local experience is vital in assessing the severity of conditions and determining priorities. Specialist expertise may be needed to tackle epidemics.

New long-term programmes should not be initiated unless there is reasonable assurance that they will be able to be sustained (with adequate personnel and financing) within the national health services after the ending of the emergency operation.

Role of UNICEF

Specific objectives

- To ensure that measures are taken to tackle any immediate health problems affecting children and their mothers, and to protect them against foreseeable health risks.

- To ensure that essential health care services for children and their mothers are provided/restored as quickly as possible and in a way to encourage and facilitate further development and improvement through subsequent long-term programmes.

Possible programme interventions

If previous EPI operations have been disrupted:
— Assist the re-establishment and re-inforcement of those operations, including the cold chain.
— Ensure the supply of necessary vaccines, vehicle fuel, etc.

If there is significant (perhaps seasonal) risk of widespread measles and/or other preventable child diseases, but there was no previous EPI operation:
— Promote and assist the initiation of immunizations (measles first, DPT, polio and BCG later) as an accelerated development of a long-term national programme, including cold chain.
— Include yellow fever, Japanese encephalitis and, perhaps meningitis *if* there is a very high risk locally *and* vaccination capacity exists.

If there is widespread and serious diarrhoea and dehydration among children:
— Promote and assist the use of oral rehydration therapy in the home and in clinics — training, health education, ORS, home-prepared solutions.
— Strengthen capacity and facilities to rehydrate very severe cases in health centres.

If the existing health services have been disrupted:
— Assist any necessary repairs, re-equipping and resupply of PHC and MCH facilities.
— Ensure transport and fuel for supervision of village-level workers and any mobile clinic operations.
— Assist the (re)training of community-level health workers and their supervisors.

If drugs and other expendables are lacking:
— Complement the inputs of WHO and others in respect of a limited number of essential drugs.
— Anticipate any seasonal increases in malaria, respiratory infections, etc. and ensure delivery of necessary drugs in advance to field units/workers.
— Offer reimbursable procurement services to the government and others (if problem is lack of foreign exchange).

If there is a current epidemic:
— Complement the inputs of WHO and others to ensure treatment of victims and actions to remove/control the causes — drugs, chemicals, operating costs for public health measures.

If there are clear risks of communicable disease outbreaks and/or if previous vector control programmes have been disrupted:
— Assist the (re-)establishment and operation of control operations.

77

If the existing health services are over-stretched, unable to cope with the situation:
  —Assist the strengthening of overall management of health services.
  —Ensure necessary technical assistance.
  —Support the operation of any necessary, special medical teams.

UNICEF would normally have no role in respect of casualty management—apart possibly from diverting/providing some basic drugs, dressings, etc.— but might, if necessary, assist later in respect of prosthetics for injured children.

Only in exceptional circumstances should UNICEF be involved in directly sponsoring or administering foreign medical teams although, in agreement with the government, UNICEF supplies may be made available to Red Cross and NGO teams and/or there be collaboration in joint projects, e.g. for acceleration of immunization operations.

UNICEF actions should be planned in close consultation and co-ordination with WHO which is responsible, within the UN, for technical aspects of health care including advising on and co-ordinating emergency health care assistance.

Health

Baseline data:

☐ What diseases are normally prevalent in the area? What seasonal variations?

☐ What kind of health services exist? What manner of community involvement?

☐ What hospitals, dispensaries and other health care facilities exist? Where? What staff?

☐ What immunization programmes normally operate? What coverage? What staff?

☐ What special disease control programmes? What coverage? What facilities?

☐ What reporting and surveillance systems? What lines of communication between field and central units?

☐ What effects do cultural/social influences have on the utilization and effectiveness of existing health services?

☐ In instances of population displacements, were the same diseases prevalent in the areas from which the people have migrated?

Impact of events

☐ What specific effects on the health of survivors? What casualties?

☐ How have health services been affected:
   —Premises, equipment?
   —Staff?
   —Supplies?
   —Transport?

☐ How have pre-existing control programmes been affected?

☐ To what extent have stockpiles of drugs and essential supplies been affected: locally—nationally?

☐ Has local production of drugs and essential supplies been disrupted?

Present situation

☐ Who is in charge of emergency health/medical services and any special teams?

☐ Is capacity sufficient to handle immediate needs? What extra measures are being taken?

☐ What reporting and surveillance systems are operating?

☐ Do reported mortality and morbidity rates differ significantly from the seasonal norm? (Not simply due to increased medical coverage and reporting.)

☐ Is there any evidence of abnormal (for the time of year) prevalence of:
—Serious dehydration?
—Frequent diarrhoeas?
—Measles?
—Respiratory diseases?
—Malaria?
—Neo-natal tetanus?
—Other communicable diseases?
[Cross-check any reports of epidemics.]

☐ What are the probable causes? Are people living in unusually crowded/squalid conditions?

☐ What is the present effectiveness of:
—Community-level (PHC), MCH and other basic health services?
—Referral services?
—Immunization programmes? Is there a functioning cold chain?

☐ What actions have already been taken to re-establish services? What constraints remain?

☐ What personnel (qualified, trainees and experienced auxiliaries) are available? Do they have the facilities to live and work effectively? What other personnel might be mobilized?

☐ What quantities of essential supplies—dressings, ORS, basic drugs, vaccines—are available? Where? For how long will stocks last?

☐ What actions/plans have already been taken/prepared (by the government or others) to provide personnel, supplies, and to rehabilitate/reinforce pre-existing services?

Probable evolution

☐ What evolution can be expected in:
—The numbers of casualties requiring treatment?
—The prevalence of disease?

☐ What climatic/seasonal and environmental factors are to be considered?

☐ To what extent will existing stocks, already-planned inputs and any local production of drugs and other supplies meet expected requirements?

☐ How will logistics considerations and constraints influence operations?

Conclusions for action

☐ The main health problems and hazards:
  —At present are . . .
  —Which can be anticipated are . . .

☐ Priority measures necessary:
  —To prevent further spread of disease are . . .
  —To tackle current health problems are . . .

☐ The restoration/provision of basic community-level health care and MCH services requires the *immediate* provision of . . .
  [E.g. temporary shelter/repairs for health premises—emergency drugs and other supplies—vehicles, fuel, vehicle repairs—additional personnel.]

☐ To then consolidate and re-establish reasonable community-level and essential referral services requires . . .
  [E.g. reconstruction—re-equipment—resupply—retraining. Specify feasible targets and means for implementation.]

☐ Priorities and practical possibilities for immunization operations are . . .
  [E.g. measles vaccination of all children—full immunization (EPI) of children—tetanus vaccination of pregnant women. Specify numbers, schedules and include cold chain requirements.]

☐ The (re-)establishment an effective disease surveillance system requires . . .

☐ Overall health management and administration can cope/needs to be reinforced by . . .

☐ More detailed, expert investigations/surveys are needed to plan operations for . . .
  [E.g. reconstruction, re-equipment, retraining.]

Sources of information: ministry of health—hospitals, clinics, etc.—special medical relief teams—local administration—WHO—other organizations involved in health care and community development in the area—community leaders—the people themselves.

CHAPTER 10

WATER

Possible problems/needs

- **Insufficient safe water for domestic and hygiene purposes — and thus a health hazard.**

- **Lack of water for animals and irrigation — and thus a threat to food production and supplies.**

N.B. Water availability can vary enormously between areas and over quite short distances.

Insufficient quantities of water may result from:
- Drying up of surface water sources—rivers, lakes (droughts);
- Reduction in yield or complete drying up of wells or springs (droughts, possibly earthquakes);
- Blockage of open wells, or (temporary) loss of access to them (earthquakes, floods, conflicts);
- Reduced flow in piped water systems due to damage to pipes, pumping installations, reservoirs, etc. (earthquakes, storms, conflicts); and/or

—Increases in the demand for water beyond the capacity of available systems/sources in specific localities (population displacements).

Unsafe (poor quality) water may result from:

—Contamination of open wells or other surface water sources by polluted water, bodies or faecal matter (floods, conflicts); and/or

—Contamination of (damaged) piped water systems, e.g. by sewage (earthquakes, storms, conflicts).

Problems are compounded if facilities to store, conserve and distribute available supplies are damaged or otherwise insufficient.

General aims and priorities

- To save life and preserve health by making at least minimum quantities of reasonably safe water available for household use, for institutions and community services.

- To provide supplies, where possible, for livestock and irrigation purposes.

- To restore previously existing sources, pumping, storage and distribution systems where possible. To develop alternative arrangements where necessary.

The need is usually for practical, expedient measures to make minimum supplies available fast. Initial emphasis should be on storage and conservation measures for available supplies. Drilling and developmental approaches to exploit possible new sources may come later.

In all cases:

—Protect available water sources and any functioning storage and distribution systems from possible contamination (by restricting access by people and animals).

—Ensure arrangements—including funding, materials, fuel and personnel—for the ongoing operation and maintenance of all systems, and prompt repairs (or replacement) in the event of breakdown.

Where quantities are inadequate:

—Conservation measures: establish storage tanks—control storage and distribution—minimize waste and promote recycling for sanitation and irrigation where possible—enforce rationing where necessary.

—Restore pre-existing sources, pumping, storage and delivery systems wherever and as quickly as possible.

—Seek and exploit new/alternative sources where necessary, using technologies which are simple and already familiar in the area and for which the capacity for operation and maintenance can be assured.

—Ensure supplies for health and other institutions and any special feeding centres.

—Deliver water by truck if necessary, but only as a strictly short-term, stop-gap emergency measure to ensure survival while other arrangements are made.

Where available water is contaminated:

—Remove the causes of contamination where possible.

—Disinfect wells, storage and distribution systems.

—Ensure adequate chlorination of supplies in municipal systems and the improvement of water quality elsewhere by storage, filtration and/or chemical treatment if necessary and supervision can be assured.

—Ensure arrangements for regular testing of water quality at distribution points.

After floods:

—Pump out flooded wells once flood water recedes.

General principles

An adequate quantity of reasonably safe water is preferable to a smaller quantity of pure water.

The community itself must be involved as much as possible in planning and implementing arrangements.

In all situations, the national and/or local authority responsible for water resources should normally be responsible and must in any case be involved in all phases of operations. Existing equipment and organizational structures should be used to the extent possible, and reinforced if necessary.

Special attention must be given to ensuring supplies for hospitals, health and feeding centres.

At least minimum quantities of reasonably safe water should be provided as close as possible to homes, and in any case not further away than other, polluted sources which look and taste acceptable.

Provide as much safe storage as possible at community and household levels. Try to minimize the risk of water being contaminated (in household containers) after collection from sources or distribution points.

The investment of resources (time, effort and material) in "interim" solutions must be kept to a minimum. As a last resort, people may have to be moved to locations where water is available.

Appropriate technical expertise must be mobilized:
— Water engineers to exploit available sources.
— Sanitarians to test and if necessary organize the treatment of supplies.
— Hydrogeologists to assess ground water potential.
— Hydrologists to assess surface-water potential.

Measures to ensure reasonable domestic hygiene and general environmental sanitation require as much attention as the provision of safe water itself. Keep water supplies and sanitation facilities well-separated.

Table 14

Estimating water requirements

Minimum needs depend on the situation but, as a general indication, the following amounts are desirable:

Individuals: 15-20 litres per person per day (absolute minimum of 3-5 l/day for survival);

Health centres: 40-60 litres per patient per day;

Feeding centres: 20-30 litres per beneficiary per day.

Additional quantities may be needed for:
— Sanitation facilities (2-5 l/day/person for many latrine systems).
— Other community services.
— Livestock (perhaps 30 l/day/head for cattle; 5 l/day/head for small animals).
— Irrigation (perhaps 5-6 l/day/sq.m = 50-60 cu.m/day/ha, but get local advice for crops concerned).

Individuals' needs increase with air temperature and physical exertion. In all cases, the more convenient the supply, the higher will be consumption.

People who have been displaced or concentrated into camps for any reason require more water than they previously managed on (because of crowding and other environmental factors).

Where water is short, waste water after domestic use may, at least initially, be recycled—used in latrines or (if free from soap/detergents) for growing vegetables. Large-scale irrigation is a matter for expert investigation and advice.

Role of UNICEF

Specific objectives for UNICEF

- To ensure the availability of sufficient safe water for hygiene and domestic use at household level and for institutions and services benefiting children.

- To ensure the availability and efficient use of water for household or community-level food production.

Possible programme interventions

In all cases:

—Ensure sufficient supplies of safe water for feeding centres, communal kitchens, health clinics, etc., and train staff to prevent contamination.

—Ensure that households have suitable containers for collecting and storing water.

—Ensure quality testing wherever contamination is suspected and/or diarrhoeal diseases prevalent.

—Promote conservation of available supplies and recycling wherever feasible.

—Ensure the ongoing maintenance of all pumps and delivery systems.

If yields from existing wells are reduced and/or insufficient for an enlarged population:

—Get good hydrogeological advice, promote expert surveys and, *where found appropriate,* assist deepening of existing wells and/or sink new wells.

If surface-water sources are reduced/dried up:

—Ensure protection and the conservation of available surface water (by controlling access, constructing small dams, retention pits, etc.).

—Assist digging wells in/near normal surface flows, possibly in conjunction with sub-surface dams.

If wells are blocked, damaged or contaminated:

—Assist cleaning/re-sinking where possible, then pumping out and disinfection.

—Assist construction of replacements nearby where necessary.

If piped distribution systems have been damaged:
— Assist the setting up of standpipes and/or distribution tanks as immediate, temporary measures.
— Assist repairs and disinfection of the system based on expert surveys.

If available water is unsafe and of a quality less than the people are habituated to:
— Assist rainwater collection where possible and the search for and exploitation of alternative sources (especially ground water).
— Assist the improvement/treatment of unsafe water until better quality water is available.

If, after all other possible short-term measures, the quantities available are still insufficient for survival:
— Assist in delivering supplies by truck to ensure survival until other sources can be found, water be piped in, or the population be moved.
— Assist in setting up any tanks necessary to receive and store such water at strategic locations: ensure arrangements to control its use.

Where UNICEF is already involved in water supply activities—especially in rural and/or underprivileged urban areas—expand/adapt those activities to meet the particular needs created by the emergency situation.

Where WHO, the World Bank and/or bilateral aid projects and personnel are substantially involved in water supply and water resource development activities in an area—particularly in urban areas—they may be expected to take a lead in assisting the relevant local authorities in assessing and responding to needs.

In the event that sufficient technical personnel are not immediately available, help (pending the arrival of needed expertise) to: inspect, protect and where necessary disinfect currently used sources—assess possibilities of restoring other previously used sources and systems—investigate any alternative possibilities—ensure the ongoing operation of existing systems—initiate storage and filtration treatment where necessary, etc.

Evaluate very carefully any proposals for large investments—e.g. in drilling rigs—and programmes with major long-term implications. Do not rush into them hastily.

Water supplies

Baseline data

☐ What are the normal sources and arrangements for distribution and any treatment of water for drinking and hygiene purposes:
  —In rural areas?
  —In urban areas?

☐ What authorities control the supplies and maintain distribution systems, pumps, etc.?

☐ How, by whom are new wells normally dug/installed? What equipment is normally used and available in the area?

☐ What hydrogeological (ground-water) and hydrological (surface-water) data are available for the area?

☐ What are the normal seasonal variations in water levels, etc.?

☐ To what quality of water is the population habituated?

☐ What awareness is there of the importance of safe water and sanitation? What habits, attitudes and beliefs affect the use of water?

Impact of events

☐ In what ways have water sources and/or distribution systems been affected (damaged, contaminated, etc.):
  —In rural areas?
  —In urban areas?

☐ Has the capacity for operation, repair and maintenance of systems been affected?

☐ Has severity of impact varied between areas?

Present situation

☐ From where are people obtaining water at present:
  —For drinking?
  —For domestic hygiene purposes?
  —For animals and irrigation?

☐ How much water is available and being used per household?

☐ How much is actually required:
  —For basic human needs?
  —For institutions?
  —For animals and agriculture?

☐ Which, if any, population groups do not have access to sufficient quantities of water? What proportion of the total population? How many people?

☐ Is the water now being used for drinking safe, of acceptable quality?
— Has it been tested?
— How does it compare with that available and used previously?
— Is there evidence of widespread diarrhoea or skin disease?
— Are any supplies being treated?

☐ Are available sources sufficiently protected to avoid contamination? Are contaminated wells or distribution systems being disinfected?

☐ What stocks of chlorine chemicals are on hand? How long will they last?

☐ Are existing pumps operating and being maintained? What stocks of fuel are on hand? Is resupply assured?

☐ What action is already being taken to repair damaged, distribution systems, pumps, etc.?

☐ What stocks of repair materials are on hand? How many technicians? Transport?

Potential supplies

☐ What more can be done to conserve and/or recycle available supplies? Who can do it?

☐ What possibilities are there for restoring previously used sources and delivery systems?

☐ What other (private) supply sources and systems existed in the area? Are they functioning and accessible?

☐ What possibilities for finding and exploiting other/new sources in the vicinity?

☐ What equipment, materials and expertise would be required? What yields might finally be expected?

☐ What capacity exists—and how long will it take—to organize and implement such measures:
— In the short term?
— In the longer term?

Probable evolution

☐ What weather is forecast? What are the implications for water supplies?

☐ What changes in supply are now expected due to seasonal variations? When?

☐ Are (further) population movements anticipated?

☐ What other changes in demand for water might be anticipated?

☐ What further supplies are likely to be restored—and when—with currently available resources?

☐ What actions are being taken or planned by the government and others:
   —To meet any short-term needs?
   —To meet longer term needs?

Conclusions for action

☐ Water supplies are/will be adequate/inadequate/unsafe for . . .
[Specify for each distinct area/community the number of people concerned and the amount and quality of water which will be available to them during particular periods.]

☐ Where supplies are inadequate or unsafe, *immediate* action is required to:
   —Protect sources and distribution systems against contamination by . . .
   —Make minimum quantities available (while repairs or other actions are being organized) by . . ..
   —Conserve supplies and re-cycle waste water by . . .
[Specify actions required in particular areas, how and by whom they can be organized on an emergency basis.]

☐ The restoration of previous sources/systems requires . . .
[Specify actions and the time required for implementation.]

☐ Measures required to develop alternatives sources/systems . . .
[Specify actions and the time required for implementation.]

☐ Assistance is needed in respect of . . .
[E.g. equipment—materials and spare parts—transport and fuel—technical advice/expertise.]

☐ The following more detailed investigations are required to determine water needs and supply possibilities more specifically: . . .

Possible sources of information: local administration, especially officials responsible for water resources, agriculture, local government—community leaders—community organizations, NGOs, WHO—engineering consultants and contractors.

CHAPTER 11

HYGIENE AND SANITATION

Possible problems/needs

- **Contamination of water supplies and the environment in general by human excreta, especially faeces.**

- **Proliferation of disease-bearing insects and rodents.**

- **Inadequate personal and domestic hygiene.**

These factors may create actual or potential threats to the health of individuals and the community as a whole.

Contamination may result from:
  —Damage to sewerage systems (earthquakes, conflicts);
  —Human faeces or bodies being swept into wells and other water sources (floods, storms); and/or

—Overcrowding and disruption of previous arrangements for the disposal of human excreta (displaced populations).

Vector proliferation from:

—Disruption of previous vector control activities; and/or

—Creation of habitats and conditions in which the vectors multiply—especially the accumulation of refuse and waste/stagnant water (floods, storms, earthquakes, conflicts).

Inadequate hygiene from:

—Loss of necessary utensils and supplies (e.g. soap) and/or insufficient water.

In cases of displaced populations in camps/settlements, overcrowding and an unfamiliar environment often lead to general insanitary conditions.

Emergencies do not normally create any new problems of sanitation in rural areas unless people are concentrated into camps.

General aims and priorities

- To prevent the spread of disease and promote the establishment of a safe environment.

- To provide the means for reasonable personal and domestic hygiene.

In all cases, but especially in densely populated urban areas after storms and floods, and in cases of displaced populations:

—Ensure the (re-)establishment and operation of suitable arrangements within the community for the safe disposal of human faeces.

—Organize the removal and sanitary disposal of refuse, the disposal of corpses in a culturally appropriate manner, and the draining off of waste or stagnant water.

—(Re-)Establish activities to control the carriers of common vector-borne diseases (insects and rodents).

—Ensure necessary water supplies and facilities for personal and domestic hygiene.

In droughts and cases of displaced populations in dry areas:

—Control dust.

General principles

Public education campaigns emphasizing the importance of sanitation and focusing on practical measures which people can take are essential. Sanitation measures must be closely co-ordinated with those for water supply and health services.

The rapid establishment of a basic excreta disposal system is better than delayed provision of an improved one! Where there are large numbers of people and no (functioning) sewerage system, communal trench latrines are often the best immediate measure—with strict arrangements to ensure proper use and cleaning of them.

In all cases, community participation is essential. Arrangements must be culturally as well as technically appropriate—even if circumstances necessitate a departure from traditional practices. Systems, once established, must be able to be operated with a minimum of external involvement, but ongoing monitoring of conditions must also be assured.

In cases of displaced populations, rapid pilot projects can yield valuable lessons on what should be done, and how.

Role of UNICEF

Specific objectives

- As above, realizing that young children are the most vulnerable to the diseases which arise from inadequate sanitation.

Possible programme interventions

If households lack the means to ensure reasonable personal and domestic hygiene:
- Ensure the provision of necessary facilities, soap, utensils, etc.;
- Ensure the availability of clean household water containers; and
- Promote other practical measures and education to achieve feasible improvements in hygiene.

If pre-existing sewerage systems have been disrupted and are contaminating the environment:
- Ensure immediate repairs and disinfection where possible.

—Promote the establishment of temporary alternative arrangements where necessary.

If there are large numbers of people and no functioning sewerage system:

—Assist the prompt establishment of appropriate arrangements—possibly trench and/or family latrines—which are suitable for children to use;

—Ensure arrangements to regularly clean communal latrines; *and*

—Promote relevant health education.

If there is an accumulation of refuse, stagnant or waste water:

—Assist community-based arrangements to remove, compost and/or burn refuse.

—Promote action to drain away or recycle waste water from households and institutions and, where/when possible, to drain off stagnant water.

If particular disease-bearing insects or rodents are—or are likely to—proliferate:

—Ensure the (re-)institution of appropriate vector control measures; *and*

—Promote public awareness and action to reduce health hazards.

Sources of information for assessment: local water authority personnel—public health workers (governmental and NGO)—community leaders—WHO.

Hygiene and sanitation

Baseline data

☐ What are traditional arrangements for defecation, anal cleaning and disposal of excrement:
— In rural areas?
— In urban areas?

☐ What cultural/religious considerations influence arrangements for defecation?

☐ How high is the water table level? What seasonal variations? What other physical considerations affect means of disposal of excrement? Is it ever composted?

☐ How is refuse disposed of?

☐ What vector control programmes operated in the area? What methods? Equipment? Staff?

☐ Which authorities are responsible for environmental sanitation?

Impact of events

☐ What effects on:
— Urban sewerage systems?
— Arrangements for defecation in rural areas?
— Accumulation/disposal of waste water?
— Accumulation/disposal of solid refuse?
— Facilities for personal hygiene (washing, etc.)?

☐ How have vector control programmes been affected?

Present situation

☐ What weather conditions prevail? What are ground conditions and the water table level? Any stagnant water?

☐ Where are people defecating now? Are there health hazards arising from the inadequate disposal of faeces:
— In urban areas?
— In rural areas?

☐ What is being done with solid refuse? With waste water?

☐ What standards of personal and food hygiene are people able to maintain?

☐ Is there evidence of:
 —Diseases likely to be related to poor sanitation or particular vectors?
 —Significant problems with insects or rodents?

☐ How well are existing vector control operations functioning?

☐ What are the perceptions of the people themselves: is sanitation seen to be important, a "problem" or not?

Probable evolution

☐ What weather is forecast, with what implications for environmental conditions including water table level?

☐ Are health hazards likely to increase:
 —Is there a danger of contamination of water supplies by excreta?
 —Are insects and/or rodents likely to proliferate?

☐ To what extent do existing services/authorities have capacity to handle to the situation?

☐ What can the communities be expected to do themselves in the immediate future?

Conclusions for action

☐ The main environmental health hazards are caused by ...

☐ To reduce health hazards, *immediate* action is necessary to ...
 [E.g. control defecation—dispose of faeces—dispose of damaged food stocks. Specify actions which are technically *and* culturally feasible, how and by whom they should be organized on an emergency basis.]

☐ *Further* measures to then be taken include: ...
 [Specify actions, how and by whom: e.g. repairing previous latrines/sewerage systems—improving interim/emergency arrangements for excreta disposal—(re-)establishing facilities for personal hygiene—disposing of waste water and solid refuse—draining away stagnant water—(re-)activating vector control activities.]

☐ Personnel and material resources which can be mobilized locally include ...

☐ Assistance will be needed in respect of ...

☐ More detailed investigations should be undertaken by ... to determine needs and medium/long-term solutions for ...

CHAPTER 12

SHELTER AND HOUSEHOLD FUNCTIONING

Possible problems/needs

- **Lack of adequate shelter.**

- **Lack of essential personal and household items — clothing, blankets, utensils, etc.**

Shelter may be lacking as a result of
   —Dwellings having been destroyed or rendered unsafe (earthquakes, storms, conflicts); and/or
   —Abandonment of homes—either forced or voluntary (displaced populations).

Essential personal and household items may be lacking as a result of:
- Loss or damage (floods, conflict);
- Abandonment (displaced populations); and/or
- Exchange for other more essential items, e.g. food (drought, conflict, displaced populations).

Separately or jointly these factors may directly endanger life—through risk of exposure in harsh climates and the inability to prepare food—or at least render normal family life impossible with consequent social and psychological effects, but:
- Don't overestimate the need for emergency shelter or the speed with which materials can be delivered from outside and distributed.
- Don't underestimate the capacity of the stricken community to cope and help itself.

People often manage to arrange temporary shelter—using the remains of their previous homes and/or through kinship ties—and perhaps even make a start towards permanent reconstruction, in the first few days following a disaster.

In the particular instance of *earthquakes*, however, people generally do *not* wish to start reconstruction immediately (for fear of further shocks) but prefer to remain for a while in light-weight, temporary structures adjacent/close to their property. Temporary shelter may then also be needed, during this "waiting" period, by people whose own dwellings have not (yet) been damaged.

General aims and priorities

- **To save lives and facilitate the resumption of normal patterns of life by ensuring at least the minimum necessary provision of shelter, clothing and other essential household items.**

In all cases:
- Ensure the ability of households to prepare food.
- Organize communal kitchens as an immediate emergency measure where necessary.

Where lack of shelter and/or personal protection items is an immediate threat to health and survival (in cold and wet climates):
- Ensure availability of materials to enable people to make rapid, temporary repairs or constructions.

—Encourage reconstruction as early as possible, as below.

—Ensure provision of appropriate blankets or clothing to those most in need.

Where dwellings have been damaged and personal protection items lost, but there is no immediate threat to survival:

—Promote full community participation in planning assistance to reconstruction. Ensure the delivery of inputs according to the communities' own priorities and schedules, and attention to questions of land ownership, structural design, financing, etc.

—Ensure the availability of suitable cloth and the means to make up clothing locally.

When evacuation of communities is unavoidable (in cases of severe flooding or when major secondary disasters are anticipated):

—Ensure necessary services as well as temporary accommodation.

—Facilitate as rapid a return as possible to previous homes/lands.

Where there is no alternative to permanent resettlement:

—Ensure (thorough advance investigation and planning) the re-creation of viable communities with necessary services as well as housing.

General principles

Evacuation of people from their homes, temporary camps and re-settlement elsewhere should be avoided if at all possible. "Survivors" must not be turned into "refugees". Children must not be separated from their families.

Arrangements for shelter should be planned on the basis of assessed human *needs* rather than a detailed survey of physical *damage*. The people themselves must be the principal participants in the reconstruction process, including the establishment of priorities.

Maximum effort and resources should be directed to encouraging, assisting and accelerating local reconstruction efforts from the earliest possible moment.

When provisions do have to be made for temporary, emergency shelter:

—Provide materials which can be reused later in permanent reconstruction.

—Make maximum use of materials which can be salvaged from damaged buildings.

—Give highest priority to roofing.

—Avoid "temporary" and prefabricated/relief housing.

Facilitate the re-establishment of normal household operations as soon as feasible: communal kitchens, etc. only as stop-gap measures where necessary.

99

Give particular attention to fuel for cooking, especially in droughts and cases of displaced populations. Try to avoid further degradation of the environment by too much collection of firewood.

Items provided for personal and household use, if needed at all, must be delivered quickly. They must be culturally appropriate and durable. Second-hand clothing from other countries is rarely appropriate.

Role of UNICEF

Specific objective

- To safeguard the lives of young children by ensuring the availability of necessary shelter, clothing and household items essential to their survival and the satisfactory functioning of the family units to which they belong.

If lack of shelter and personal protection is an immediate threat to the survival and health of children:
- Ensure rapid availability of suitable materials to improvise emergency shelter, e.g. plastic sheeting, nails.
- Ensure timely provision of blankets and/or suitable clothing (child sizes).

Where dwellings have been damaged and personal protection items lost, but there is no immediate threat to survival:
- Ensure the materials and facilities for children's clothing to be made within the community.
- Consider limited, catalytic inputs to support community reconstruction efforts.

Where households are unable to prepare food:
- Ensure provision of necessary household utensils, sanitary water carriers, efficient stoves, cooking fuel, etc. as soon as possible.
- Assist the rapid establishment and operation of communal kitchens where necessary in the mean time.

UNICEF should not normally be involved in housing reconstruction programmes. Very limited, catalytic inputs may, however, be provided where necessary to break bottlenecks inhibiting communal efforts (and when such inputs cannot be supplied quickly enough by others).

Shelter and reconstruction of dwellings

Baseline data

☐ What types of construction are commonly used for private dwellings and public buildings:
  — In the urban areas?
  — In the rural areas?

☐ What was their general condition before the disaster?

☐ What is the average family size and occupancy rate of dwellings?

☐ How many days does it take to construct a typical dwelling? Who normally does the work? What total cost?

☐ What construction materials are normally available in the area:
  — Natural products?
  — Locally manufactured?
  — Brought in from outside?

☐ What arrangements have communities previously/traditionally made to establish emergency shelter and reconstruct dwellings after similar disasters?

☐ What structures/organizations exist, or were created in the past, to allocate materials and/or organize temporary shelter?

Impact of events

☐ What has been the effect on the various types of structures?

☐ What proportion — thus how many — family dwellings no longer offer safe shelter?

☐ What materials can be salvaged?

☐ What effects on stocks and any local production of construction materials?

☐ What has been the immediate reaction/response of the population: voluntary evacuation (to where) — erection of temporary shelters — immediate start towards permanent reconstruction?

Present situation

☐ Where are families whose dwellings have been destroyed now living? What temporary arrangements have already been made privately or officially?

☐ What proportion (how many) families are still without even temporary shelter?

☐ What is the weather like? What is the temperature at night? Is improved shelter immediately necessary to preserve life? What priority do the people themselves give to arranging better temporary shelter?

☐ What construction materials are currently available locally? Where? In what quantities? What price?

☐ What craftsmen, other manpower and equipment are available for salvage and reconstruction work?

☐ What stocks of materials suitable for improvising emergency shelters and making repairs to dwellings are available: in the locality—in the country?

Probable evolution

☐ What weather is forecast for the immediate future? What secondary disasters are anticipated? What implications for shelter arrangements?

☐ If families have been forced to evacuate homes/villages temporarily, how soon might they be able to return?

☐ What arrangements for temporary shelter and long term reconstruction do the people intend/hope to make for themselves?

☐ What could they do with limited assistance:
   —In the next few days?
   —In the longer term?

☐ What are the policies of the government and other agencies with regard to shelter and reconstruction? What plans and inputs are already envisaged?

Conclusions for action

☐ **If** it is considered necessary to evacuate people temporarily:
   —Why? The reasons are ...
   —The number of people affected in each location is ...
   —Basic needs (shelter, food, water and services) should be provided as follows ...

☐ **If** the immediate provision of improved shelter is necessary to preserve life:
   —Emergency shelter is required by ...
   [Specify number of families in particular locations.]

— The best inputs would be . . .
[E.g. plastic sheeting, tents.]
— They should be obtained from . . . and be delivered and distributed by/on the basis of . . .

☐ Local reconstruction efforts should be supported and accelerated by . . .
[Specify priority inputs, implementation mechanisms and schedules.]

☐ Further detailed investigations to assess long-term reconstruction needs and possibilities should be undertaken by . . . and focus on . . .
[Specify issues e.g. land ownership/tenure, alternative ways of financing private reconstruction and distributing materials, etc.]

Household functioning/personal protection

Baseline data

☐ What type of clothing is normally worn (by children)?

☐ How many and what types of blankets and sleeping mats are normally used?

☐ What type of cooking stoves, fuel, and utensils are used?

☐ What type of containers are used for collecting and storing water?

☐ Are blankets, mats, utensils, etc. produced locally—in the household, by artisans or industrially? What market prices?

Impact of events

☐ Have clothing and blankets been lost?

☐ Have essential household items—stoves, utensils, etc.—been lost or damaged beyond use?

☐ What has been the effect on living arrangements and household functioning in general? Are families still able to live and prepare food as individual units?

☐ What effects on local production and marketing of clothing, utensils, cooking/heating fuel, etc.

Present situation

☐ What proportion/how many children do not have adequate clothing, blankets to protect their health in the prevailing conditions?

☐ What proportion/how many families no longer have the essentials for collecting water and cooking? What communal arrangements have been made?

☐ Have certain sub-groups within the community been more severely affected than others? If so, which?

☐ What stocks of clothing, blankets, buckets, utensils, etc. exist in the area? Where? What prices? What quantities/current production rates?

Probable evolution

☐ What climatic conditions are anticipated? Will additional clothing and blankets be essential?

- [ ] What arrangements are being made for water and food supplies? Will additional utensils, cooking fuel, etc. be required? What kinds (for communal facilities and/or household use)?

- [ ] How soon, if at all, will local production be able to meet the needs? Are necessary raw materials available?

- [ ] What are the policies of the government and other agencies? What relief inputs are already arranged/envisaged?

Conclusions for action

- [ ] **If** clothing and blankets are:
  - —Necessary immediately to protect the health of children, the quantities required for particular communities are ...
  - —Desirable to restore reasonable living patterns, but not immediately life-saving, ...

    [Specify needs and whether finished products should be provided or raw materials to be made up locally.]

- [ ] **If** family units are unable to prepare food individually, the establishment of temporary communal kitchens requires:
  - —Stoves, fuel, utensils as follows ...
  - —These items should be immediately borrowed/purchased from ...
  - —Kitchens should be organized by ... and will need funds, etc. as follows ...
  - —Such arrangements should be able to be phased out by ...

- [ ] To enable household units to function adequately:
  - —Utensils, cooking fuel, etc. should be provided as follows ...
  - —These items should be obtained from ...
  - —They should be sold/distributed by ...

    [Specify criteria/special arrangements to ensure receipt by those most in need.]

- [ ] More detailed investigations should be undertaken by ... to determine needs, define appropriate means of distribution, restore local production, etc. as follows: ...

CHAPTER 13

CHILD CARE AND PSYCHO-SOCIAL NEEDS

Possible problems/needs

- Unaccompanied children who, having lost or become separated from their parents and other close adult relations (or guardians), are without proper care and protection.

- Women who have lost/become separated from their husbands and face difficulties in providing for their children.

- Men who have lost/become separated from their wives and need help in caring for their infants and young children.

- Young women who are without family support and protection and need help in arranging a safe place to live.

- Individual children and families experiencing social, psychological and/or emotional problems as a result of or increased by the recent events.

● Individuals who are physically handicapped or mentally disordered, isolated old people and ethnic minorities may face particular problems and be less able to help themselves than others.

Such needs are possible in all emergencies. They are likely to be especially pronounced in cases of population displacements—when families may become separated and community resources and services are lacking—and/or when casualties have been high (some earthquakes, floods and conflicts).

Children may be traumatized by sudden, cataclysmic events, separation from their families, extreme deprivation, or—in conflict situations—being tortured/abused or seeing parents and others being tortured/killed.

Traditional arrangements and any pre-existing social services for coping with social and psychological needs and problems may be disrupted or over-extended and unable to respond adequately to these particular needs.

Breakdown of normal education and other community services—due to damage to premises, loss of materials and/or loss/absence of staff—may itself disrupt normal community life and retard the general process of recovery.

Returnees—individuals and families returning to their previous homes after being displaced for a time elsewhere—may also face major problems of reinstallation when housing, crops, employment and community services have been lost.

General aims and priorities

● To prevent the separation of families where possible, and quickly reunite families whose members have become separated.

● To provide, in a culturally appropriate manner, necessary protection and special care/services for individuals and groups with special needs.

● To expedite the normalisation of community life and re-establishment of essential community services.

Where family members have become separated (especially in population displacements and conflicts):
—Ensure appropriate interim care for unaccompanied children and others with special needs.
—Establish tracing systems to facilitate family reunion.

107

In all cases:
- —(Re-)Establish traditional mechanisms and community-based social services to meet the particular, priority needs of the population.
- —Ensure that the psychological and emotional needs of individuals are recognized and provided for as well as their physical needs.
- —Ensure that those with special needs are identified and helped to receive and use assistance which is available to them.

General principles

Priority needs should be determined by rapid surveys/enquiries by experienced, local social work professionals where such are available. Otherwise the determination should be made by local people recognized for their commitment to the well-being of all within the community, e.g. traditional and religious leaders, teachers.

Decisions and actions must follow quickly to safeguard the needs and interests of the most vulnerable, and to capitalize on the community solidarity which often exists immediately after a disaster but may dissipate quickly.

Care and services should be arranged in a culturally appropriate manner to serve the best interests of the individuals concerned. They should be decentralized with workers assigned to specific localities. Any necessary special accommodation/centres should be small and integrated into the local community.

Continuity of all personnel is essential so that stable relations of trust are built up with those being helped.

Personnel from within the community—or at least having the same cultural and linguistic background—must be mobilized to provide social services. Personal qualities, capability and acceptability to the local community are at least as important as formal qualifications as a basis of selection. Rapid basic training should be organized for previously untrained personnel, including volunteers.

As few outsiders as possible should be involved, and their role be limited to overall co-ordination, support, training and liaison with local authorities and other bodies.

All social service programmes should have the approval and backing of the local administration and community leaders, but are often best organized and implemented by NGOs using local staff and volunteers, subject to appropriate professional guidance and supervision.

Protection of refugees and civilian populations

UNHCR seeks to ensure protection and the provision of appropriate care for groups recognized as "refugees". The UNHCR Handbook for Emergencies and Handbook for Social Services outline the principles and practices for dealing with refugees. They are similar to those reflected here, especially for the care of unaccompanied children.

The ICRC endeavours to ensure the protection of civilian populations in conflict situations in accordance with the Geneva Conventions, and provides a tracing agency service to try to find and establish contact between family members who have become separated. This includes but is not limited to children separated from their families.

Many NGOs also seek—by their presence and/or programmes—to provide some protection to communities likely to be discriminated against or victimized.

Unaccompanied children

Prompt action is needed to identify children who are unaccompanied and ensure that they are cared for in ways which best meet their individual emotional and developmental needs, helped to trace or be found by their families, and protected from possibilities of abuse.

Arrangements for the care of unaccompanied children should ensure that each child:

—Benefits from the individual and sustained care of at least one adult, and continuity in community and cultural ties to the extent possible;

—Is enabled to maintain his/her existing relationships with other adults and children as much as possible; *and*

—Is helped to overcome any particular, individual problems.

This applies both to temporary, interim care while family tracing efforts are made, and to long-term care for those for whom family reunion is not achieved within a reasonable period of time.

Children should be fostered with other families wherever possible, not isolated from their communities in institutions. The should not be moved around any more than absolutely necessary between different care arrangements. Sibling groups should be kept together, and older children participate in decisions regarding arrangements for themselves and their younger siblings.

Role of UNICEF

Specific objectives

- To preserve/restore stable family environments for children, and normal community life and services for their benefit.

- To ensure appropriate care and protection for children who are unaccompanied, and rehabilitation training and services for those who are disabled.

- To ensure that other children with special needs — physical, psychological or emotional — are provided the particular help and assistance they need.

- To (re-)establish any special support services necessary to help parents — especially single parents and those who are destitute — to care for their children.

Possible interventions

In all cases:
- Advocate policies and programmes which contribute to the preservation or re-establishment of stable family environments: resist any proposals which run counter to this.
- Promote and assist the rapid re-opening of schools and other community services to meet children's basic needs.

For unaccompanied children:
- Ensure the rapid identification, adequate documentation and medical screening of unaccompanied children;
- Assume that reunion with parents or other family members is possible and ensure the establishment of arrangements for tracing and family reunion;
- Promote and assist appropriate arrangements for the temporary — emergency and interim — care of unaccompanied children while family tracing is undertaken;
- Ensure arrangements for the long-term care of any children who remain unaccompanied after reasonable tracing efforts have been undertaken;
- Ensure supervision of all care arrangements by adequately qualified social work personnel; *and*
- Determine the causes of separation and promote/assist measures to prevent further family separations (particularly focusing on single-parent families).

For children who have been traumatized or are suffering other emotional or psychological problems:

— Ensure screening to identify children suffering from such problems; *and*

— Ensure the provision of culturally appropriate, community-based help for them and their families.

For children who have been disabled:

— Ensure the expansion/establishment and operation of appropriate community-based rehabilitation services; *and*

— Promote the maximum possible integration of disabled children in normal schools and other community activities.

For women, destitute and single-parent families:

— Promote and assist relevant education/training wherever appropriate and feasible; *and*

— Promote income-generating and other services/activities to enhance their ability to support themselves and care for their children.

If informal/traditional arrangements do not meet the needs for children to be cared for while parents are working or engaged in other essential activities:

— Promote mutual support groups among mothers to care for young children; *and/or*

— Assist the re-establishment of previous day-care services, where necessary and appropriate.

Child care and psycho-social needs

Baseline data

☐ Who normally assumes responsibility for children in the absence of the mother and father?

☐ What are the traditional arrangements for:
— Care of children while parents are working?
— Care of unaccompanied children?

☐ To what extent were unaccompanied children present in the community before the emergency? For what reasons were they separated from their families? How did they live? Who cared for them?

☐ What child care facilities/services existed in the area: official, other (community/religious/voluntary)?

☐ What other welfare services? What community centres existed? What activities took place there?

☐ How many primary schools? Where? What percentage of children attended, from what age?

☐ Did schools act as centres/locations for activities in addition to formal schooling?

Impact of events

☐ What effects on children who were already unaccompanied and/or on-the-street?

☐ Have more children become "unaccompanied"? How and why have they become separated from their families?

☐ What has been the effect on traditional child care arrangements and organized social services?

☐ What has been the effect on schools and other education activities?

☐ Have children been abducted, abused, tortured?

☐ Have children been traumatized by what they have seen/experienced?

Present situation

☐ How many children are now "unaccompanied"? What ages? Any sick/injured?

- [ ] What arrangements (formal/informal) have already been made for the care of any or all of them? Do they meet the emotional and psychological as well as physical needs of the children?

- [ ] How are other unaccompanied children surviving? Where are they?

- [ ] Are arrangements (either legal or customary) established for the guardianship/representation of the unaccompanied children.

- [ ] What self-help arrangements are operating for care of children while parents work? What proportion of families/children benefit from such arrangements?

- [ ] What priority do the people themselves attach to reviving:
  —Child care services?
  —Other social services?
  —Primary schooling and other education?

- [ ] What competent agencies are available to provide appropriate social services? What trained/experienced staff are available:
  —Social workers?
  —Teachers?
  —Community/religious leaders?

Probable evolution

- [ ] Are any (further) population movements likely? Are more family separations likely? Why?

- [ ] What will need to be done to try to trace the families of unaccompanied children and reunite families?

- [ ] Are arrangements made (by the community and other bodies) for the care of unaccompanied children likely to be in the best interests of the children?

- [ ] To what extent will needs for day care of children and other social services be able to be met by existing community mechanisms and resources?

- [ ] What are the policies of the government and others with regard to arrangements for unaccompanied children and other social services?

- [ ] What efforts are foreseen to (re-)start primary schools?

- [ ] What inputs and programmes are already arranged or envisaged by the government and other agencies?

Conclusions for action

☐ Special services are required for:
  —Unaccompanied children ...
  —Disabled children ...
  —Children with emotional and psychological problems ...
  —Destitute and single-parent families ...
  —Others with special needs ...
  [Estimate numbers in particular areas/communities.]

To ensure appropriate care and protection of unaccompanied children:

☐ Children who are unaccompanied should be identified and documented by ...

☐ Parents who are looking for children should be documented by ...

☐ Tracing and matching up children and families should be organized by ...

☐ Emergency and interim care of the children (stable adult care, shelter, food, clothing, medical examinations and psychological screening) should be provided by ...

☐ Protection of the children's interests and supervision of care arrangements should be assured by ...

☐ Existing expertise, facilities and resources which can be mobilized include ...

☐ Additional guidance and assistance is required for ...
  [Specify how and by whom the various operations should be organized, the resources required, etc.]

Other social service needs

☐ To prevent further family separations, help should be provided to destitute and single-parent families as follows ...

☐ Rehabilitation training and other assistance for disabled children requires ...

☐ Children with particular emotional and psychological problems (including those traumatized) should be helped by ...
  [Specify the how and by whom appropriate services will be provided.]

☐ The protection of children against (further) abuse should be assured by ...

☐ Existing informal and/or formal arrangements for the day-care of children are adequate/require support as follows: ...

☐   To (re-)establish primary schools and other normal community activities for children requires . . .

☐   Assistance required for other social services includes . . .

☐   More detailed investigations should be undertaken by . . . to determine specific needs and design programmes for . . .

[E.g. unaccompanied children and family tracing—other child care services—primary schools—teacher training institutes.]

Sources of information: local administration—social welfare, health and education departments—social workers (government and NGOs)—health workers—teachers—community leaders—relief workers.

CHAPTER 14

LOGISTICS AND OVERALL MANAGEMENT

Possible problems/needs

- **Insufficient logistic capacity (transport and warehousing) to receive and/or deliver the required quantities of assistance to the communities in need.**

- **Lack of management capacity and/or expertise to organize and control the overall operation (particularly the management of logistics).**

Insufficient logistic capacity may be a major constraint, at least initially, if:
- Roads and/or rail lines have been cut; bridges, tunnels or wharves damaged; *and/or*
- Trucks, rail wagons and locomotives, river boats or ferries have been damaged, or fuel is lacking (earthquakes, storms, floods, landslides, conflicts).
- Large numbers of people are to be reached in areas never well-served by normal transport (droughts, displaced populations).

Problems will be exaggerated if management and control systems are not adequate to ensure that available capacity and resources are used to best effect.

Lack of capacity/experience is possible if a major emergency of any kind overtakes a small poor country, or if experienced personnel are taken for other functions or have fled (e.g. in conflicts).

General aims and priorities

- **To mobilize/develop the logistic capacity necessary to deliver assistance to the communities in need.**

- **To ensure the efficient management of the overall emergency operation.**

- **To re-establish normal communications and transport possibilities to facilitate the re-establishment of normal economic life.**

Logistics for the emergency operation itself requires action to:
- Ensure facilities to receive/discharge and store (temporarily) at ports and airports any supplies to be imported;
- Organize the transport within the country of supplies through to the points of final use/distribution;
- Organize storage for operational and any necessary contingency stocks at appropriate locations, and transit storage at any transshipment points;
- Ensure fuel supplies, maintenance and repair for all vehicles, boats, aircraft being used (and food and water for any animals used for carrying supplies);
- Establish operational budgets and ensure the availability of cash when and where needed to pay for fuel, maintenance, labour and other operating expenses; *and*
- Appoint suitable personnel for all management functions and ensure facilities for them to live and work.

Where transport and storage capacity is inadequate for the planned operations (perhaps as a result of damage to existing facilities) it might be necessary to:
- Repair and/or replace damaged roads, rail lines, bridges, ferries, vehicles, locomotives, etc.
- Provide additional transport units.
- Repair and/or establish new warehouses, including necessary handling equipment and stock control systems.

117

In the mean time, careful co-ordination—possibly central control—of all logistic operations is essential to make the optimum use of the facilities/capacities which are available. This includes:

—Establishing priorities for the delivery of various supplies;
—Controlling the allocation and use of available means of transport and storage; *and*
—Avoiding competition between agencies for facilities, or unnecessary duplication of logistical services.

In all cases, effective management requires:

—Clear definition of responsibilities, procedures and lines of communication;
—Provision of appropriate guidelines, forms and training for personnel in various functions;
—Reliable means of (tele-)communications between all key locations: ports, airports, transshipment points, major warehouses; *and*
—Continuous monitoring and control of all stocks of essential supplies and transport.

(See also Table 9, p. 46.)

Continuity in management—especially of logistics—is essential. Technical expertise, local knowledge and managerial ability are needed.

Wherever transport routes are vulnerable to natural, political or military actions within or outside the country:

—Use the most advantageous routes as long as they are available but don't rely exclusively on them;
—Develop and make some use of alternative routes at the same time.

Continuously monitor actual requirements and logistic capacities. Adapt plans and take new actions in response to any changes—expected and unexpected.

Monitor the state of roads, bridges and ferries. See that any necessary repairs and reinforcements are made in good time—before roads become impassable. (Sometimes it may be necessary to suspend operations for a few days to make repairs in order to avoid the possibility of much longer and more damaging interruptions.)

Provide 30% spare capacity wherever possible to allow for maintenance, breakdowns, unplanned peaks in deliveries and other unexpected occurrences.

Consider airlifts only as a last resort—except for the movement of personnel and high value, low volume supplies such as drugs and spare parts.

Role of UNICEF

Specific objectives

● To ensure the timely delivery to the target communities/institutions of supplies for programmes assisted by UNICEF or otherwise of importance for children.

● To ensure efficient management of overall operations so that programmes benefiting children are able to be implemented efficiently.

Possible interventions

Where means are lacking to receive, transport and store supplies for programmes of concern to UNICEF:

—Ensure in-country transport capacity by contracting road, river and/or air transport for particular deliveries and/or borrowing, renting, repairing and/or buying trucks, boats, etc.;

—Ensure fuel supplies, spare parts and maintenance for vehicles involved in programme operations;

—Ensure suitable warehousing for programme supplies;

—Ensure efficient use of available transport means—organizational and technical assistance; *and*

—Ensure timely actions to repair or prevent further deterioration of vital roads (including local access roads to needy communities), bridges, airstrips.

Where overall management capacity needs strengthening:

—Ensure funding for employment of locally available expertise and operational personnel;

—Arrange any other necessary technical assistance; *and, if necessary*

—Assist directly in the organization of operations.

Ensure that the logistic requirements of programmes of concern to UNICEF are properly co-ordinated with those of the operation as a whole. UNICEF should, however, not normally be involved in logistics for the overall emergency operation.

UNICEF should not normally be involved in repairing roads, bridges, etc., but may act to break any bottlenecks in repair operations necessary for the continuation of programmes of concern to UNICEF. **119**

Logistics

Logistic requirements

☐ What quantities of what supplies need to be received and delivered? From where? When? To where?

☐ If there are major peaks in the required delivery schedule, can these be spread out over time?

☐ What intermediate storage and contingency stockpiles are needed? Where?

☐ What other priority supplies will be competing for the same transport possibilities at the same time?

Port and airport capacities
(*See also Annexes 31 and 32*)

☐ What kind of vessels/aircraft can be received?

☐ At what rate can cargo be unloaded and dispatched? What handling equipment is available? Any limits on the size and weight of individual items able to be handled?

☐ What facilities are there for temporary/transit storage?

☐ What constraints are there on the operation of the port/airport?

☐ What means of transport are available for on-forwarding? What are current off-take rates? Can sufficient capacity be guaranteed for the intended programme supplies?

☐ What possibilities are there for increasing the unloading and off-take capacities, if necessary? What would they cost? How long would it take?

Border crossings

☐ What type of trucks and/or rail wagons are able and allowed to cross? How long does a round trip take?

☐ What quantities of different types of supplies can each truck/wagon carry? How many will therefore be required? Will sufficient units be available?

☐ What constraints are there on cross-border movements, including customs operations?

☐ What facilities are there for temporary/transit storage?

☐ What actions might be possible to accelerate movements?

In-country transport routes

☐ What routes are available? At what points are transshipments necessary?

☐ What particular constraints are there on each route: weight limits on damaged and other bridges — ferry capacities — restricted depths (rivers) — adverse weather (aircraft operations)?

☐ What was the volume of traffic previously? What is present capacity? Will emergency traffic be in addition to or in place of normal traffic?

☐ What seasonal/weather factors must be considered? Will any routes become impassable? During what periods?

☐ Are there significant security risks on any of the routes?

☐ What type and size of cart/truck/wagon/boat/aircraft can be used on each route? How long do round trips take, including loading and unloading? What is the cost of each round trip?

☐ What bottlenecks exist? What possibilities are there for re-opening routes and/or increasing movement capacities? What materials, equipment, expertise would be required? What would it cost? How long would it take?

In-country storage/transshipment locations

☐ What government stores are available? What others might be requisitioned, rented or improvised?

☐ What quantities of different items can those warehouses hold?

☐ Are they well-located, close to the arrival and departure points of the transport routes to be used?

☐ Are they secure? Well run? Clean? Are there sufficient staff? Do effective records and control systems exist?

☐ At what rate can cargo be received and handled? What handling equipment is available? Any limits on the size and weight of individual items able to be handled?

☐ What particular constraints are there on capacity and operations? What might be done to improve the situation: Repairs? Generators? Lighting? Equipment?

☐ What alternatives are there? What arrangements could be made to improvise other/additional storage? What would it cost? How long would it take?

Fuel and maintenance

☐ Are supplies of fuel available at all locations? What stocks of petrol and diesel are held? Is replenishment assured?

☐ Where are fuel depots? How could supplies be obtained directly, transported and stored in field locations?

☐ What maintenance facilities exist? For what types of vehicles? For boats and other equipment? What range of spare parts are available?

Available transport units

☐ What trucks, rail wagons, locomotives, barges, tugs, boats, etc. are available in running order? How many of each type/capacity?

☐ What quantities of different types of supplies can each unit carry? Where? Who owns/controls them?

☐ What other demands will there be for the use of these units? What can realistically be expected to be available for the programme?

☐ What additional units are on hand but out-of-service? What parts and expertise would be needed to repair them? What cost? How long?

Conclusions for action

☐ The most reliable and economical ways of moving the required quantities of supplies are . . .
[Specify means of transport for all areas and routes concerned.]

☐ The main bottlenecks are . . .

☐ Actions which would most quickly and efficiently increase capacity are . . .
[Specify how, by whom and within what period such measures could be implemented.]

☐ Communications between all locations will be assured by . . .

☐ Co-ordination and control of the logistics for the overall emergency operation will be assured by . . .

☐ Deliveries to final distribution sites will be made by . . .?
[Specify the means, possibly including animals, and how it will be organized.]

☐ Necessary budgets for operational costs at all levels will be established and the flow of funds be assured by . . .

Sources of information: local and national administrations (including public works departments and the military)—transport and bus companies; other commercial companies—oil companies—organizations working in the area.

If there is good knowledge of what facilities, capacities and constraints existed before, attention can be focused on checking whether and to what extent key elements have been affected by events.

N.B. In some situations (war, civil disorder, etc.) some of this data may be considered as "classified" or "strategic". In such cases, seek information from official sources and be discrete in making direct observations.

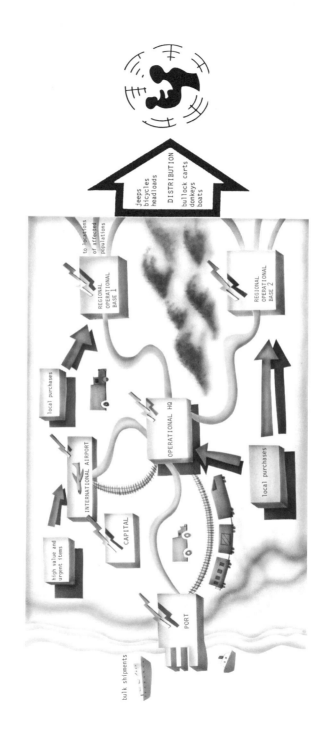

DISTRIBUTION

jeeps
bicycles
headloads
bullock carts
donkeys
boats

to locations
of affected
populations

REGIONAL
OPERATIONAL
BASE 1

REGIONAL
OPERATIONAL
BASE 2

local purchases

OPERATIONAL HQ

local purchases

INTERNATIONAL AIRPORT

CAPITAL

high value and
urgent items

PORT

bulk shipments

Part 4 FIELD OFFICE OPERATIONS

This Part provides guidelines and reminders for things which may need to be done to assure an efficient UNICEF response. It includes a brief summary of relevant organizational rules and procedures and actions to support public information and the mobilization of funds.

The attention necessary to the various aspects will depend on the particular situation, the role being taken on by UNICEF and the size and capacity of the existing UNICEF office.

In all aspects, refer to the Emergency and other books of the *UNICEF Field Manual* for full details of procedures.

Chapter 15

MOBILIZING AND MANAGING PERSONNEL

Organizing the office

(Manual 3.2)

- **Designate a focal point for the co-ordination and control of** *all* **emergency-related actions.**

- **Define work priorities within all concerned offices in respect of (a) emergency actions, and (b) continuing regular programme activities.**

- **Specify the authority delegated to any outposted staff.**

Individual responsibilities and lines of communication must be clearly defined. The designated "focal point" must receive at least copies of *all* emergency-related reports and communications.

Managing personnel

(*Manual 8.4*)

- **Ensure the best use of available staff; monitor the performance and reactions of all individuals.**

Personnel should be assigned taking due account of personal capacities as well as functional skills and experience.

National staff should not be placed in situations where they may be subjected to undue political, nationalistic or other pressures.

Staff in particularly difficult field postings should take short breaks regularly — whether they feel the need or not!

Individuals should be re-assigned if it seems advisable for their own good or that of the operation.

All staff must, at all times, have valid contracts, visas and required vaccinations — and take reasonable precautions with their own health.

A performance evaluation report should be prepared in respect of all personnel who serve for three months or more in the operation.

Overtime

Personnel will often be required to work long hours, seven days a week. Professional staff do not receive overtime payments but may, exceptionally, be granted compensatory time off subject to approval by DOP/NYHQ.

Regular GS staff are entitled to compensatory time off (the same number of hours off as those worked in excess) or overtime pay at 1.5 times their hourly rate. Overtime payments should be charged to the emergency BAL, if any.

Mobilizing additional personnel

(*Manual 8.3*)

- **Actions required:**
  1. **Define requirements.**
  2. **Determine funding possibilities.**

3. **Inform HQ and get approval.**
4. **Seek candidates locally.**
5. **Ask HQ to assign personnel if necessary.**

In the meantime, redeploy existing staff to make maximum use of available capacity and expertise in the face of new priorities.

Sources of personnel

Personnel may be obtained:
- —From the staff roster (for up to 3-6 months);
- —On loan from government or other organizations;
- —By direct recruitment locally or internationally.

Assistance in programming, supply and other aspects of internal UNICEF operations will normally be met, initially, by temporary re-assignment of staff from other offices.

Requirements for technicians and personnel for field operations may be most quickly met by finding locally available candidates, otherwise NYHQ will try to second or recruit suitable personnel.

Except for HQ and regional office staff (and other current staff re-assigned for very short missions), the *salaries* as well as travel and DSA costs of staff seconded for temporary assignments will normally be charged to the emergency operation. An appropriate CCF must be raised.

Family members: A spouse may be engaged provided he/she meets all recruitment requirements, will not be in the same line of management as the staff member, and no internal candidates are available. Children, parents, brothers and sisters of current staff cannot be recruited unless it is proven that their skills and expertise are not otherwise available inside or outside UNICEF.

Defining requirements

Table 15 lists the aspects to be defined for each additional, temporary post required. Complete the normal job description form 309 rev.I(8-79) to the extent possible.

Where several staff will be required to work together, ensure the necessary balance of complementary skills for the particular situation: constitute a team with a designated team leader.

Additional, temporary personnel may be required to assist in assessments, the initiation and/or ongoing implementation of emergency assistance. Programming, management and administrative skills might be needed; possibly functional specialists and field assistants. See Annex 45.

Table 15

Aspects to be defined for each required post

☐ The specific functions/tasks to be fulfilled;

☐ The minimum period for which the services may be required, and what should therefore be the length of the *initial* assignment;

☐ The level of responsibility, whether working independently or as a member of a team;

☐ The proposed level of the post (international professional, L-; national professional, NPO-; international GS-; or national GS-);

☐ Whether (for international posts) suitable candidates are available locally or candidates should be sought and assigned by HQ;

☐ The conditions under which they will have to live and work; any consequent special considerations; *and*

☐ The budget (CCF) provision—or at least proposal of how the post/assignment should be funded.

Informing HQ of requirements:

● **Telex details of requirements to HQ. Use the format in Annex 39.**

Include full details of each professional-level post individually. List GS-level posts with functional title, location, proposed level and duration.

Describe responsibilities and required qualifications particularly clearly if candidates are to be sought and assigned by HQ. Requests simply for persons "with experience in emergency situations and UNICEF procedures" are *not* adequate.

In some instances, technicians may be sought through UN Volunteers. All negotiations with UNV must be undertaken by RSDS-DOP/NYHQ who will also advise concerning the cost to be covered from the programme budget.

Local candidates for professional-level posts

If a suitable individual is already employed by government or another organization, try to arrange a joint project or a loan of their services to UNICEF. This protects their long-term employment.

Otherwise, ask the individual to complete a P11 (personal history form) and get medical clearance, see Table 16. Telex details and recommendation for recruitment to NYHQ (for internationals) or the Regional Director (for national professional officer posts) using the format in Annex 40. Pouch the P11 and medical certificate.

In case of either a *joint project* (employer contributes the individual's services) or a *loan* (UNICEF reimburses employer), make clear, formal agreements with the individual and the employer. Specify supervisory, reporting and administrative responsibilities, including responsibility for insurance and travel costs.

Inform EOU and Regional Director of proposals for joint projects. Obtain DOP/NYHQ approval for obtaining services of non-nationals "on loan".

For *recruitment*, any candidate proposed must have skills and/or experience appropriate to the level of post for which he/she is proposed. They should be qualified to the same extent as if being recruited as a regular staff member at the same level.

For internationals: DOP/NYHQ, if satisfied, telexes an offer through the Representative and, if accepted, issues the contract. The candidate should sign the necessary insurance forms immediately on accepting the offer, not wait for receipt of the Letter of Appointment. Any extensions are also issued by DOP, on recommendation of Representative.

Table 16

Medical clearances

All staff being considered for appointments must have medical clearance.

Anyone being appointed—on a basis other than an SSA—**for less than 6 months** should submit a certificate issued by a qualified medical doctor stating that he/she has been in good health for the preceding 9 months.

Anyone being proposed for an appointment of **6 months or longer** should have a full medical examination by a designated UN examining physician. Their appointment will be contingent on clearance by the UN Medical Service.

For national professionals: on receipt of the Regional Director's approval, a short-term (for less than 6-months) or fixed-term (6 months or more) letter of appointment is issued locally.

For GS-level staff

Once HQ approval is received for the number and level of extra posts, seek, interview and appoint candidates as quickly as possible consistent with:
— Ensuring satisfactory calibre of personnel;
— Normal criteria (Admin. Instruction 358); *and*
— Medical clearances (see Table 16).

If assignment is expected to exceed 6 months, issue a Fixed-Term letter of appointment. If less than 6 months, issue a Short-Term letter of appointment. (N.B. personnel appointed for less than 3 months have no medical insurance cover.)

Establish normal working hours according to operational requirements. Specify conditions for overtime on similar basis to other involved UN organizations.

Casual/manual workers

For labourers and any other workers required on a casual basis, follow local practices — pay cash daily at local rates for the job.

Give Special Service Agreements (SSAs) to watchmen and others responsible for the security of UNICEF offices and programme materials, and to other, selected manual workers whose services are found particularly valuable and required beyond 2 months.

If casual labourers and other daily-hire workers will frequently be required to work in a UNICEF-operated warehouse or workshop, make every effort to obtain local insurance to cover such workers against accidents at work in these locations.

Chapter 16

ASSURING CAPACITY AND SUPPORT SERVICES

Communications

(*Manual 9.2*)

- **Ensure/establish fast, reliable communications — both telex and letters — between UNICEF offices and the affected area(s), and between the country office and the outside world (NYHQ, GEHQ and the regional office).**

- **Ensure efficient use of all communications; establish discipline, regular schedules for contacts, etc.**

For relatively minor emergencies in countries where there is a well-established UNICEF office, there may be no particular difficulties and no need for special arrangements. Major emergencies, especially in countries having poor communications at the best of times can, however, demand urgent and imaginative attention to this aspect.

In-country

Try to establish telephone, telex and/or cable contacts between out-posted staff and the country office. Seek permission to use police and/or Red Cross radios if necessary.

Set regular schedules for contacts with out-posted field staff.

Arrange for the delivery of mail and packages to outposted field staff, e.g. through airlines, bus companies and/or arrangements with other organizations.

International telecommunications

Use phone, but with discretion; set regular schedules with EOU if necessary; record all key points; confirm important decisions and requests by telex.

Get out-of-hours phone numbers for EOU staff NY and GE; give them phone numbers for key field personnel.

Get the use of a telex—rent/buy a machine if necessary; ensure rapid transmission and collection of messages. Use UN network where available; check delivery delays; ensure rapid local delivery and collection.

Ensure a cable address exists for use if necessary.

In the event of a total breakdown of telecommunications:
— Request an embassy to transmit messages, and/or ask reliable travellers to carry messages out.
— If no alternative, send a staff member as courier.

International pouches

Check delays on delivery through existing UN pouch.

If necessary: use airmail, courier services, or make special courtesy arrangements with an airline which flies directly to NY, Geneva or the regional office.

Confidentiality and other considerations

Avoid sending sensitive information or opinions by telex or cable. Be discrete in remarks on telephone.

Ensure confidentiality within each UNICEF office.

Avoid unnecessary communications; do not use phone when telex could serve as well or better.

Be sure each message is clear and complete.

Clear/consolidate messages through the country office focal point; address to HQ focal point.

Ask the UNDP Resident Representative to send coded messages through the UN radio system if absolutely necessary and the facilities are available.

Security

(*Manual 8.2*)

The UN Resident Co-ordinator (UNRC) is responsible for the security of all UN personnel and dependents.

All personnel must always:

—Know the UN security plan for their location, and who their "warden" is;
—Complete the household and personal effects inventory; *and*
—Follow the instructions of the UNRC and wardens unless other specific instructions are received from the UNICEF Representative.

If there are foreseeable risks:

—Maintain contacts on a regular schedule between all out-posted and travelling staff and the country office;
—Inform the wardens of all personnel movements;
—Advise personnel to keep essential personal documents and some money with them at all times; *and*
—Keep EOU and DOP/NYHQ informed of the situation and arrangements made in consultation with the UNRC.

If, when an emergency strikes, contact with the warden or UNICEF Representative is impossible, any staff up-country should:

—Consult with local government and security personnel, and/or any local representatives of the International Red Cross and other international agencies;
—Use own judgement whether to stay put or move elsewhere; *and*

135

—Re-establish contact with the Representative or any other UNICEF office as soon as ever possible.

Evacuation of international personnel

UNICEF international staff must follow any instructions received from the UNICEF Representative or the UN security wardens for the evacuation of dependents, initially, and of themselves, later.

Based on consultations between the UNICEF Representative and the UNRC and, if possible, with NYHQ, some UNICEF international staff *may* continue to work even if most other international UN personnel leave.

A refusal to comply with an evacuation instruction may be considered as an act of defiance and could lead to suspension pending investigation. The individual then stays on at his/her own risk, it may not be possible to include them in subsequent evacuation arrangements, and UN/UNICEF can take no further responsibility for their protection.

An evacuation allowance is paid to staff and dependents evacuated from their duty station. Reasonable compensation is paid for personal effects irretrievably lost or damaged as a result of the performance of official duties provided personal inventory forms had been properly completed in advance.

Arrangements for national staff

National staff should be helped to ensure their own security within their own country. See Table 17.

The provisions for evacuation and compensation for international staff may be applied to national staff in only the *most exceptional cases* in which their security is endangered, or their property lost or damaged, as a direct consequence of their employment by the organization.

UNICEF property and programme supplies

(*Manual 9.3*)

In the event of any major risk or situation in which the office cannot continue to operate at all:

—Store UNICEF files, vehicles and non-expendable property as securely as possible, preferably in premises which are clearly identified as belonging to UN/UNICEF. Keys should normally be left with the most senior national staff member.

136

Table 17

Security of national staff

Keep up-to-date lists of all national staff, their dependents, home address/location and nearest contact point outside the place of work, and any other relevant information. Give copies to the UN Resident Co-ordinator.

In the event of specific security risks:

1. Alert national staff in the same manner as internationals.
2. If internationals are advised to remain as home, nationals are not required to report to work.
3. If internationals are advised to "concentrate", national staff should be advised to remove themselves from any city area likely to be an area of disturbance. In agreement with the Designated Official for UN security, the head of the office may give UNICEF national staff up to two months salary in advance and, if needed, a special grant to allow them to transport themselves and their families to a recognized home location elsewhere within the country if they wish.
4. If international staff are being regrouped within the country or are evacuated, national staff may absent themselves from the duty station on special leave with pay, provided they give the acting head of the office a contact address at which they can be reached within a reasonable period of time.

Depending on the nature of any evacuation, it may be necessary to place the care of the UNICEF office in the hands of senior national staff.

—Cash and cheque books should be deposited with a bank if at all possible.
—Programme supplies still in the custody of UNICEF should also be protected to the extent possible.

Keep a record of all action taken. Try to get a receipt for any property/supplies handed over for safe keeping or taken over by any party.

UN flags and UNICEF decals should be used to identify office and residential premises. Consult with the UN Resident Co-ordinator. Ask EOU/UNIPAC for more flags and/or decals if required and not available from UNDP.

UNICEF vehicles should be immobilized if they are being parked and there is a danger of them being taken for inappropriate purposes. Staff members' personal safety should not, however, be put in jeopardy.

Administrative support services

(*Manual 9.3*)

- Ensure necessary administrative capacity and systems to efficiently support field operations, including assurance of all necessary local formalities.

- Ensure adherence to basic UNICEF rules and procedures.

Permits

— Get any permits necessary for personnel and/or vehicles to visit the area (valid for multiple/extended visits if posssible).

Visas

— Check and advise HQ of any change in visa regulations.

— Monitor visa expiry dates (especially for temporary personnel) and apply for extensions in good time.

Maps

— Get good maps. If sufficient are not available locally, ask EOU to help— provide publishers' references if possible (check with major embassies).

Identity cards

— Issue ID cards/certificates to persons working for UNICEF (except those on a casual/daily basis). Include photos and expiry dates. Keep a record of cards issued.

Accidents; thefts

— Report all significant accidents, losses, thefts to the local police and, through the country office, to NYHQ.

Travel authorizations (TAs)

— Representatives may issue "blanket" TAs valid for one month at a time for staff required to travel extensively for emergency operations. The total number of days travel foreseen must be specified and claims be submitted at the end of each trip or month.

Support to outposted personnel

Arrange to send food and essential personal supplies to outposted field staff in need. Operate special personal cash accounts for them to pay for such supplies separate from normal office accounts.

138 Ensure that inventories of personal effects are deposited with UNDP.

Transport for staff operations

(*Manual 9.4*)

- **Borrow or otherwise rapidly arrange necessary vehicles for field surveys and operations.**

- **Ensure necessary insurance and proper control of the use of all official vehicles.**

Provision of vehicles
—Borrow from existing offices/projects if possible, at least initially.
—If additional vehicles are required for continuing operations, hire or purchase depending on costs, expected duration, etc. and agreement of EOU/NYHQ.
See Annex 48 regarding choice/specification of vehicles.

Insurance of office vehicles
—Telex the make, model, year, serial and engine numbers to Chief AS/NYHQ for inclusion in global third party policy. (Include *any* vehicle/motorcycle used by UNICEF personnel for project/administrative purposes.)
—Arrange additional, comprehensive insurance locally if possible.

Use of official vehicles

- **Put log books and first aid kits in all vehicles.**

- **Monitor use and fuel consumption, and arrange regular preventive maintenance.**

Vehicles are always assigned to an office, not an individual, and to be used for official/project purposes only. They should normally be driven only by locally recruited drivers—never by anyone who does not have a licence valid locally.

Drivers should, if possible, be assigned to and responsible for specific vehicles. Establish a safe driving bonus scheme if feasible. Insist on using seat belts.

Representatives may, exceptionally, authorize certain staff on temporary assignments to use particular vehicles for personal purposes against payment per km/mile of such use. Staff using vehicles for personal purposes are advised to arrange their own comprehensive insurance.

Chapter 17
MANAGING FUNDS

Programme commitments and documentation

(*Manual 10.2*)

- **Agree allocations/budgets with EOU and programme desk/NYHQ. Place call-forwards by telex if necessary, but ensure that proper documentation is prepared and sent as soon as possible thereafter.**

BAL and call-forward documentation

Specify which staff are authorized sign call-forwards (CFs) ; notify EOU and programme desk/NYHQ.

Amend G BAL for any general resources reprogrammed. Issue addenda to the latest G BAL for emergency reserve allocations; addenda to S BAL for any special contributions.

Assign "M" codes for short-term "relief" assistance; "R" codes for interventions which are primarily contributions towards long-term rehabilitation.

Specify donor and form 300 number in CFs if a specific donor contribution to be charged.

Inform EOU/NYHQ of any "diversions" and issue amendments to CFs with appropriate new codes.

Monitoring programme commitments

Ensure that all CFs issued are within established BAL provision and approved CF ceiling: use TAD/SIMS Table I.

Cross-check local records against HQ reports.

Adjust any unspent CF balances as early as possible.

For major operations:
- Telex to EOU/NYHQ each week a list of CFs and LPOs issued or amended, and major payments made.
- Prepare periodic summaries of receipts/pledges of special contributions against total appealed for, and the amounts called-forward and actually expended.

Local financial arrangements

(*Manual 10.3*)

- Foresee requirements for disbursements by UNICEF in field locations—the likely magnitude and where payments will have to be made—and determine how these can best be arranged.

- Ensure necessary cash flow from HQ, expeditious action and proper control of all local financial transactions.

- Advise Comptroller of the arrangements envisaged/being made. Get his approval for any new accounts and/or increases in ceilings, considered necessary.

Ensuring cash flow and management

Check time taken for transfers from NYHQ to be credited to local account.

Foresee cash needs for all purposes each month and request replenishment from NYHQ in good time.

Ensure transactions in the country office will not be delayed by absence or travel of authorized signatories: telex Comptroller to add new signatories if necessary.

Is available finance/adminintrative manpower and experience sufficient? Request additional assistance if necessary.

When payments are made through UNDP, notify Comptroller in good time to transfer funds to UNDP to cover payments of more than $10,000 against any CCF/SCF during any month.

Arrangements for disbursements in the field

If disbursements will have to be made directly by UNICEF in field locations, arrangements to ensure adequate funds and accounting might include:

a. Increase in existing petty cash/imprest ceilings;
b. Establishment of new Special Imprest Bank Accounts, Special Petty Cash accounts and/or designation of new petty cash holders; *and/or*
c. Opening of new, official UNICEF bank accounts.

Actual arrangements will be determined by:

—The level of disbursements which will have to be made, and where;
—Whether there is a sub-office and petty cash account already on the spot;
—Whether any staff are going to be assigned there and, if so, for how long;
—Whether any banks are operating in the area.

'a' may be appropriate when disbursements are to be made in areas close to an existing UNICEF office and/or no staff is being outposted; 'b' when a particular staff member will be out-posted for the emergency operation and/or be required to disburse funds during official travel.

'c' will normally be appropriate only if expenditures totalling $10,000 or more each month are anticipated over an extended period *and* there will be capacity for the preparation of full accounts on-the-spot.

Table 18 provides some guidelines for outposted staff responsible for funds (designated as petty cash holders).

Table 18

Handling and accounting for cash in the field

Responsibilities of petty cash holders:
—Keep funds separate from personal monies/accounts;
—Make payments only for actions covered by an approved budget and CCF or SCF;
—Get invoice/receipt or make out and sign a Petty Cash Disbursement Voucher (or similar slip) for each payment; *and*
—Submit accounts promptly and account for or refund everything before end of assignment.

General guidelines for operating a special imprest bank account or special petty cash:
—If at all possible, avoid carrying or keeping large amounts of cash. Use bank accounts, transfers and payments by cheque whenever possible.
—If cash must be held: do not advertise the fact; keep it in a secure safe; do not take any unnecessary risks or endanger personal security.
—Always carry blank petty cash disbursement vouchers/slips.
—Record all payments/expenditures in cash or bank book.
—Prepare and submit accounts regularly (monthly), or whenever needed to ensure replenishment before funds run out.

Annex 51 outlines a suitable accounting system.

Advances to authorized petty cash holders are held as special petty cash under the individual, not as an ARL against the staff member.

Control of advances

● Give only to government or other collaborating agencies and for clearly defined purposes in the context of an agreed Plan of Action (or exchange of letters).

● Monitor receipt of accounts carefully (record on form 153).

● Give further advances only if a reasonable proportion of those previously given has been satisfactorily accounted for.

Advances should not normally be given to suppliers, but see *Manual 11.6*. Personal advances to staff only for travel/DSA; recorded as ARLs. Staff are not **143** permitted to advance funds to themselves. NYHQ approval is required for salary advances to international staff.

Personal finances

DSA should normally be paid/advanced to short-term or seconded international staff on regular schedule.

Personal funds in sealed envelopes may be placed in UNICEF office safes, but UNICEF cannot be responsible for them.

Comptroller must authorize the receipt for exchange of residual local currency from departing international staff.

Receipt of contributions

Advise Finance Section/NYHQ of any cash contributions received. See p. 154 regarding unsolicited contributions.

Chapter 18

ORDERING AND RECEIVING SUPPLIES

Preliminary actions

(*Manual 11.2*)

Check the practical aspects listed in Table 19 and advise Supply Division, EOU and the Regional Office concerning:

—Ports, airports and border crossing points for reception of imported emergency supplies;

—Consignee and document distribution requirements (if different from the standard list held by UNIPAC);

—Kinds of supplies which *might* be required from offshore sources and local procurement; *and*

—Any information on possibilities for cheap airfreight.

Depending on the likely nature and scale of UNICEF emergency supply assistance:

● **Ensure adequate supply manpower and experience: request additional assistance if necessary.**

● Ensure that the local contract review committee (CRC) is able to meet at short notice whenever required.

● Request increase in limits on local procurement authority (from UNIPAC) and contingency SL/SCF (from NYHQ) if required.

Ensure that supply records are up to date and stocks of forms sufficient.

Table 19

How and where can imported supplies be received?

☐ What sea- and air-ports are functioning?

☐ What direct road and rail links are open from neighbouring countries? To where could supplies be conveniently delivered directly with proper inspection on delivery?

☐ What government department(s) will be responsible for receipt and clearance of emergency supplies? What arrangements exist for customs clearance?

☐ What information is available locally concerning possibilities for cheap airfreight from Europe, North America, Japan or elsewhere?

Calling-forward supplies

(*Manual 11.3*)

● Send copies of SLs/SCFs simultaneously to UNIPAC and EOU/NYHQ. Use existing number series and "M" codes for relief inputs, "R" for rehabilitation.

● For urgent requirements, telex all necessary details to UNIPAC and EOU. Use format in Annex 41. Send SLs/SCFs as soon as possible.

● Use "G" BAL contingency SL/SCF for small value items (up to $100 per item, $500 per order) or similar SL/SCF issued against any "S" BAL for special emergency funds.

For local procurements in excess of delegated authority, give sufficient reasons and justification.

For offshore orders, provide as much information as possible concerning specifications and required TADs; also shipping, packing and marking arrangements to facilitate field operations. See Table 20.

Table 20

Ordering supplies from UNIPAC (offshore)

Specifications
—For items not in the UNIPAC catalogue, provide as full technical specifications as possible, and explain the intended use.
—Ensure that tools, utensils, clothing, etc. are culturally appropriate.

Cost estimates
—State your estimates/assumptions regarding costs. Refer to UNIPAC catalogue (blue pages). Ask UNIPAC for estimate in advance if necessary.

Required TADs
—Specify and explain the required TAD (not just "urgent" or "as soon as possible").
—If certain items will be useless unless delivered before a certain date (e.g. seeds), say so.
—If certain items must be delivered before other supplies can be used or activities be started, say so.
—Request phased deliveries if this will help field operations.

Shipping: air or surface
—Request airfreight of at least initial quantities if felt necessary—but explain justification.

Packing
—Is set-packing required to facilitate rapid distribution (at least for UNIPAC inventory items)?
—Are "partial shipments" acceptable? If appropriate, state in SCF/telex: "complete sets requested: advise if any items delaying completion and delivery."
—State any limits (e.g. "no pkgs over 50kg") if packages will have to be unloaded/moved manually.

Markings
—Specify any special marks required on outer packages (in addition to normal references).
—Specify if colour-coding is required—see Annex 49.

Ensure close liaison between local programme and supply staff, and establish a dialogue with UNIPAC to ensure the best possible response.

Be sure the information is sufficient for the procurement officer to (a) understand exactly what is needed without having to ask further questions, and (b) weigh the often competing considerations of delivery time, price and quality.

Standardization can be important, but insistence on a particular manufacturer or other very tight specifications reduces the flexibility available to UNIPAC to obtain what is quickly available, and may therefore delay delivery.

See Annex 48 for special considerations regarding vehicles; Annex 50 for criteria for local procurement.

Monitoring the supply pipeline

(*Manual 11.4*)

Ensure that supply records are kept up-to-date. (Table 5A's; shipment status board; local procurement status lists, etc.)

Request UNIPAC and supply division/NYHQ to provide telex advice of all emergency shipments effected.

For major operations, prepare regular summaries of the status of the "pipeline".

Receiving supplies

(*Manual 11.5*)

- **Plan for the clearance and on-forwarding of supplies *before* each ship/aircraft arrives.**

- **Whenever possible, be present to verify arrival, supervise sorting/stacking and initiate clearance of consignments.**

- **Obtain government receipts for all supplies delivered.**

Clear sea shipments on a letter of guarantee if necessary documents (Bills of Lading) are delayed.

Ensure landing rights for charter flights; co-ordinate with other organizations to seek waiver of royalties, landing fees, fuel tax, etc. Advise UNIPAC and supply division/NYHQ of any concessions.

Remember to obtain outturn reports, short-landing certificates, etc. and file notices of any loss or damage within a few days of arrival. If losses appear to be substantial, arrange an independent survey.

Vehicles and other major items of non-expendable equipment may, at the Representative's discretion, be issued initially on loan agreements for specified emergency purposes.

Use of staging areas

If, exceptionally, a "staging area" in a neighbouring country is to be used to receive, consolidate and onforward supplies, liaise with Supply Division to ensure arrangements for appropriate reporting and documentation.

Buying supplies locally

(*Manual 11.6*)

General considerations

Before requesting local procurement:

- **Get good technical advice (especially if items are beyond the normal experience of available staff);**

- **Check costs;** *and*

- **Ensure that appropriate items can be delivered quickly and without adversely affecting the local market.**

Where purchases could disrupt the local market, supplies should be purchased and brought in from outside the immediately affected area. Annex 50 lists the general criteria for local procurement.

Representatives' authority

Representatives can authorize local procurements, without prior reference to UNIPAC, as follows:

— SLNs of which the total value is less than $5,000 and no item costs more than $1,000 provided no similar order has been or is expected to be made within 6 months; *and*

Table 21

Expediting local procurement

Preliminary research
- —Get best possible technical advice;
- —Make rapid survey of local availability of suitable items of satisfactory quality.

Request for PA
- —Explain reasons/justification in telex: see Annexes 41 and 50.

Bidding
- —Orders less than $5,000: get at least 3 offers (by phone if necessary, but get written confirmation later and make note for the record).
- —Larger orders: ask a wide range of known potential suppliers to sumbit written/telex offers within 24-48 hours if necessary; publicly open bids at the stipulated time.
- —Ask for unit prices (offers) for total required quantity *and* smaller quantities.

Specifications and delivery
- —Include full packing, marking and delivery as well as product quality specifications in both invitations to bid and final LPOs.
- —Consider including a penalty for late delivery.

Evaluation of offers
- —Verify ability of tenderers to deliver on time.
- —If necessary to ensure fast delivery and reduce risks/effects of any default, consider splitting total required quantity between different suppliers.

Quality control
- —Ensure necessary inspection on delivery. Engage superintendence company if necessary for large orders.

Advances
- —Payment terms should normally be "on satisfactory delivery." Advances should be given to suppliers only in special circumstances and then not more than 30% of the total order value.

Forms and CRC
- —Ensure adequate stock of forms and ability of CRC meet at short notice.

—Other SLNs up to a cumulative value of $15,000 per year for countries with annual CF ceiling below $1m; $25,000 per year if ceiling more than $1m.*

For larger orders, telex details with request and justification for local procurement to UNIPAC to obtain a "PA" (procurement authorization): see Annex 41.

Request a specific increase in the above authorities if believed to be necessary and justified. Telex a specific proposal to Chief Procurement/UNIPAC repeated to Directors Supply and Programme Divisions and Chief EOU/NYHQ.

Procurement procedures

Orders should normally be placed following competitive bidding procedures, and using the standard Local Purchase Order (LPO) form. (For small purchases against the Contingency SCF an LPO need not be issued.)

Contract Review Committee (CRC) should decide on contracts of $10,000 or more. (For certain regional offices a higher limit is established.)

Table 21 provides a brief summary of the main aspects. See Emergency and Supply Manuals for details of rules and procedures, and further practical guidelines.

Ensure that all decisions taken and the reasons for them are recorded—either as a note for the record signed by the responsible staff member, or as a formal CRC minute. Copy/inform EOU and UNIPAC.

In only very limited and exceptional circumstances may exceptions be made to these processes: see *Manual 11.6.*

---

* These limits are in addition to the $10,000 supply list per current BAL which may be established each year for procurement of small value items costing less than $100 each. **151**

CHAPTER 19

PROMOTING EXTERNAL RELATIONS

Public information

(*Manual 12.2, 12.3*)

- **Keep DIPA/NYHQ and GEHQ informed of all actions and developments likely to be of interest to the media.**

- **Establish arrangements and responsibilities for servicing the media locally.**

- **Help to provide written material and photographs (35mm black and white) to HQ for information and fund-raising use internationally. Co-operate with HQ requests to assist visiting jounalists.**

Ask assistance from the regional information officer or request the assignment of information staff locally if necessary. Especially in major/complex emergencies, get information policy guidance from EOU-DIPA/NYHQ

Formal relations with media

- Decide local policy on use of press releases or press briefings. Telex the text of any press releases to NYHQ and GEHQ: consult with DIPA/NYHQ in advance when feasible.

- Do not distribute internal reports, e.g. sitreps.

- Avoid quoting data from other agencies unless they have already released it themselves.

- In any statements, stick to facts. Be objective.

Formal statements on behalf of UNICEF at field level should be given only by the Representative or an information officer deputed to handle the task. (Formal statements include press releases and on-the-record responses at press conferences and in interviews. In some situations a Representative may delegate this responsibility to a senior programme officer.)

Informal/unplanned contacts with journalists

Annex 52 provides general guidelines for handling contacts with journalists. Where information personnel are available, refer journalists to them.

Working with donor representatives

(*Manual 2.3, 2.4*)

Fund raising

Once assistance proposals and funding strategy have been agreed by NYHQ:

- Provide information to donor representatives on your assessment, UNICEF's response and any outstanding funding requirements.

- Give copies of any formal documents/appeals issued by HQ. Prepare informal briefing notes if possible. Don't distribute internal reports (sitreps etc.).

- Inform PFO and EOU/NYHQ and GEHQ of all contacts with potential donors, and possible outcomes. Leave formal negotiations to HQ.

153

Co-ordinate closely with HQ (NY and GE) in all contacts with potential donors. Clear with PFO/NYHQ any plans by staff to engage in fund-raising activities while on visits to donor countries.

"Unearmarked" contributions to the overall UNICEF emergency programme are preferred to ones which are tied to specific inputs.

NGOs may sometimes wish to contribute to UNICEF programmes. Advise HQ to follow up with the agency HQ or get PFO/EOU approval to conclude an agreement locally if the NGO representative has full negotiating authority.

Reports to donors

Issued by PFO/NYHQ. HQ may have to ask the field office to provide special reports for earmarked contributions.

Unsolicited and in-kind contributions

- **Notify EOU/NYHQ of any offers. The Executive Director decides whether to accept.**

- **Ensure that any supplies offered are of appropriate type and quality, and that both international and in-country transport costs have considered (in general, paid by the donor). Check drug expiry dates.**

Offers of supplies or funds for specified kinds of activities which do not correspond to UNICEF's priorities and proposed programme should, in general, be politely declined.

Take the initiative to suggest, in the early stages of any operation, any specific kinds of items which might be welcome as in-kind contributions (although possibly not being a high priority for the allocation of UNICEF funds directly). Telex your suggestions, if any, to EOU/NYHQ and GEHQ.

The *Handbook for donors,* ICRC, Geneva (1983), provides technical guidelines for donations in kind to ICRC relief operations. The indications of specifications and packing requirements are equally relevant and useful for in-kind contributions to other agencies/programmes.

Part 5 GUIDELINES FOR PROGRAMME INTERVENTIONS

This Part, made up of a number of separate "annexes", provides guidelines for specific kinds of programme interventions which might be appropriate in particular circumstances (as defined in Part 3).

Possible objectives are indicated and guidelines given for the aspects which need to be considered in planning and supervising each kind of activity.

Subject to the considerations indicated in Parts 1-3 of this *Handbook*, UNICEF should co-operate with and assist the responsible government authorities and other concerned organizations in planning and implementing programmes appropriate to the needs of the particular situation.

An attempt has been made to reflect key aspects of organizing the various kinds of programme, i.e. to outline the overall process with which UNICEF should co-operate. This is not to be taken as implying that UNICEF should do it all itself! Substantial emergency assistance is usually available from other donors/organizations, and responsibility for implementation rests with the government: see Chapter 1.

Individuals involved in actually implementing programmes in the field should refer to the appropriate practical and technical guides and reference materials listed.

(Within each annex, cross references to other publications are to those listed at the end of the annex concerned.)

PREPAREDNESS AND ANTICIPATION

Objective

- **To minimize the impact of potential disasters/emergency situations on vulnerable communities by:**
  a. **Ensuring that the communities themselves, the government and UNICEF field offices are prepared to respond effectively if and when an emergency occurs; *and***
  b. **Establishing arrangements to alert populations to impending hazards and recognize the early signs of slow-onset situations.**

How to be prepared

Assign responsibilities
  —Designate a focal point for preparedness and recognition-surveillance.

Know:
  —Which areas are prone to particular types of disasters, and any seasonal/cyclincal patterns;

157

—The consequences of previous disasters, and which have been the most vulnerable communities;

—The results of previous post-disaster assistance.

Have (or have access to):

—Base-line data on the vulnerable areas and communities, see Table 1/1;

—Information on available in-country resources.

Table 1/1

Base-line data on vulnerable areas

☐ Demographic details: the location, size and socio-economic characteristics of communities.

☐ General climatic conditions, including day- and night-temperatures at different times of year.

☐ Local food habits—including weaning practices—of the various socio-economic groups.

☐ "Normal" nutritional status of children—including any normal seasonal variations.

☐ Diseases endemic to the area: prevailing patterns of mortality and morbidity.

☐ Normal sources of water: type(s) of sources; methods of extraction, treatment and distribution (if any).

☐ Food production: types, seasonal production cycles and normal yields—major crops and small gardens.

☐ Services operating (official and non-official): health, education, rural development, public works, social welfare, etc.; the location and specific nature of the services provided and personnel employed.

☐ Coverage and general condition of infra-structure: roads, telecommunications, electricity supplies, etc.

☐ Location, capacities and normal stock levels of any food and medical stores.

☐ Normal transport routes and facilities; likely logistic problems if supplies have to be moved into the area.

☐ Any particular social/religious considerations—any taboos or traditional community support processes.

Sources of information: local administrations, extension workers, and organizations active in the areas concerned.

Up-to-date information should be to hand on:
—Potential suppliers of items commonly required for emergency programmes, including tarpaulins, blankets, utensils, tools, drugs, vehicles, etc.
—Transport routes and capacities, and reliable transport contractors.
—Persons in public and private organizations with expertise in relevant fields, including water supplies, nutrition, logistics, social anthropology, etc.

Helping to develop national capacity to cope

Collaborate with government, UNRC and others to:
—Develop Early Warning systems;
—Define general policies for emergency assistance; *and*
—Develop emergency response capacity. See Table 1/2.

Recognizing a deteriorating situation

The aim is to detect—and correctly interpret—early signs of deteriorating conditions and potential problems, to determine who is adversely affected (by geographic area and socio-economic group), and to *trigger timely action.*

For areas prone to drought, large fluctuations in crop output, or where administrative breakdown might be envisaged:

● **Data on selected "indicators" must be collected regularly;**

● **Data from several indicators should be presented and interpreted together, not individually;**

● **Results must be fed into an appropriate decision-making body to produce action.**

Select "indicators" which are:
a. Relevant to the characteristics of the particular circumstances, and the kind of problems anticipated; *and*
b. Feasible—for which data can in fact be obtained from existing reporting systems and limited additional arrangements.

Table 1/3 suggests some indicators which might be appropriate. A limited number should be selected.

159

Data from existing health reporting systems should be sampled either in the field units or centrally before analysis. Additional arrangements might include reports

Table 1/2

Developing national capacity to cope with emergencies

Promote early warning systems:
- —Broadcast warnings to areas being threatened by a cyclone or flood; *and*
- —Provide guidelines and training to officials and communities on what to do.

Establish general policies for emergency assistance:
- —Roles of local leaders and institutions, national NGOs and outside assistance agencies;
- —"Whether or not" and "how" regarding: vaccinations; prophylactic distribution of drugs; the care of any unaccompanied children; salvage of materials; etc.
- —Whether material relief should be provided free, on a sale or credit basis. The kind of allocation and selection criteria which might be appropriate.
- —Particular objectives and standards to be applied: e.g. ration scales for food and water; *and*
- —Kinds of food and other commodities which would be appropriate inputs—and those which would not.

Develop emergency response capacity:
Anticipate what will probably need to be done, and what kind of resources be required. On that basis:
- —Define who is (will be) responsible for what, and the lines of communication;
- —Arrange for available personnel and transport to be quickly mobilized in a co-ordinated manner;
- —Establish arrangements by which appropriate quantities of selected, relief supplies can be mobilized at very short notice: this *may* include the maintenance of stockpiles in strategic locations;
- —Establish arrangements for the control of available supplies (especially medical supplies and food); *and*
- —Provide concise guidelines and training to officials and community leaders on what they should do in particular foreseeable circumstances.

from NGOs, regular "sentinel group" surveys, ad hoc surveys, and informal means including keeping "ears-to-the-ground". Try to separate the data for distinct population groups.

Table 1/3

Possible indicators for recognition-surveillance

- ☐ Rainfall (or evapotranspiration rates).
- ☐ Water levels—in rivers and selected "index" wells.
- ☐ Crop growth rates and yield expectations.
- ☐ Livestock—state of herds, prices, migrations.
- ☐ Availability and price of essential foodstuffs.
- ☐ Nutritional status of young children.
- ☐ Birth weights.
- ☐ Infant and young child mortality rates.
- ☐ Morbidity—diagnoses or symptom complexes.

Observations should, if possible, also be made of any:
- —Unusual out-migrations to towns and other regions;
- —Unemployment and purchasing power among labourers and artisans;
- —Levels of household and commercial food stocks;
- —Changes in food habits—consumption of items normally ignored; domestic animals, seed stocks;
- —Increases in distances and time for daily water collection;
- —Increases in sales of family possessions—jewelery, furniture, tools, animals, land;
- —Development of a "black market" in essential supplies;
- —Observable deterioration in the sanitary state of the environment; *and/or*
- —Decline in the effectiveness of local administration and services.

Use of data: graded response

Data must be analysed and interpreted on the basis of a good understanding of local social and economic processes. Reports and conclusions should be submitted to an appropriate executive, inter-ministerial body to take action when necessary as follows:

161

1   Response to the first signs of problems may be to initiate more detailed and specific data collection and analysis, possibly special surveys.

2   Later interventions should focus on removing the causes (if possible) or on mitigating the eventual effects on the vulnerable population groups.

3   If the earlier interventions have failed to fully arrest the deteriorating situation of certain groups, organize targeted relief measures *before* the situation becomes acute.

Role of UNICEF

UNICEF co-operates and collaborates with the UN Resident Coordinator and other interested organizations in promoting and assisting the development of national preparedness and recognition-surveillance systems.

The UNICEF office should itself also be well informed at all times of the situation of the most vulnerable population groups in areas likely to be affected, and be prepared internally to respond quickly when necessary.

Further references

a.   *UNICEF Field Manual Book E, Emergencies,* chapter 4.

b.   *Disaster prevention and mitigation* vol. 11, *Preparedness aspects*—UNDRO (1984) E/F/S

c.   *Disaster prevention and mitigation,* vol. 12, *Social and sociological aspects*— UNDRO (1986) E/F/S

d.   *Disasters and Development,* F. Cuny—Oxford University Press (1984) E

e.   *Guide to food and health relief operations for disasters,* Protein Advisory Group—UN (1977) E/F/S

Concerning preparedness only:

f.   *Guide to effective cyclone awareness programmes,* E. Ressler—WHO/UNDRO/LRCS (expected 1988) E

g.   *Medical Supply Management after Natural Disaster,* PAHO Scientific Publication No. 438—PAHO (1983) E/S

h.   Role of the Resident Representative in respect of pre-disaster planning and disaster relief, UNDP/PROG/FIELD/110/Rev.1, Oct. 1983—UNDP.   E

i.   *Shelter after Disaster*—UNDRO (1982) E/S

Concerning recognition-surveillance only:

j.   *UNICEF Field Manual Book E, Emergencies,* reference note R5.

k.   *Nutrition Surveillance,* J. B. Mason et al.—WHO (1984) E

ANNEX 2

ACCESS TO BASIC FOOD SUPPLIES

Objectives

- To restore self-reliance in basic food supplies—through local production and/or market exchange—as early as possible; *and*

- To assure, in the mean time, that all population groups have access to sufficient basic food to maintain reasonable nutritional health.

Overall priorities and the food chain

An approach is needed which flexibly integrates:
  —Local food production possibilities (including protection and storage of crops);

163

—Food exchange/marketing arrangements for basic commodities;

—Cash employment opportunities;

—Food-for-work programmes; *and*

—Free distributions (general to whole population groups or selective to only the most needy).

Ensure that people have access to food in the most efficient and rational manner, and avoid any disincentive to local production and self reliance. This requires an analysis of both supply and demand aspects:

—Food stocks available in the locality and surrounding regions;

—Size and timing of anticipated harvests;

—Consumption requirements; *and*

—Purchasing power (present and future expected) of different population groups.

Avoid the kind of situation which has occured in the past when traders have trucked locally produced food *out* of a striken area to sell it elsewhere in the country while, at the same time, the government and assistance agencies have paid high transport costs to move donated/relief food into the same area to give to people who had no money to buy what had been available!

Employment and self-help rather than "relief"

The free distribution of food/meals *may* be required in the immediate aftermath of some traumatic events but is not always necessary.

Assuring the availability of basic commodities for purchase at fair—possibly subsidized—prices together with action to ensure that income-earning opportunities and therefore purchasing power are available to otherwise destitute households, is preferable to prolonged free distributions. Self-respect is preserved and able-bodied manpower mobilized for useful, productive activities.

Any provision of food through free distribution (if required at all) and/or food-for-work projects should be reduced or phased out completely when locally produced crops become available or access to adequate food can be assured by cash income and market mechanisms.

UNICEF should normally concentrate on:

—Promoting small-scale, community and household level food production;

—Operations to provide income for the most deprived households/population groups; and

164 —Co-operating, where necessary, in assuring food for the most vulnerable.

In some instances limited inputs may also be appropriate to complement those of FAO, WFP and others in relation to larger scale food production and distribution operations.

Reasonable preparatory actions/efforts by the community itself should be a prerequisite to the delivery of any relief inputs.

Food production

National/regional policies should encourage production of food for local consumption. Actions should facilitate the more intensive use of land—especially for cereals, root crops and pulses—and exploitation of possibilities for increasing food yields from gardening, fish and small animals.

The use of available but normally little-used sources of food—including insects and birds—should be promoted and facilitated where appropriate, but having due regard to any known risks. All organic waste material should be systematically used to feed animals or fish (or for composting).

Give priority to actions which can produce early returns in terms of usable nutrient yields. Stengthening of extension service infrastructure to support these actions and provide practical guidance and training will often be needed.

Staples and other main food crops

Following floods, storms, droughts and other events which have interrupted normal agricultural activity, late (re-)sowing of usual crops is sometimes possible, e.g. following the recession of flood waters. Otherwise alternative "catch" crops may be able to be planted (e.g. sorghum instead of maize in southern Africa or beans instead of rice in Asia when rains have been delayed).

Prerequisites are:
  —Capacity to prepare and till the land—sufficient manpower and hand tools, draught animals and ploughs, and/or tractors and fuel;
  —Sufficient seeds of varieties appropriate to the local conditions and familiar to the farmers: see Table 2/1;
  —Adequate water (irrigation) and necessary complementary inputs of fertilizer and pesticides; *and*
  —Mechanisms to allocate and distribute seed and other inputs in good time; credit facilities may be needed.

165

Table 2/1

Ordering seeds

Local varieties of seed should be bought wherever possible. If seed has to be ordered from outside the country, try to provide the following information:

—Type and variety of seed normally used;

—Usual source/supplier;

—Growing season, rainfall and temperature in the particular location;

—Any local epidemic diseases; *and*

—Packaging arrangements to suit distribution.

For irrigation, needs may include: repairs to existing channels—repair/replacement of pumps and assurance of fuel supplies—the design and construction of new small scale water retention/irrigation systems.

The aftermath of a disaster is generally *not* the time to attempt the introduction on a large scale of new crops or "improved" varieties of seeds which require significant changes in previous farming practices and demand extra irrigation and fertilizer. It may, however, be an opportunity to introduce changes on a small, demonstration scale with adequate explanation and supervision by extension workers.

In some instances, e.g. Kampuchea 1980, donated food grains have been given to peasant farmers in exchange for local seed grains which might otherwise have been eaten. The seed grain is then stored by local government or co-operative organizations to be sold/released when needed for planting.

Livestock

Apart from assuring fodder and water, action to vaccinate livestock against prevalent diseases if often a priority.

In droughts, it is often impossible to keep all livestock alive and in reasonable health. Programmes to buy dried meat—or buy cattle at fair prices and dry the meat—which is then used in special feeding programmes can help both herders and children. Give careful attention to quality control and the process of drying. Training and supervision may be needed. (Such projects, organized through co-operatives and schools and financed by UNICEF, were successful in Ethiopia and Mali in 1984.)

Mixed gardening

Gardening—in small household plots, schools or at community/co-operative level—can make an important contribution to the household diet in both rural and urban areas during dry seasons and droughts, and may provide some income *if* marketing arrangements have been assured.

Emphasize vegetables which not only grow well in the local conditions but also provide vitamins and minerals otherwise lacking in local diets. Give priority to dark green leafy vegetables (especially local varieties), carrots, other root crops and pulses. Orange and yellow-coloured fruits (especially mangoes and papaya) are also valuable as sources of vitamin A.

Ensure that:
— Households have access to sufficient water, adequate soil and rights to use of the land;
— Seeds and any other required inputs reach households in time for the planting season;
— Clear, local-language guidelines are provided on row spacing, water and any other requirements; *and*
— Practical extension workers are mobilized and trained.

Try to avoid dependence on distributing fertilizer.

Fishing/fish farming

Where there is potential for increasing fish catches in the sea, rivers and lakes:
— Repair/provide nets, boats, etc.
— Provide training and basic materials for appropriate (possibly improved) drying/preservation methods.

The (re-)establishment of fish farming in ponds and lakes can give quick returns. Requirements are:
— A suitable pond (natural or specially dug) or carefully constructed enclosure in a lake;
— Fish fry (young) of suitable, fast growing species (e.g. tillapia, carp);
— Suitable food to be put into the pond (e.g. kitchen waste, human excreta from latrines);
— Nets of suitable mesh sizes for enclosures and selective catching; buckets, etc.; *and*
— Provision of appropriate guidelines, training and ongoing extension services—expertise.

Poultry and small animals

Where adequate edible material and roughage can be provided (including from domestic scraps), poultry and small animals raised at household or co-operative/small community level can convert otherwise waste material into useful protein-rich food.

After dairy cattle, pigs and poultry generally give the best return in useful calories per unit of starch equivalent consumed. Rabbits breed quickly in all climates, can be inexpensively housed and fed largely on weeds, crop residues. etc.

If new animals/practices are being introduced, appropriate guidelines, training and extension services should be provided.

Food storage, preservation and processing

Wherever food supplies are and/or will be short, give special attention to minimizing losses through spoilage and rodent attack in village-level food stores:
— Repair community level grain stores and/or introduce improved storage practices;
— Replace equipment necessary for processing local crops at community level (to improve storage properties and/or before they can be used in the household); *and*
— Promote household/community-level methods for preserving vegetables, etc.

Storage arrangements for grain and other foods should be based on proven designs, using a maximum of materials accessible (available and affordable) to the communities themselves.

Clear, local-language guidelines, training, ongoing extension services and technical expertise may be needed.

Food exchange/marketing arrangements

When staple foods are short, it is often found necessary for governments to control—or at least directly influence—the movement and trading of such commodities within the affected region or the country as a whole. This might involve special laws or administrative action to:

- —Introduce and enforce price controls, subsidies and/or rationing (using existing official food marketing structures, co-operative shops and/or private traders);
- —Prevent hoarding by traders;
- —Prevent thefts from available stocks; *and*
- —Control the movement of basic foods out of the area and the use of grains for the manufacture of non-essential products.

New, temporary government structures may be needed to manage such administrative measures.

Employment opportunities

Projects should:

- —Provide work for people—including women—from those population groups who most lack resources, other income-earning opportunities and, therefore, the ability to buy sufficient food and other necessities;
- —Yield benefits to the community as a whole, not to particular, priviledged individuals, e.g. land owners; *and*
- —Contribute towards reducing future vulnerability.

E.g. development of communal land and water resources—dams, embankments, irrigation and erosion-prevention works—or (re)construction of communal infrastructure—wells, sanitation works, clinics, schools, etc.

In all cases, careful planning is essential:

- —Materials, tools and technical supervision necessary for the work must be available/provided in time;
- —Any equipment and trained personnel necessary for the operation of the resulting facilities must be available as soon as the work is completed;
- —Community participation in determining priority works as well as organizing participants is essential; *and*
- —The timely availability of cash and/or food for payment must be assured.

Where sufficient food will be available in the area if purchasing power exists, payment should normally be *in cash.* Even where supplies of basic foods must be brought in, payment in cash and ensuring the availability of food at affordable prices (see above) is generally preferable.

In some situations—including where food, not cash, is the resource available and donors are unwilling to allow it to be sold to generate funds—payment of part (or as a last resort all) of the wages may be made in food.

169

Food-for-work (FFW) projects may be particularly useful for subsistence farming communities until the next harvest, but must be scheduled to permit timely tilling and planting. They are also "self-selecting"—those not really in need may choose not to participate. Regular deliveries of all food items *must* be assured (by WFP or others).

UNICEF has financed successful "cash-for-work" projects (e.g. Ethiopia, 1984) and collaborated with WFP in FFW projects (e.g. Bangladesh, 1972).

Efforts may be made to persuade food donors to allow food to be sold within such programme operations—with proceeds being used to finance cash-employment projects and/or relevant investments—rather than insisting on all being distributed free.

General food distributions/grants

Free distribution of basic food for whole families, if necessary at all, should normally be a very *short-term*, gap-filling measure. Only in cases of severe famine should such "general" distributions be envisaged for an extended period.

Aspects to be defined include:
—Whether total feeding is necessary or only supplementation of what the population is otherwise able to provide for itself;
  [Define the quantity of energy—kilocalories—which should be provided daily, the quantity of protein and, finally, the vitamins and minerals otherwise lacking: see Annex 7.]
—The period during which distributions will be required—until local production or employment plus food marketing will meet the need;
—Whether cooked food or dry rations should be provided and the mechanisms for distribution, rationing, etc.

Food Commodities

To the extent possible, commodities should be provided which can be prepared in a traditional manner, meet nutritional needs and economise on scarce fuel. Avoid items which the people cannot easily (or will not) use themselves, and any which may create new tastes (thus long-term dependency on external sources) or disrupt local markets.

The "food basket" provided by WPF and the other major donors usually includes a staple/cereal, fat/edible oil and a source of protein (usually either beans or milk powder). Where people are dependent on food distributions for long periods, small quantities of other items are necessary to add variety, flavour and nutritients otherwise lacking. This may include locally purchased vegetables, fruits, salt, spices, sugar, tea, etc.

If such additions to the diet are not possible, it may be necessary, in a long-running emergency, to seek donated commodities which are reinforced with the vitamins/minerals required.

Note that whole grain cereals are generally preferable to flours—having higher nutritional value and longer shelf lives—but local availability of grinding/milling equipement and/or sufficient fuel for cooking must be assured.

Cooked food

The provision of cooked food *may* be necessary:
—For short periods immediately after some traumatic disasters; and
—For new arrivals in concentrations of displaced persons where families do not have the facilities or utensils to cook for themselves, or where there is insufficient cooking fuel (firewood).

Bread is easy to distribute and has often been useful. Temporary communal kitchens, if needed, require good organization and close supervision to assure reasonable hygiene (see also Annex 5, p. 216).

Take measures to enable households to cook for themselves—or in small groups— as quickly as possible.

Dry ration distributions

Practical aspects to be defined are listed in Table 2/2. Arrangements must ensure that the most needy receive priority in distributions and that any "general" distributions are carefully co-ordinated with any "supplementary" feeding/distribution operations—see Annex 5.

Ration cards and strict procedures are usually necessary to ensure a reasonable measure of control over distributions. Refs. k, l, m and Annex 5, p. 213 provide more detailed guidelines.

Annex 7 provides information on daily nutrient requirements. Table 2/3 provides figures to help in calculating quantities of food needed: the figures shown do *not* make any allowance for losses/wastage. Final figures may be rounded up or down within 5%.

171

As a rule of thumb, each person requires 5-600 g of food per day. 15-18 tons of food are therefore required each month to meet the "maintenance" needs of a population of 1,000 which has access to no other supplies. 30-36 cubic metres of storage space are needed to store this quantity—perhaps 20 m² of floor space on a warehouse: see Table 34/2, p. 444.

Where rations have to be distributed to large numbers of people in difficult circumstances, it can be useful to pre-pack certain items before taking them to the distribution site. E.g. for distributions to displaced persons on the Thai/Kampuchea border, rice was packed into plastic bags of 12.2 kgs being equivalent to daily rations of 350 gms for 7 days for 5 persons.

Table 2/2

Aspects to be defined for food distribution programmes

☐ **Criteria**: who should be entitled to receive taking account of both need and the availability of supplies;

☐ **Allocation system**: ration cards and arrangements for the issuing and control of them;

☐ **Commodities**: must be acceptable to beneficiaries and able to be prepared with the facilities/fuel they have available: see p. 170;

☐ **Rations**: based on the commodities obtainable and taking account of the quantity and type of foods available to households from other sources;

☐ **Schedules**: when and where distributions will be made—must be regular and announced in advance;

☐ **Logistics**: how supplies will be moved from point of origin to distribution sites; how and where stocks will be stored;

☐ **Organization**: personnel to unload trucks, control stores and make actual distributions: containers beneficiaries must bring: any prepacking arrangements;

☐ **Facilities**: organization of premises or corrals of local construction to facilitate the distribution process;

☐ **Utensils and fuel**: must be assured for households—see Annex 25;

☐ **Demonstrations**: to show women how best to use/prepare meals with available foods, especially any with which they are not familiar; *and*

☐ **Monitoring** and control systems.

Where communities are small, separate and well organized—with established allocation mechanisms and accepted leadership—allocations may be made to communities without individual family ration cards.

Cash-for-food

In some instances where food is available within the country, local community institutions (e.g. co-operatives) may be able to arrange to buy and transport commodities more quickly and efficiently than government or outside agencies. Cash grants to carefully selected institutions might then be considered. UNICEF provided such "cash-for-food" in Ethiopia in 1984.

Such cash relief leaves the recipients a measure of choice, mobilizes local resources including transport, and supports the infrastructure of markets rather than making the region rely on continued *ad hoc* arrangements for food supplies.

Monitoring and the use of food

Monitoring must ensure that:
—Food reaches the specified distribution points in the right quantities at the right time;
—Distributions are properly conducted and controlled: that those elligible receive and not others;
—Programme criteria and processes are modified as and when necessary; *and*
—"Leakage" is kept to a reasonable minimum.

See also Chapter 6 ("monitoring").

In situations involving conflict, all reasonable efforts must be made to ensure that internationally donated food goes only to civilian populations, not to combatants.

Food which is provided through food-for-work or free distributions is intended to be eaten by the recipients and their families. Beneficiaries may, however, be allowed some discretion to determine how they use resources made available to them. A limited degree of trading of commodities at the household level may therefore be accepted *provided* there is no evidence of large scale diversions of assistance or detrimental affects on the nutritional status of the community.

In many cases, people have exchanged small quantities of relief foods against locally available items to be able to prepare a more paletable meal. Some cash, intended for household food purchases, has been wisely used to acquire tools and other agricultural inputs.

Table 2/3

Computations for food requirements

Average daily ration (g)	Feeding days	Total intake in period per beneficiary (kg)	Total quantity required (in metric tons)					Number of beneficiaries fed by:			
			For 500 people	For 1,000 people	For 2,000 people	For 5,000 people	For 10,000 people	1 metric ton	50 metric tons	100 metric tons	200 metric tons
10	90	0.9	0.45	0.9	1.8	4.5	9.0	1 111	55 560	111 110	222 220
	120	1.2	0.6	1.2	2.4	6.0	12.0	833	41 670	83 330	166 670
	180	1.8	0.9	1.8	3.6	9.0	18.0	555	27 780	55 560	111 110
20	90	1.8	0.9	1.8	3.6	9.0	18.0	555	27 780	55 560	111 110
	120	2.4	1.2	2.4	4.8	12.0	24.0	417	20 830	41 670	83 330
	180	3.6	1.8	3.6	7.2	18.0	36.0	278	13 890	27 780	55 560
30	90	2.7	1.35	2.7	5.4	13.5	27.0	307	18 520	37 040	74 070
	120	3.6	1.8	3.6	7.2	18.0	36.0	278	13 890	27 780	55 560
	180	5.4	2.7	5.4	10.8	27.0	54.0	185	9 260	18 520	37 040
40	90	3.6	1.8	3.6	7.2	18.0	36.0	278	13 890	27 780	55 560
	120	4.8	2.4	4.8	9.6	24.0	48.0	208	10 420	20 830	41 670
	180	7.2	3.6	7.2	14.4	36.0	72.0	139	6 940	13 890	27 780
50	90	4.5	2.25	4.5	9.0	22.5	45.0	222	11 110	22 220	44 440
	120	6.0	3.0	6.0	12.0	30.0	60.0	167	8 330	16 670	33 330
	180	9.0	4.5	9.0	18.0	45.0	90.0	111	5 560	11 110	22 220
60	90	5.4	2.7	5.4	10.8	27.0	54.0	185	9 260	18 520	37 040
	120	7.2	3.6	7.2	14.4	36.0	72.0	139	7 140	13 890	27 780
	180	10.8	5.4	10.8	21.6	54.0	108.0	92	4 630	9 260	18 520
80	90	7.2	3.6	7.2	14.4	36.0	72.0	139	7 140	13 890	27 780
	120	9.6	4.8	9.6	19.2	48.0	96.0	104	5 210	10 420	20 830
	180	14.4	7.2	14.4	28.8	72.0	144.0	69	3 470	6 940	13 890
100	90	9.0	4.5	9.0	18.0	45.0	90.0	111	5 560	11 110	22 220
	120	12.0	6.0	12.0	24.0	60.0	120.0	83	4 170	8 330	16 670
	180	18.0	9.0	18.0	36.0	90.0	180.0	56	2 780	5 560	11 110
125	90	11.25	5.6	11.3	22.5	56.3	112.5	89	4 440	8 890	17 780
	120	15.0	7.5	15.0	30.0	75.0	150.0	67	3 330	6 670	13 330
	180	22.5	11.3	22.5	45.0	112.5	225.0	44	2 220	4 440	8 890
150	90	13.5	6.75	13.5	27.0	67.5	135.0	74	3 700	7 410	14 810
	120	18.0	9.0	18.0	36.0	90.0	180.0	56	2 780	5 560	11 110
	180	27.0	13.5	27.0	54.0	135.0	270.0	37	1 850	3 700	7 410

Possible UNICEF inputs

Depending on the assessment of actual needs and possibilities, some of the following inputs might be considered:

— Vegetable and other seeds for household, school and small community gardens; plus hand tools, buckets, watering cans, etc.

— Materials and/or local costs to repair/construct wells and small irrigation systems for gardens.

— Replacement/provision of animals for ploughing (through co-operative groups).

— Poultry stocks; fish fry; rabbits; plus nets, materials and/or local costs to repair/construct enclosures, fish ponds, etc.

— Materials, equipment and/or spare parts to (re-)establish community-level facilities for food storage and processing.

— Expertise and funds for the training and operations of local extension workers; preparation and distribution of guidelines for all the above activities.

— Equipment and/or limited local costs for employment programmes and/or to complement the inputs of WFP (and others) for food-for-work projects.

— Funds to recruit, train and support the field operations of local women demonstrators to show mothers how to prepare nutritious meals with available items.

— Household (and possibly communal) cooking utensils, and assurance of fuel for cooking.

Wherever possible, actions should be planned in close consultation with FAO, WFP and other concerned organizations—including ILO for employment and food-for-work projects. Where necessary, UNICEF might also seek to mobilize/provide funds for cash-for-work projects and/or the purchase and distribution of locally available foods until WFP and other organizations can organize deliveries.

Where materials are required, concentrate on providing those not otherwise available to the communities themselves.

Further references

a. *Food and nutrition procedures in time of disaster*, G. Masefield—FAO (1967) E/F/S
b. *Poverty and famines: an essay on entitlement and deprivation*, A. Sen—Oxford, Clarendon Press (1981) E

(Summary paper: *Food entitlement and food aid programmes* in report of the WFP-Government of the Netherlands seminar on food aid, October 1983   E)

c.   *Famines*, a report to the independent commission on international humanitarian affairs—Pan (1985)   E/F/S

Concerning food production:

d.   *The UNICEF home gardens handbook* (for people promoting mixed gardens in the humid tropics)—UNICEF (1981)   E

e.   *Gardening for food in the semi-arid tropics*, a handbook for programme planners—UNICEF/WHO (1985)   E

f.   *Home gardening in international development—what the literature shows*, L. Brownrigg—League for International Food Education, Washington DC (1985)   E

g.   Better farming series—FAO   E/F/S simple practical guides, especially:
No. 11, *Cattle breeding* (1977)
No. 12, *Sheep and goat breeding* (1977)
No. 13, *Keeping chickens* (1977)
No. 27, *Freshwater fish farming: how to begin* (1979)
No. 29, *Better freshwater fish farming: the pond* (1981)
No. 30, *Better freshwater fish farming: the fish* (1981)

h.   *Fruits and vegetables in West Africa*, H. Tindall & F. Sai—FAO (1965)   E

i.   *The Samaka guide to homesite farming*, 4th edition—Samaka Service Centre, Manila, Philipines (1973)   E

j.   *Small-scale irrigation*, P. Stern—Intermediate Technology Publications, London (1979)   E

k.   *Irrigation practice and water management*, rev.1, L. Doneen & D. Wescot—FAO (1984)   E/F/S

Concerning general/emergency feeding:

l.   *A guide to food and health relief operations for disasters*, Protein Advisory Group—UN (1977)   E/F/S

m.   *Management of nutritional emergencies in large populations*, C. de Ville de Goyet, J. Seaman & U. Geijer—WHO (1978)   E/F

n.   *Management of group feeding programmes*, FAO food and nutrition paper 23—FAO (1982)   E/F/S
and the companion training kit *Group feeding programme management—a training pack*, 2nd edition—FAO (1980)

o.   *Field programme management: food and nutrition—a training pack*—FAO (1982)   E/F/S

p.   *Logistic guidelines—distribution and monitoring*, R. S. Stephenson—International Disaster Institute, London (1984)   E

Concerning food storage and preservation:

q.   *Handling and storage of food grains in tropical and subtropical areas*, D. Hall—FAO (1977)   E

r.   *Processing and storage of foodgrains by rural families*, E. O'Kelly & R. Forster—FAO (1983)   E/F/S/A

s.   Rural home techniques series—FAO—multilingual E+F+S
simple practical guides, especially:
Food preservation, series 1: *fish, meat, equipment* (1976)
Food preservation, series 2: *vegetables, cooling, outside storage* (1977)
Labour saving ideas, series 3: *sanitation, food, water* (1977)

176   t.   *Food storage manual*, 2nd edition—WFP (1983)   E

ANNEX 3

INFANT FEEDING

Objective

- **To ensure the best possible nutritional health of infants by: facilitating breast-feeding — providing for infants whose mothers have been lost or cannot lactate — assuring that mothers can prepare suitable weaning foods.**

For the treatment of those already severely malnourished see Annex 6.

Breast-feeding and
breast milk substitutes

Breast-feeding is even more important in emergencies than in normal times to ensure the health of infants.

- **Encourage mothers to breast-feed for as long as possible, while gradually introducing complementary weaning foods from 4-6 months.**

177

- Include mothers in supplementary feeding programmes if necessary to improve their health and ensure adequate production of breast milk, see Annex 5.

- Promote the restimulation of lactation of any mothers not producing sufficient milk — even those who may themselves be sick and malnourished — by feeding the mother and frequently putting the child to the breast.

For infants whose mothers cannot lactate — or whose mothers have disappeared or died:

—Seek substitute mothers ("wet nurses") from among women who have recently breast-fed their own infants. Their milk production can be reinstituted by letting an infant suck frequently at both breasts. (Provide supplementary rations to substitute mothers as to other lactating women.)

—Arrange for breast milk substitutes to be prepared and fed, by cup and spoon, until a substitute mother is found and her lactation restimulated.

Table 3/1

Locally-prepared breast milk substitutes

	Full cream milk powder (FCM)	Dried skim milk powder (DSM)	Evaporated milk
Milk	15 g (1½ tblspns)	10 g (1½ tblspns)	50 ml (3 tblspns)
Water, boiled	200 ml (1 teacup)	200 ml (1 teacup)	150 ml (¾ teacup)
Sugar	15 g (1 tblspn)	15 g (1 tblspn)	15 g (1 tblspn)
Oil	—	5 g (1 teaspn)	—

All measures are "level". Tblspn = tablespoon. Teaspn = teaspoon.

Determine the capacities of commonly used local measures (e.g. milk tins) for each of the items concerned and issue instructions expressed in terms of those measures.

150 ml of the mixture is required per kg body weight per day.

If these substitutes are to be relied on for more than a few days, add vitamin concentrates. As an emergency measure, add a few drops of fruit juice or citric acid.

(Adapted from ref. a)

Breast milk substitutes

Infants require a total of 120 kcal per day per kg of body weight—best given in 5 feeds per day (each providing 24 kcal/kg body weight).

— Use infant formula that is formulated in accordance with applicable Codex Alimentarius Standards where available, otherwise prepare simple milk-based substitutes: see Tables 3/1 and 3/2.

— Ensure that clear instructions on preparation and feeding are given to and understood by mothers/attendants.

— Ensure that clean, boiled water is always used, and cups and spoons well cleaned (boiled if possible) each time.

Table 3/2

Milk powder and infant food products

Milk powder can be very useful—mixed into gruels rather than reconstituted—where it is used under supervision for on-the-spot supplementary and therapeutic feeding programmes.

Milk—in powder or condensed form—should *not*, however, be distributed as part of food rations (unless it is a traditional part of the local diet and its correct, hygienic usage can be assured—not normally possible in emergencies).

Dried skim milk (DSM) is the most commonly available item from donor countries. Ensure that any quantities accepted are vitamin-A fortified. Shelf life is then 6 months. It is difficult to store in humid climates unless in plastic-lined bags.

DSM is high in protein but low in energy: sugar and/or oil must always be added (except when mixed into gruels). Even then it does not meet the vitamin and mineral needs of infants.

"Infant formulas" which conform to applicable Codex Alimentarius Standards contain all necessary nutrients and are appropriate as substitutes for infants for whom breast-feeding is (temporarily) unavailable or inadequate. They might also be used—where they are available and suitable local items are lacking—in the communal preparation of weaning foods. Their acquisition and use must, however, be strictly controlled to avoid any suggestion that they are preferable to breast-feeding and the use of appropriate local foods where these are available.

Ensure that different items/products are stored separately, and that appropriate instructions for the use of each are drawn up—in an appropriate local language—for feeding centre staff.

Baby bottles

- Do *not* distribute feeding bottles to mothers but actively discourage their use.

A few feeding bottles may, however, be needed for the interim feeding, under medical supervision, of any very young, motherless babies unable to take a spoon.

Weaning foods

Semi-solid supplementary ("weaning") foods should be introduced into an infant's diet starting at 4-6 months while breast-feeding is also continued. The need is to assure:

—Availability and use of high caloric density foods (containing oil, fat, sugar) and protein-rich foods to produce a weaning food low in bulk, of high nutritional density;

—Means to pound or grind ingredients to make a smooth semi-liquid food (since the child cannot yet chew);

—Facilities to prepare food separately, outside the family pot (requiring more fuel or an extra cooking pot and a stove capable of accomodating it); *and*

—Regular feeding—3 meals/day between breast-feeding both morning and evening—and avoiding spoilage.

Traditional weaning practices and beliefs must be observed, understood and, if appropriate, supported. Consult local public health personnel including health workers, traditional birth attendants, nurse-midwives, paediatricians and nutritionists. (Note that fermentation of cereals and milk can increase digestability and the nutrient density of foods.)

If mothers are not able to obtain and prepare foods normally used for weaning—or if those foods are not appropriate for the children's needs:

—Arrange demonstrations to show mothers how to prepare suitable weaning foods using items which are available to them from local sources and/or from any food distribution programmes.

—Make appropriate foods available if necessary.

If supplementary feeding programmes are being organized for other "vulnerable groups" including lactating women (see Annex 5), the preparation and provision of suitable weaning foods should be a part of the larger SFP. Otherwise, arrange for weaning food provision alone, perhaps with communal preparation (see below).

Foods

Weaning foods should be prepared, to the extent possible, from locally available/familiar foodstuffs. They must not be spiced. Sample recipes can be found in refs. a and c.

Table 3/3 shows the quantities of various staples and protein-rich foods which, when mixed together with 10g oil—or 5g oil plus 10g sugar—or 20g sugar—provide approximately 350 kcal with the equivalent of 5-6g reference protein (about one third of the daily needs of a 2-year-old child, see Table 7/4, p. 242).

Instructions to mothers must be given in locally available measures: Table 3/4 shows the volume equivalents of some raw foods.

If necessary, imported blended foods like ICSM (Instant Corn-Soya-Milk which needs only to be mixed with cooled boiled water) may be used initially and on an interim basis. If ICSM is required, ask WFP locally and inform EOU—but note that deliveries can rarely be obtained in less than 3 months.

Commercial weaning foods should *not* be distributed. Offers of such "baby foods" should normally be declined. Glass packaging and water usually make up a high proportion of the total weight and bulk. Very little food value is delivered for all the time, money and effort it takes to transport, store and handle such products.

Demonstrations

Recruit and train women who have raised their own children locally to demonstrate—at health clinics, supplementary feeding centres and in villages—the preparation of weaning foods using available ingredients. They should also follow up by visiting homes to check that food is being properly prepared and give further advice and demonstrations if necessary.

Communal preparation

The preparation of weaning foods at community level may be encouraged:
—When fuel and other necessities for appropriate food preparation are not readily available to individual households;
—In the immediate aftermath of a sudden disaster (especially, but not only, if the communal preparation of food for the general population is necessary); *or*
—If mothers have difficulty in accepting and using unfamiliar items or changing habits.

181

Quantities of staples and protein-rich items to prepare weaning foods

All figures are for edible portions of raw food in grams

Supplement \ Staples	Oats		Wheat		Rice		Sorghum, millet		Maize		Potato		Sweet potato		Yam		Taro, coco-yam		Banana		Plantain		Cassava flour, gari	
Legume	75	5	80	10	65	25	75	10	55	35	320	20	125	50	165	40	150	45	105	55	85	55	40	55
Soybeans	60	10	60	15	55	20	55	15	50	25	250	20	150	25	175	20	150	20	140	25	115	30	50	30
Dried skim milk	65	5	65	10	65	15	60	15	60	15	280	15	175	20	190	15	180	15	165	20	150	20	60	20
Dried whole milk	55	10	55	15	45	25	45	20	40	25	220	20	100	30	115	30	115	25	100	30	90	30	35	30
Chicken/lean meat	65	10	65	20	65	25	65	25	65	35	300	25	180	35	210	35	195	30	185	40	160	45	70	45
Fresh fish	65	15	70	30	70	30	70	25	70	20	310	25	210	35	240	35	220	40	210	40	180	45	75	50
Eggs	65	10	65	25	65	30	60	30	65	25	300	25	180	35	220	25	190	25	190	30	150	45	60	50

The basic mixes have been calculated to give the best possible protein value (i.e. amino-acid score). The least amount of protein is used to supplement the staple to provide the basis of a meal for a child of about two years of age.

To each of the basic mixes, 10 g oil — or 5 g oil and 10 g sugar — or 20 g of sugar — should be added. Each mix then provides about 350 kcals (approximately one-third of the daily needs of a two-year-old child).

The volumes of most of the basic mixes are between 200-300 ml when the water absorbed by the food is taken into account.

(Reproduced from ref. a)

The mothers themselves should be largely responsible for any such operations, guided by trained women demonstrators.

Health/nutrition personnel should provide overall supervision and also relevant health and nutrition education. This might include the use of growth charts if literacy levels are reasonably high, if scales and appropriately trained community health workers are available, and if there are reasonable prospects that the use of charts will become part of an ongoing growth monitoring and nutrition surveillance programme.

Table 3/4

Volumes and equivalent weights of some raw foods

Food	Weight (in grams) of: 500 ml	200 ml	100 ml	1 level table-spoon (= 15 ml)
Staples				
Rice	450	180	90	..
Wheat noodles (small)	450	180	90	..
Rolled oats	200	80	40	..
Wheat flour: whole grain	275	110	55	..
refined	300	125	65	..
Cassava flour, gari	350	150	75	..
Legumes/oil seeds				
Large, e.g. kidney beans, cow peas	..	150	75	..
Small, e.g. mungbeans, chickpeas	..	175	90	..
Split, no skin, e.g. lentils	..	175	90	..
Groundnuts, whole	..	145	75	..
Bean flour	..	170	85	12
Sesame seeds	..	140	70	10
Other foods				
Vegetable oils	..	200	100	15
Sugar	..	200	100	15
Milk, liquid	..	200	100	15
Dried skim milk (DSM) powder	..	90	45	8
Dried skim milk granules	..	70	35	4
Full cream milk (FCM) powder	..	100	50	9

Example: a measured volume of 100 ml rice weighs 90 g. To obtain the volume of a particular weight of *rice*, say 200 g:
divide by 90 and multiply by 100: e.g. 200 ÷ 90 x 100 = 222 ml.

Possible UNICEF inputs

Depending on the assessemnt of actual needs and possiblities, some of the following inputs might be considered:

- —Local operating costs for substitute programmes and the appointment, training and subsequent operations of food preparation demonstrators.
- —If necessary, some suitable food items (locally purchased or ICSM) may be provided for distribution through appropriate channels.
- —Materials to (re-)establish community-level facilities for the storage and preparation—e.g. grinding—of food for weaning.
- —Local costs for the preparation, production and distribution of education materials on the feeding of infants and young children.

Further references

a. *Manual on feeding infants and young children*, 3rd edition, M. Cameron & Y. Hofvander—Oxford University Press (1983)   E
    (2nd edition, UN Protein Advisory Group, 1976, E/F/S)
b. *Guidelines for training community health workers in nutrition*—WHO offset publication no.59 (1981)   E/F
c. *How to feed young children*, Children in the tropics No. 138-139-140—International Children's Centre, Paris (1982)   E/F
d. *The use of artificial milks in relief actions*—ICRC & LRCS (1985)   E/F/S
    (To be superseded by *Guidelines for relief feeding,* expected 1986)

ANNEX 4

DETERMINING NUTRITIONAL STATUS

Purposes

- **To obtain objective measures of and monitor the nutritional status of specific communities (for recognition-surveillance, determining priorities and/or evaluating nutrition interventions).**

- **To select malnourished children for admission to special, selective feeding programmes.**

Techniques

A malnourished child is wasted—abnormally thin and underweight for his/her height—and body measurements provide a good indication of nutritional status. (Strictly speaking they indicate the probability that the child is suffering from a particular degree of malnutrition.)

185

Weight-for-height

This is the preferred method for screening and surveying in emergencies. The weight of the child is expressed as a percentage of that of a well-nourished child of the same height as given in international reference tables.*

Using tables:

1. Weigh and measure the child: length is measured instead of height for children under 2 years (less than 85 cm) or any unable to stand.
2. Calculate the percentage of weight-for-height or simply classify the child according to the ranges given in the reference tables (e.g. Tables 4/2 and 4/3 pp. 198, 200):

    (120 per cent and over = overweight)
    90-119 per cent = adequately nourished
    80- 89 per cent = slightly malnourished
    70- 79 per cent = moderately malnourished
    Less than 70 per cent = severely malnourished.

    (Some nutritionists count 70-84 per cent as moderately malnourished.)

Using weight-for-height charts:

— Weigh the child, stand him/her in front of the chart (UNIPAC 01-455-70 sometimes called a "Nabarro" or "thinness" chart) and read off the status category directly from the colour-coded bands: see Figure 4/d.

The chart avoids the need for tables and calculations, and may be more easily understood by mothers.

A child suffering from oedema (see p. 237) should not be categorized in terms of weight-for-height measurements but automatically be considered as severely malnourished.

Mid Upper-Arm Circumference (MUAC)

The thinness of the upper arm provides an approximate indication of the degree of malnutrition of children without the need for weighing scales, and can be very useful for rapid screening in emergencies. Reference tables are available relating MUAC to age and height for well-nourished children (e.g. refs. b and f).

Arm circumference alone:

— *For children 12-60 months only*: the arm circumference measured at the mid-point of the upper left arm should normally be approximately 16 cm.**

---

* There is little evidence of any difference between the weight-for-height values for well-fed children of different races or ethnic origins.

** MUAC changes little at this age as growth in muscle is almost compensated for by loss of fat.

The following categories are now used by many field-experienced nutrition-ists: MUAC more than 13.5 cm = adequately nourished
MUAC 12.0—13.5 cm = moderately malnourished
MUAC less than 12.0 cm = severely malnourished

(Earlier recommendations of WHO propose the cut-off at 12.5 cm instead of 12.0 cm.)

Arm-circumference-for-height tables:

MUAC is expressed as a percentage of reference value for a child of the same height. The percentages corresponding to degrees of malnutrition similar to those given above for weight-for-height are:

More than 85 per cent = adequately nourished
75-85 per cent = moderately malnourished
Less than 75 per cent = severely malnourished.

(Some nutritionists categorize as severely malnourished any child less than 80%.)

Using a "Quac" stick:

— An height stick/board is calibrated in terms of selected cut-off values of MUAC (usually 75 per cent and 85 per cent).
— MUAC is measured and compared with the values on the stick level with the top of the child's head to determine the category (per cent rank) directly.

(This eliminates the need for measuring height and referring to tables. See Figure 4/i and refs. b and e.)

Weight-for-age and height-for-age

Weight-for-age and height-for-age comparisons are valuable in long-term surveil-lance programmes—and regular measurements of weight and height provide a measure of an individual child's progress over time—but these methods are *not* appropriate for screening or one-off surveys in emergencies.

Ages are often not known with sufficient accuracy, and no distinction is made between children who are currently malnourished and any who are small/stunted due to earlier periods of under-nutrition but now reasonably healthy—of a weight appropriate to their height.

Screening—selection of the severely malnourished

If sufficient time, trained personnel, scales and charts are available, WHO and most nutritionists recommend using weight-for-height.

187

If large numbers of young children have to be screened and categorized very quickly with few staff and little equipment, use the simple MUAC classification.

If screening is to include significant numbers of children over 5 years and weighing is not feasible, prepare and use Quac sticks with scales corresponding to the chosen cut-off percentages of MUAC-for-height.

Where there is much oedema and/or children suffer from heavy infestations of intestinal parasites, weights may be inflated by sub-clinical (unrecognized) oedema and the weight of the parasites themselves (up to 2 kg). Some nutritionists then prefer the Quac stick even to weight-for-height.

Whatever technique is used, any child with clinically evident oedema is classified as such and automatically counted as severely malnourished. (Weight should still be measured and recorded if possible for monitoring the child's future progress.)

Two-stage screening and selection may be considered where there are large numbers of children and sufficient personnel resources to organize it (see Figure 4/a):

Figure 4/a **Two-stage nutritional screening**

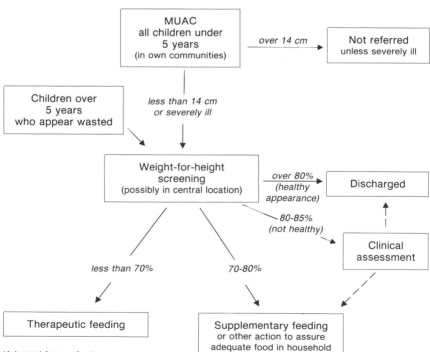

(Adapted from ref. c.)

1. Measure MUAC of all children under 5 years.
2. Refer those having MUAC less than 14 cm to be weighed.
3. Also refer any older children obviously malnourished.
4. Make weight-for-height classification of those referred.

If possible, public health nurses (or doctors) should be present and clinically examine those referred.

In all cases:

—Community leaders must understand the purpose of and be involved in organizing the screening.

—The purpose of the exercise must be clearly explained, to mothers—a few days in advance if possible.

—All sick children must be screened: house-to-house searches may be necessary and/or children be mobilized to find and bring them forward.

Nutritional status surveys

Community leaders should be involved in organizing the survey. The purpose of the exercise must be clearly explained.

If possible, use weight-for-height charts and scales. Otherwise Quac stick or simple MUAC. Look for oedema. Figure 4/b suggests a format for recording survey results.

Measure only children 12-60 months. Their status is also a good indicator of that of the community as a whole. If there is doubt about childrens' ages, take all children who can walk without stooping under a horizontal stick fixed at 115 cm. (This allows a safety margin: some older children will be included, but none less than 5 years will be missed.)

Try to ensure that a "representative sample" of *all* children in the community is measured—not just those who are readily accessible or who appear to be thin.

Get personnel with field survey experience—from statistical or demographic units—to plan the exercise and train those who will do the sampling. The notes in Table 4/1 provide only an indication of what may in practice need to be done. It is more important to ensure that proper sampling procedures are followed than to measure large numbers of children.

If feasible, record the results separately for a limited number of ranges of height (e.g. less than 75 cm; 75-94 cm; 95-114 cm; 115 cm and over), calculate the totals and percentages separately within each height range and then a weighted average of all these ranges for each category of malnutrition. This will help to compensate for any under representation of any agegroup in the sample, and identify any significant differences within the 1-5 age group.

Figure 4/b

Sample nutritional survey report

Location .... Date ....

Survey by:

Estimated total population .... *Number measured:*

Estimated No. children U-5 .... Boys ....

Sampling method used: Girls ....

Boys + Girls ....

	Oedema		*Less than 70% wt/ht (or MUAC <12.0 cm)*		*70-79% wt/ht (or MUAC 12-13.5 cm)*		*80% and over wt/ht (or MUAC >13.5 cm)*	
	Boys	*Girls*	*Boys*	*Girls*	*Boys*	*Girls*	*Boys*	*Girls*
<75 cm								
75-94 cm								
95-114 cm								
>115 cm								
Totals								
Percent-ages								

Remark:

Signature:

The percentage in each column is obtained by taking the column total, multiplying by 100 and dividing by the total number of children of that sex measured.

The refinement of recording and calculating totals and percentages in each column separately for selected height ranges is desirable, but optional. See p. 189.

Table 4/1

Some suggestions for taking representative samples

Take "cluster" samples:

1. Identify distinct geographic sub-sections within the total population of interest.

2. Take a random sample of children within each cluster.

If there are a large number of clusters (e.g. villages) take a random sample of the clusters first—by numbering them and using a random number table—and then of the children within those selected.

To get a "random sample" within a cluster:

1. Estimate the total number of children 12-60 months.

2. Line up *all* such children—boys and girls separately—and measure every 5th one until 50-100 of each have been measured.

Or: Number each house on a sketch map and then select houses using a random number table: measure *every* child normally living in the first house selected, then the second, etc. until a total of 50-100 boys and 50-100 girls have been measured.

Or: Go to the centre of the cluster, spin a bottle, identify the house towards which it points and go there: measure *every* child normally living there, and in every 2nd or 3rd nearest house in a similarly selected direction until a total of 50-100 boys and 50-100 girls have been measured.

If less than 200 young children in total in the cluster, measure all of them. If total population in the cluster is more than 10,000, measure 100 boys plus 100 girls.

Note: For more complex surveys, not only do questionnaires need to be carefully designed and pre-tested but preliminary, pilot surveys must also be made to determine the size of the sample required to give the desired accuracy of results for the particular data concerned.

Monitoring a child's status

The nutritional progress of an individual child—once admitted to a special feeding programme—is monitored by regular weighing. The date and weight (to the nearest 100 g) should be recorded each time. If the child does not gain weight progressively, medical examination and/or checking on actual food consumption in the household and feeding centre is needed.

191

Growth ("road-to-health") charts should be used if the personnel concerned are able/can be trained to make entries accurately.

If weight-for-height charts are used, the child's classification (percentage/colour band) can be recorded on a similarly colour-coded record card—a simplified growth chart. This has the advantage of being directly linked to the admission and discharge criteria for the feeding programmes, is easier for poorly trained personnel to do, and may be more readily understood by mothers.

Try to ensure that all involved organizations agree with the ministry of health on the use of a common system!

Equipment and procedures for measurements

Weighing children

Hanging scales with pants (UNIPAC 01-455-50) are convenient for young children. Local beam balances might also be used if accurate to 100 g, see Figure 4/c.

Figure 4/c **Weighing a young child**

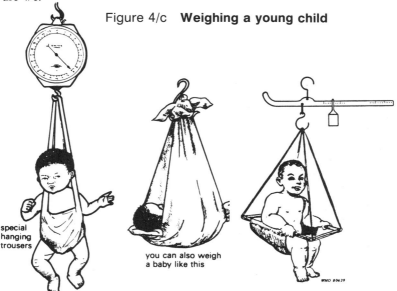

special
hanging
trousers

you can also weigh
a baby like this

(Reproduced from *Primary child care, a manual for health workers,* M. & F. King & S. Martodipoero, Oxford University Press, 1978 and ref. d.)

If older children (more than 25kg) are to be weighed, beam balances are preferred: they must be robust and simple to use. Bathroom scales are often used but not recommended for field use where they tend to be inaccurate. Spare scales should be available wherever possible.

— Personnel must be trained to read scales accurately and consistently.
— Scales must be checked for accuracy before every session using a standard weight.
— The zero setting must be checked before each child is weighed.

Using the weight-for-height chart

The zero (ground level) line of the chart must be at the level of the floor where the child stands. The chart must hang straight with no bumps: see Figure 4/d.

If charts are to be used in field surveys, in clinics which don't have solid walls or have uneven/earth floors, mount the chart on a large flat board and fix a small board at right angles at the bottom for the child to stand on.

Measuring height/length

If weight-for-height charts are not used, measuring sticks/boards should be obtained/constructed, preferably with foot-boards attached: see Figure 4/e.

Figure 4/e **Measuring height**

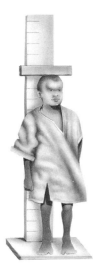

The child must be looking straight ahead with knees straight, feet flat, heels almost together, shoulders relaxed and the heels, buttocks, shoulders and back of the head all touching the board/chart.

193

Figure 4/d   **Weight-for-height chart in use**

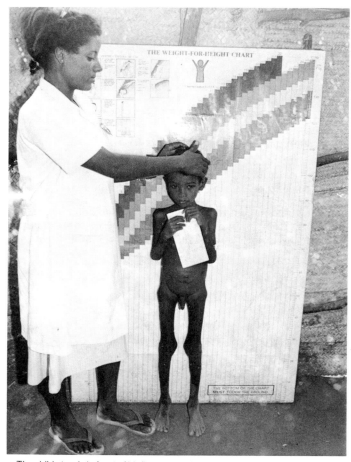

Photo. LRCS/de Toledo

The child stands in front of his/her own weight column on the chart. If the child weighs 13.5kg, the 13.5kg mark at the bottom of the chart should be visible between the child's feet.

Whether being measured against a weight-for-height chart or an height stick, a sliding head board—or at least a piece of wood held against the top of the head and the chart/stick—is necessary to get an accurate reading.

A length board is needed for measuring children less than 2 years (less than 85 cm): see Figure 4/f.

If infants are laid on a weight-for-height chart, note that approximately 1.5 cm should be subtracted from the measured length to obtain their equivalent standing "height".

Figure 4/f   **Measuring length**

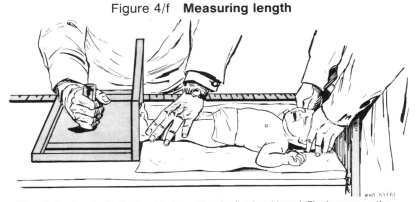

The child is placed with the head just touching the fixed end-board. Firmly press on the knees and slide the movable board up to touch the whole surface of the feet. Read off the length. (The child should be as relaxed as possible. The mother should help to hold the child and at least maintain eye contact, not stand behind the child's head!)

Measuring arm circumference

A tape measure may be used, but greater accuracy is likely to be achieved using specially made strips or insertion tapes. Any tape/strip must be of non-stretch material, e.g. plastic. (X-ray film cut into strips has been used to improvise strips in the field; marks can be scratched on.)

Figure 4/g   **Measuring MUAC**

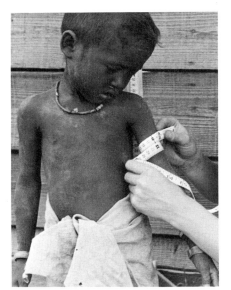

Photo. LRCS/de Toledo

The left arm must be hanging loosely and the tape not be pulled tight. The measurement should be made at the mid-point between the shoulder and the elbow but, with inexperienced personnel, it may be better to tell them to measure at the broadest point.

This boy's arm circumference is 22.0 − 10.0 = 12.0 cm.

(Most people find it easier to take an accurate measurement like this than to try and hold the zero end of the tape against the arm and the other long part of the tape.)

195

Details of how to prepare and use a "Quac" stick are provided in Figure 4/i. They are adapted from refs. b and e which also include figures for 80 per cent of reference arm circumference for height in case it is decided to use that as one of the cut off points.

Figure 4/h **MUAC tapes**

Improvised tape from x-ray film

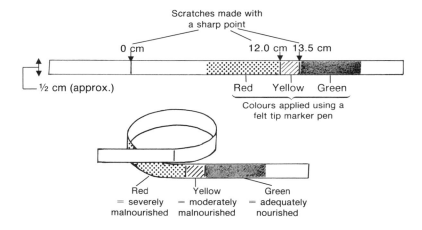

An insertion tape

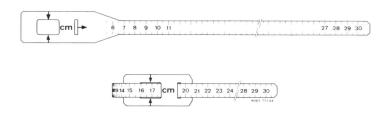

(Reproduced from ref. b)
From Zerfas, A. J., *Am. J. clin. Nutr.*, No. 28 (1975)

Figure 4/i   **Quac stick**

85% (cm)   **75%** (cm)

```
17.5    -134-    15.5
        -132-
17.0    -130-    15.0
        -128-
16.5    -126-    14.5
        -124-
16.0    -122-    14.25
        -120-    14.0
15.5    -118-    13.75
        -116-    13.5
        -114-    13.25
15.0    -112-
        -110-
14.75   -108-    13.0
14.5    -106-    12.75
        -104-
        -102-    12.50
14.25   -100-
        - 98 -
14.0    - 96 -
        - 94 -
        - 92 -    12.25
        - 90 -
13.75   - 88 -
        - 86 -
        - 84 -    12.0
        - 82 -
13.5    - 80 -
        - 78 -
        - 76 -
        - 74 -
13.25   - 72 -    11.75
        - 70 -

        - 2 -
        - 0 -
```

Centimetre rule temporarily taped to stick during preparation

Preparing a Quac stick

1. Obtain a straight pole/piece of wood about 140 cm long and at least 4 cm wide.
2. Smooth one surface to take marking by a felt tip pen. Attach a foot board if possible.
3. Tape a centimetre rule down the middle of the stick so that it will not move during marking. The 0-cm end of the tape must be level with the surface of the foot board (end of the stick).
4. Measuring from the bottom, make a mark on the *right* side of the tape corresponding to each of the heights listed below for the 75% scale. Make marks on the *left* side corresponding to the heights listed for the 85% scale.
5. Remove the centimetre rule.
6. Extend the height marks to the right and left edges of the stick with bold, horizontal lines using different colours for the two sides (scales).
7. Just above each line write clearly the arm-circumference measurement corresponding to that height on each scale.

Height (cm)	AC 85% (cm)	Height (cm)	AC 85% (cm)	Height (cm)	AC 75% (cm)	Height (cm)	AC 75% (cm)
132	17.50	106	14.50	132½	15.50	113	13.25
129	17.00	101	14.25	129	15.00	108	13.00
126	16.50	96	14.00	125	14.50	105	12.75
122	16.00	88	13.75	122½	14.25	100	12.50
117½	15.50	80	13.50	120	14.00	92	12.25
112	15.00	72	13.25	117½	13.75	84	12.00
109	14.75			116	13.50	72	11.75

Using a Quac stick

1. Stand the child against the stick.
2. Measure the arm circumference of the child (e.g. 13.5 cm).
3. Find the figure you have measured (e.g. 13.5) on the 75% scale and put your finger on it. See where the top of the child's head is in relation to your finger:
   - If the top of his/her head is *higher* than your finger, the child falls into the "below 75%" category and is likely to be severely malnourished.
   - If the top of the head is *lower* than your finger, the child is less severely malnourished. To find out which category to place him/her in, find the armcircumference measurement on the 85% scale, place your finger against it and see where the top of the child's head is now in relation to your finger:
     - If it is *higher* than your finger, the child falls into the 75-85% category—moderately malnourished
     - If it is *lower,* the child is probably adequately nourished.

197

Table 4/2

Weight-for-length (supine) for both boys and girls

Length (cm)	Median weight (kg)	Percentages of median			Length (cm)	Median weight (kg)	Percentages of median		
		85% (kg)	80% (kg)	70% (kg)			85% (kg)	80% (kg)	70% (kg)
49.0	3.2	2.7	2.6	2.3	67.0	7.6	6.5	6.1	5.3
.5	3.3	2.8	2.6	2.3	.5	7.8	6.6	6.2	5.4
50.0	3.4	2.9	2.7	2.4	68.0	7.9	6.7	6.3	5.5
.5	3.4	2.9	2.7	2.4	.5	8.0	6.8	6.4	5.6
51.0	3.5	3.0	2.8	2.5	69.0	8.2	7.0	6.6	5.7
.5	3.6	3.1	2.9	2.5	.5	8.3	7.1	6.7	5.8
52.0	3.7	3.1	3.0	2.6	70.0	8.5	7.2	6.8	5.9
.5	3.8	3.2	3.0	2.6	.5	8.6	7.3	6.9	6.0
53.0	3.9	3.3	3.1	2.7	71.0	8.7	7.4	7.0	6.1
.5	4.0	3.4	3.2	2.8	.5	8.9	7.5	7.1	6.2
54.0	4.1	3.5	3.3	2.9	72.0	9.0	7.6	7.2	6.3
.5	4.2	3.6	3.4	2.9	.5	9.1	7.7	7.3	6.4
55.0	4.3	3.7	3.5	3.0	73.0	9.2	7.9	7.4	6.5
.5	4.4	3.8	3.5	3.1	.5	9.4	8.0	7.5	6.5
56.0	4.6	3.9	3.6	3.2	74.0	9.5	8.1	7.6	6.6
.5	4.7	4.0	3.7	3.3	.5	9.6	8.2	7.7	6.7
57.0	4.8	4.1	3.8	3.4	75.0	9.7	8.2	7.8	6.8
.5	4.9	4.2	3.9	3.4	.5	9.8	8.3	7.9	6.9
58.0	5.1	4.3	4.0	3.5	76.0	9.9	8.4	7.9	6.9
.5	5.2	4.4	4.2	3.6	.5	10.0	8.5	8.0	7.0
59.0	5.3	4.5	4.3	3.7	77.0	10.1	8.6	8.1	7.1
.5	5.5	4.6	4.4	3.8	.5	10.2	8.7	8.2	7.2
60.0	5.6	4.8	4.5	4.0	78.0	10.4	8.8	8.3	7.2
.5	5.7	4.9	4.6	4.0	.5	10.5	8.9	8.4	7.3
61.0	5.9	5.0	4.7	4.1	79.0	10.6	9.0	8.4	7.4
.5	6.0	5.1	4.8	4.2	.5	10.7	9.1	8.5	7.5
62.0	6.2	5.2	4.9	4.3	80.0	10.8	9.1	8.6	7.5
.5	6.3	5.4	5.0	4.4	.5	10.9	9.2	8.7	7.6
63.0	6.5	5.5	5.2	4.5	81.0	11.0	9.3	8.8	7.7
.5	6.6	5.6	5.3	4.6	.5	11.1	9.4	8.8	7.7
64.0	6.7	5.7	5.4	4.7	82.0	11.2	9.5	8.9	7.8
.5	6.9	5.9	5.5	4.8	.5	11.3	9.6	9.0	7.9
65.0	7.0	6.0	5.6	4.9	83.0	11.4	9.6	9.1	7.9
.5	7.2	6.1	5.7	5.0	.5	11.5	9.7	9.2	8.0
66.0	7.3	6.3	5.9	5.1	84.0	11.5	9.8	9.2	8.1
.5	7.5	6.4	6.0	5.2	.5	11.6	9.9	9.3	8.2

(NCHS/CDC/WHO references 1982)

Possible UNICEF inputs

Depending on the assessment of actual needs and possibilities, some of the following inputs might be considered:

—Expertise: field-experienced nutritionist(s) to plan and supervise the programme: possible finance for the participation of local nutrition units/institutes.

—Equipment (depending on methods being adopted): hanging scales plus pants (01-455-50)—beam scales—weight-for-height charts (01-455-70)—arm circumference tapes—baby length measuring boards—height boards or Quac sticks.

—Transport

—Stationery: pre-printed tally forms—date stamps, pens and other stationery—pocket calculators—etc.

—Operating costs: vehicle operating costs—production and distribution of forms and instructions—engagement, training and expenses of survey personnel—data processing.

Small kits of basic drugs may also be needed to enable nurses to provide on-the-spot treatment to sick children seen during the selection/survey operations.

Note: OXFAM has standard sets of nutritional surveillance equipment—a "mini" kit (OFK4) for rapid, initial surveys and a larger one (OFK1) for systematic surveys and ongoing surveillance. There are often used by Oxfam's own field teams and those of other organizations.

Further references:

a. *Measuring change in nutritional status*—WHO (1983)   E/F

b. *The management of nutritional emergencies in large populations,* C. de Ville de Goyet, J. Seaman and U. Geijer—WHO (1978)   E/F

c. *Oxfam's practical guide to selective feeding programmes*—OXFAM, Oxford (1984)   E

d. *Guidelines for training community health workers in nutrition*—WHO offset publication No. 59 (1981)   E/F

e. *Medical care in refugee camps, Disasters,* vol. 5 No. 3—International Disaster Institute, London (1981)   E

f. *Community nutrininal assessment with special reference to less technologically developed countries,* D. Jellife—Oxford University Press (expected 1986)   E
    replacing *Assessment of nutritional status in the community,* D. Jellife—WHO monograph No. 53 (1966 now out of print)   E

199

Table 4/3

Weight-for-height (stature) for both boys and girls

Height (cm)	Median weight (kg)	Percentages of median 85% (kg)	80% (kg)	70% (kg)	Height (cm)	Median weight (kg)	Percentages of median 85% (kg)	80% (kg)	70% (kg)
85.0	12.0	10.2	9.6	8.4	108.0	17.8	15.2	14.3	12.5
.5	12.1	10.3	9.7	8.5	.5	18.0	15.3	14.4	12.6
86.0	12.2	10.4	9.8	8.5	109.0	18.1	15.4	14.5	12.7
.5	12.3	10.5	9.8	8.6	.5	18.3	15.5	14.6	12.8
87.0	12.4	10.6	9.9	8.7	110.0	18.4	15.7	14.8	12.9
.5	12.5	10.6	10.0	8.8	.5	18.6	15.8	14.9	13.0
88.0	12.6	10.7	10.1	8.8	111.0	18.8	16.0	15.0	13.1
.5	12.8	10.8	10.2	8.9	.5	18.9	16.1	15.1	13.3
89.0	12.9	10.9	10.3	9.0	112.0	19.1	16.2	15.3	13.4
.5	13.0	11.0	10.4	9.1	.5	19.3	16.4	15.4	13.5
90.0	13.1	11.1	10.5	9.2	113.0	19.4	16.5	15.5	13.5
.5	13.2	11.2	10.6	9.2	.5	19.5	16.7	15.7	13.7
91.0	13.3	11.3	10.7	9.3	114.0	19.8	16.8	15.8	13.8
.5	13.5	11.4	10.8	9.4	.5	19.9	16.9	16.0	14.0
92.0	13.6	11.5	10.8	9.5	115.0	20.1	17.1	16.1	14.1
.5	13.7	11.6	10.9	9.6	.5	20.3	17.3	16.2	14.2
93.0	13.8	11.7	11.0	9.7	116.0	20.5	17.4	16.4	14.3
.5	13.9	11.8	11.1	9.7	.5	20.7	17.6	16.5	14.5
94.0	14.0	11.9	11.2	9.9	117.0	20.8	17.7	16.7	14.6
.5	14.2	12.0	11.3	9.9	.5	21.0	17.9	16.8	14.7
95.0	14.3	12.1	11.4	10.0	118.0	21.2	18.0	17.0	14.9
.5	14.4	12.2	11.5	10.1	.5	21.4	18.2	17.1	15.0
96.0	14.5	12.4	11.6	10.2	119.0	21.6	18.4	17.3	15.1
.5	14.7	12.5	11.7	10.3	.5	21.8	18.5	17.4	15.3
97.0	14.8	12.6	11.8	10.3	120.0	22.0	18.7	17.6	15.4
.5	14.9	12.7	11.9	10.4	.5	22.2	18.9	17.8	15.5
98.0	15.0	12.8	12.0	10.5	121.0	22.4	19.1	17.9	15.7
.5	15.2	12.9	12.1	10.6	.5	22.6	19.2	18.1	15.8
99.0	15.3	13.0	12.2	10.7	122.0	22.8	19.4	18.3	16.0
.5	15.4	13.1	12.3	10.8	.5	23.1	19.6	18.4	16.1
100.0	15.6	13.2	12.4	10.9	123.0	23.3	19.8	18.6	16.3
.5	15.7	13.3	12.6	11.0	.5	23.5	20.0	18.8	16.5
101.0	15.8	13.5	12.7	11.1	124.0	23.7	20.2	19.0	16.6
.5	16.0	13.6	12.8	11.2	.5	24.0	20.4	19.2	16.8
102.0	16.1	13.7	12.9	11.3	125.0	24.2	20.6	19.4	16.9
.5	16.2	13.8	13.0	11.4	.5	24.4	20.8	19.6	17.1
103.0	16.4	13.9	13.1	11.5	126.0	24.7	21.0	19.7	17.3
.5	16.5	14.0	13.2	11.6	.5	24.9	21.2	19.9	17.5
104.0	16.7	14.2	13.3	11.7	127.0	25.2	21.4	20.1	17.6
.5	16.8	14.3	13.4	11.8	.5	25.4	21.6	20.4	17.8
105.0	16.9	14.4	13.6	11.9	128.0	25.7	21.8	20.6	18.0
.5	17.1	14.5	13.7	12.0	.5	26.0	22.1	20.8	18.2
106.0	17.2	14.6	13.8	12.1	129.0	26.2	22.3	21.0	18.4
.5	17.4	14.8	13.9	12.2	.5	26.5	22.5	21.2	18.6
107.0	17.5	14.9	14.0	12.3	130.0	26.8	22.8	21.4	18.7
.5	17.7	15.0	14.1	12.4					

(NCHS/CDC/WHO references 1982)

ANNEX 5

SUPPLEMENTARY FEEDING

Objectives

- **To ensure the health of new-born infants and prevent deterioration of the nutritional condition of young children and other particularly vulnerable individuals in situations where the quantity and/or quality of available food is inadequate.**

- **To treat — improve the nutritional condition of — children already moderately malnourished.**

Preventive measures and education may also be required if cultural factors are denying infants, pregnant and lactating women adequate nourishment.

Strategies and principles

Ensuring appropriate food for vulnerable groups

The need is to ensure that young and moderately malnourished children, pregnant and lactating women receive adequate and suitable food. Priority attention and special measures are necessary whenever normal food supplies have been disrupted and levels of malnutrition—especially levels of severe malnutrition—are significantly higher than normal for the time of year.

The best strategy for ensuring appropriate food for these "vulnerable groups" must be decided locally in each case on the basis of a thorough assessment of the causes of their nutritional vulnerability and the practical possibilities for reducing that vulnerability.

In some cases special "supplementary" feeding programmes (SFPs) as described in this annex may be necessary. In others, effort might better be concentrated on ensuring adequate basic food supplies/rations for all households (see Annex 2) and the preparation of suitable weaning foods for infants (Annex 3). See also Chapter 8, pp. 63 and 65.

Table 5/1 reproduces some suggestions concerning the circumstances in which particular types of measures might need to be considered.

Note that the distribution of "supplementary" food should not be necessary if:

a) Adequate quantities of suitable foods are available to each family/household; *and*

b) That food is properly prepared and shared within the family, including appropriate preparation for very young chidren separate from the family meal.

Principles for SFP operations

Additional food is given to selected, nutritionally vulnerable individuals to compensate for specific deficiencies—in energy, protein, vitamins and minerals—in the food otherwise available. It is intended to be in addition to their normal share of household food, including any general emergency distributions.

Based strictly on nutritional need: distributions of supplementary food must always be selective and the target focus strictly maintained. They should be continued only for as long as there is a clearly demonstrated nutritional need.

(Appropriate long-term education and food production programmes should be organized in parallel and continue afterwards. Free distributions of supplementary food should be continued on a long-term basis only where they form a part of carefully considered national food and nutrition policies.)

Table 5/1

Circumstances in which certain levels of supplementary feeding may be required

Situation	Action
Over 20% of children under 5 years less than 80% weight-for-height; Proportion of children less than 70% weight-for-height significantly higher than normal; *or* Food availability less than 1,500 kcal/person/day	Urgent action to: 1. Improve general access to basic food supplies (see Annex 2), *and* 2. Provide supplementary food for *all* young children and other "vulnerable groups" (Table 5/3). Special SFP operations probably necessary until levels of malnutrition are reduced and adequate access to basic supplies is assured.
10-20% children under 5 years less than 80% weight-for-height; Proportion of children less than 70% weight-for-height higher than normal; *or* Food availability less than 1,700 kcal/person/day; severe public health problems; high prevalence of major diseases (especially measles).	High priority to provide supplementary food selectively to the malnourished. (Other "vulnerable groups" may be included to the extent that resources permit.) Special SFP operations *may* be required.
Less than 10% children under 5 yrs less than 80% weight-for-height	Provide supplementary food selectively to the malnourished through ongoing community services if possible.

N.B. The above are only general indications. The most appropriate strategy to try to assure that the nutritional needs of young children and other vulnerable groups are met must be decided in each case taking account of the particular local (including socio-cultural) circumstances.

(Adapted from *UNHCR Emergency Handbook* and ref. b)

Mothers and community leaders must understand the need for and objectives of the programme, and take as much responsibility as possible in planning and organizing it. It should be seen as a health programme not a welfare measure.

Existing resources; minimum extra demands: to the maximum extent possible: use existing structures, mechanisms and personnel—keep requirements for additional facilities and organizational capacity to a minimum—use food items already familiar locally. Keep to a minimum the number of different commodities to be supplied and stored.

Health and nutrition education must always be integrated into any SFP with the aim of improving current and future feeding practices.

Mobilize local experience—nutritionists and feeding programme organizers—at the outset to plan and initiate any SFP operation.

Planning an SFP—aspects to be defined

Target groups and nutritional needs

Estimate the nature and extent of specific deficiencies—energy (no. calories), protein (no. grams), vitamins and minerals—in the diets currently available to infants, young children, pregnant and lactating women in different communities. Thus decide/estimate:

- Which target groups should be covered, and in which geographic areas: see below, p. 207;
- The specific selection criteria and mechanisms to be used (taking account of cultural attitudes, the socio-economic characteristics and physical locations of the most needy);
- The numbers who should be covered in particular areas at the beginning of the programme;
- How the numbers are expected to evolve; *and*
- The period during which distributions will need to be continued.

Delivery mechanisms

Identify the organizational structures, premises, logistic facilities, personnel and any existing funds available for organizing a SFP.

204 Thus decide, through consultations including all interested parties and on the basis of the numbers to be covered, population density, social and organizational factors:

— Whether needs can be met through existing mechanisms (e.g. MCH clinics or women's groups) or a separate, special SFP operation is necessary; *and*

— What method should be adopted: "on-the-spot" feeding or "take-home" (dry ration) distributions.

If it is proposed to use the school system, ensure that the real target group—the malnourished and pre-school children—will be reached and not only those attending school! Existing MCH centres may be appropriate if there are many of them and the number of children to be covered is not too large.

Commodities and rations

Determine the types and quantities of potentially useful food items which are:

— Able to be provided by the communities themselves . . .

— Available from stocks held by government and others . . .

— Available for purchase in local markets now and/or in the immediate future, and at what prices: . . .

— Able to be delivered quickly by donors (when could they be delivered—what realistic ETAs?) . . .

Thus decide:

— What food items should be used (see pp. 217 and 221) . . .

— From where they are to be obtained, how and by whom . . .

— Whether weaning foods are to be provided separately from the rations for other beneficiaries . . .

— What daily rations should be received by the beneficiaries (see tables 5/2 and 5/6, also 7/4 and 7/5, pp. 242 and 243) . . .

Table 5/2

Size of supplementary rations		
	Energy content	Protein
Minimum for a worthwhile nutritional impact	350 kcal/day	10-15 g/day
Desirable when access to basic foods is less than 1,500 kcal/person/day	At least 500 kcal/day	20 g/day

N.B. Actual rations must always be decided on the basis of assessed nutritional needs and practical possibilities.

Implementation arrangements

Define the number and location of SFP centres required and the arrangements needed at each location for:

— Premises/improvised constructions . . .

— Water supplies and storage (including treatment if necessary) . . .

— Delivery, storage and accounting for food commodities . . .

— Provision of utensils and cooking fuel . . .

Define the role and contribution of:

— The community . . .

— Various government departments/agencies . . .

— Local and international NGOs . . .

— UNICEF, WFP and others . . .

In many situations the community can provide volunteers, certain food items, local construction materials, some utensils and cooking fuel; organize beneficiaries and assure security of supplies.

In respect of personnel for the operation, define:

— The type and number of personnel required for the operation of each centre . . .

— How and by whom they should be selected . . .

— The training they should be given, how, when and by whom . . .

— How, if at all, they should be remunerated (in cash or on a food-for-work basis) . . .

Many SFPs have faced problems when different organizations involved have followed different practices in using volunteers, paying local personnel with food or in cash. Ensure standardized arrangements. In practice people are often ready to work on a voluntary basis initially, but demand payment if programmes continue for more than a few weeks.

Procedures and supervision

Establish procedures to be followed including:

— The design, production and control of ration cards . . .

— Selection and registration of beneficiaries . . .

— Reporting on operations (see p. 213) . . .

Prepare and distribute guidelines to all programme personnel.

Decide the type and number of personnel needed to supervise/organize the setting up of SFP centres and provide ongoing guidance and supervision:

— Practical organizers . . .

— Doctors, nurses and paramedical workers . . .

It has been suggested that a public health or other community nurse working full-time may be able to supervise up to 5 centres if distances are short.

Determine what transport, equipment, facilities and operating funds they will need . . .

Health and nutrition education

Specify:
- —The particular behaviour modifications which are to be sought (ones which are feasible in the local situation) . . .
- —The educational methods to be used and visual materials required . . .
- —Arrangements for the selection and training of communicators/demonstrators . . .

Overall plan and budget

See Annex 43.

Target groups—admission and discharge criteria

The extra food must be provided to those specifically identified as the most vulnerable nutritionally. These are listed, in usual order of priority, in Table 5/3. If there is a need and resources permit, all these groups should be included.

Ration cards should show the category of beneficiary, and separate registration lists be kept for each category.

A mother and infant should be treated as a unit—have a combined ration card and receive food together—as long as breast-feeding is continued.

Admission and discharge criteria

Selection methods and criteria should be agreed in each situation between the local health authorities, nutritionists and community representatives.

Children may be referred from health clinics. If there is widespread malnutrition, the entire child population should be systematically screened (see Annex 4). Normally all children 70-80 per cent of reference weight-for-height or otherwise selected clinically should be enrolled.

Table 5/3

Target groups for supplementary feeding

1. Malnourished children (less than 80 per cent weight-for-height or clinically identified *except* those receiving therapeutic feeding, but *including* those recently discharged from a TFP).

2. Children in hospital (where there is no other provision) and those recently discharged.

3. All infants 5-23 months old.

3. All young children 24-60 months old (or, if ages are uncertain, less than 115 cm in height).

5. Women in the last 4-5 months of pregnancy and first 6-12 months of lactation (while breast-feeding).

6. Other individuals referred by medical personnel (including TB patients).

All children 5-10 years and others specifically identified as being vulnerable for social or other reasons (e.g. unaccompanied children, the elderly without families) are sometimes also included. It would usually be more appropriate to ensure that they/their housholds have access to adequate basic food/rations—and the means to prepare food themselves.

Women—pregnant and lactating—should be registered and admitted through medical screening in clinics, thus ensuring appropriate medical care also. If such services are inadequate, SFP supervisors may register and admit:

— Pregnant women once the baby can be felt to be kicking in the abdomen;

— Women who are demonstrably breast-feeding an infant.

Women registered as lactating may be given food for the first 4 months after giving birth, and beyond that only if they bring their infant with them to the SFP centre. This assures that the infant can also be fed (weaning food), enables the condition of the infant to be monitored, and also reduces possibilities for other women to borrow infants in order to register and receive supplementary food.

Discharges:

—Children may be discharged when they have been above 85 per cent of reference weight-for-height for two consecutive months—unless there is good reason to believe that they will relapse quickly if discharged.

—Women whenever they stop breast-feeding.

208 —Medical referrals when advised by supervising medical personnel.

Children should be retained in the programme longer only if the continuation of similar feeding forms a part of the long-term food and nutrition policy for the area — and if sufficient resources are available to continue an appropriately adapted operation on a large scale.

Phasing out of special SFPs

If special SFP operations have to be organized separate from other community services, these might be phased out when:

- — Less than 10 per cent of all children under 5 years are below 80 per cent of weight-for-height;
- — Public health and disease control measures are effective and there are no major, foreseeable health risks; *and*
- — There is good evidence that adequate general food availability is assured.

Arrangements should ensure that continued feeding/treatment of the remaining, small numbers of moderately malnourished children is provided through ongoing community services.

Types of SFP

"On-the-spot" feeding

An extra, prepared meal is provided each day (or week days only) to the selected beneficiaries who eat it on-the-spot.

"Take-home" distributions

Dry, uncooked rations are distributed — normally to mothers — at regular intervals (usually every 1-2 weeks) to be prepared and fed to the intended beneficiaries at home daily.

Choice of system

Table 5/4 lists some of the advantages and disadvantages of the two alternative systems as they have generally been organized — usually with and dependent on major involvement of outside organizations.

"On-the-spot" feeding has, in recent years, been considered by most organizations to be preferable wherever it is feasible. This is generally where the population density is fairly high (in towns, displaced persons camps) and the capacity is available to organize and supervise the necessary feeding centres. In fact, take-home (dry ration) distributions may be both cheaper and more effective in many cases. See Chapter 8, p. 63. Where the population is widely scattered, "take-home" is the only practicable system. **209**

Table 5/4

Advantages and disadvantages of alternative SFP methods

"Take-home" distributions (dry rations)	"On-the-spot" feeding (prepared meals)

Consumption of food by recipients

No guarantee that the intended beneficiary receives the food supplement. It is likely to be shared by the whole family.

Food which has high market value might be sold. Unfamiliar food might not be eaten.

The full ration is eaten under supervision. Assistance can be given to those who are ill/unable to eat.

(Beneficiaries may, however, then receive less than their normal share of family food at home!)

Infrastructure and organizational requirements

Large numbers of beneficiaries can be covered with relatively little infrastructure.
(Distribution only once a week or less.)

Facilities, utensils, cooking fuel, sufficient water, helpers and supervisory personnel required to prepare meals every day. High cost per beneficiary served.

Logistics for mothers and organizers

Little time required of mothers. Distance to centre less critical.

Appropriate schedules can be fixed for distributions. Necessary food must then always be on-site in time.

Much mothers' time taken each day.

Centres must be close/accessible and meals served on time each day, otherwise attendances are likely to be irregular.

Health considerations and monitoring of nutritional status

Hygiene of food preparation may be poor.

Less frequent and children (especially those who are sick) may not be brought to the distribution points.

Increase risks of spreading communicable diseases.

Attendance is checked daily. Frequent nutritional status and health/clinical checks possible.

Training of personnel: supervision of operations

Little training needed for field workers, but close supervision of distributions and monitoring of actual use at household level is essential.

Feeding centre staff must be trained in management, food preparation, hygiene, record keeping. Ongoing guidance/supervision of all these aspects must be provided.

Responsibility and education of mothers and the community

Mothers take full responsibility for thier own children.	Large centres organized by outsiders take responsibility away from mothers and create dependency.
Demonstrations are necessary for the use of any unfamiliar foods.	Small centres can be organized with community participation and mothers assist in food preparation.
Demonstrations and health/ nutrition education may be best organized separately in small community groups (coupled with home visits if possible).	Health/nutrition education easily organized at daily feeding sessions.

Cultural aspects and other opportunities

Customary for food to be prepared at family/household level.	Not customary. May be contrary to beliefs—e.g. in some cultures women must not be seen eating in public.
Little disruption to family life as distributions only weekly (or less frequently). Organizing other activities in conjunction with infrequent distributions requires good planning.	Relatively easy to organize other activities with daily feeding centre as focal point.

(Adapted from ref. b)

Arrangements whereby mothers are organized in small groups to receive the dry rations and prepare food for their children collectively—with minimum involvement of outside organizations but initial guidance and occasional ongoing supervision—may be appropriate in many situations.

Procedures and reporting

Organizing SFP centres

Carefully establish procedures for registration—enrolling individuals and issuing ration cards—checking cards/identities and registering attendance at each feeding/distribution session.

Plan the layout of distribution centres and synchronize the timing of opening and closing of doors/gates facilitate control of registration and distribution, and to prevent beneficiaries presenting themselves for a second time.

Minimizing possibilities for cheating helps to ensure that the limited quantities of supplementary food available are fairly shared among those identified as most in need of it.   **211**

Figure 5/a

Sample monthly SFP report format

Supplementary Feeding Centre ....

Report for the month of: ....

Category	No. enrolled end last month a	New admissions this month b	Discharges this month 85% wt/ht c	Drop-outs this month d	Total end this month =a+b−c−d	No. who, since last report:	
						have lost weight	have not gained weight
Malnourished children (<80% wt/ht) { 5-59 months......							
5 years and over							
Other children { 5-23 months......							
24-59 months....							
5 years and over							
Pregnant women..............................							
Lactating women							
Medical referrals							
Others.................................							
Totals							

For children 5-59 months

Number attending each day:

1	2	3	4	5	6	7	8	9	10	11	12	13	14	15	16	17	18	19	20	21	22	23	24	25	26	27	28	29	30	31

(Put slash / in boxes on days when SFP closed.)

Remarks

Signature:

(Adapted from ref. b)

Ration cards

Ration cards should incorporate: name—beneficiary category—ration entitlement—distribution centre—issue and expiry dates. They should be produced centrally, printed and possibly perforated to make local forging difficult.

Cards should be marked or punched at each distribution, and may incorporate a weight/growth record for children. Examples are provided in refs. a, b.

Registrations

Registrations at neighbouring locations should be conducted simultaneously (to prevent double registrations).

Reregistrations should be made at regular intervals, especially if there are continuing population movements or the situation is changing rapidly.

Monitoring and reporting in SFPs

Ensure that responsible personnel at each SFP centre are able/trained to:
— Keep a register of all individuals selected/enrolled;
— Record those present at each session in the register and on their individual cards;
— Weigh children regularly, every 1-2 weeks if possible, and record the weight in the centre's records and on any card/chart kept by the mother;
— Make enquiries—home visits if possible—to determine and remove causes of any absenteeism and/or reasons for a child not gaining weight;
— Bring to the attention of supervising medical personnel any child not gaining weight and/or obviously sick; *and*
— Fill in simple reporting formats at the end of every month: Figure 5/a provides a sample format.

Trained health workers should be present to clinically examine beneficiaries as frequently as possible.

Organizing an "on-the-spot" SFP

Several small centres serving local communities are better than a few large centres. If centres are not within easy walking distance of the intended beneficiaries, **213** attendance will be irregular and the value of the feeding substantially reduced. 200 is a convenient number of beneficiaries for a centre, 500 the absolute maximum. It is often appropriate to serve beneficiaries in two shifts.

Facilities at each centre:

The following will be required:

—A building, or compound with shade/shelter, with space for the planned number of beneficiaries to sit and eat, a separate area for waiting, and adequate drainage.

—A separate (perhaps fenced-off) kitchen area.

—A secure store for food and equipment (with watchmen if necessary).

—Latrines for centre staff and beneficiaries.

—Sufficient clean water for food preparation, drinking, washing utensils and, if at all possible, for all beneficiaries to wash their hands before eating (Ideally 10-20 litres/day/beneficiary).

—Assured supplies of fuel for cooking.

—Utensils: depends on the type of foods to be prepared, see Figure 5/c and Table 5/5.

In a large camp, food may be prepared in a large, central kitchen and be delivered, hot, to several feeding centres.

Figure 5/b Layout of a typical "on-the-spot" feeding centre

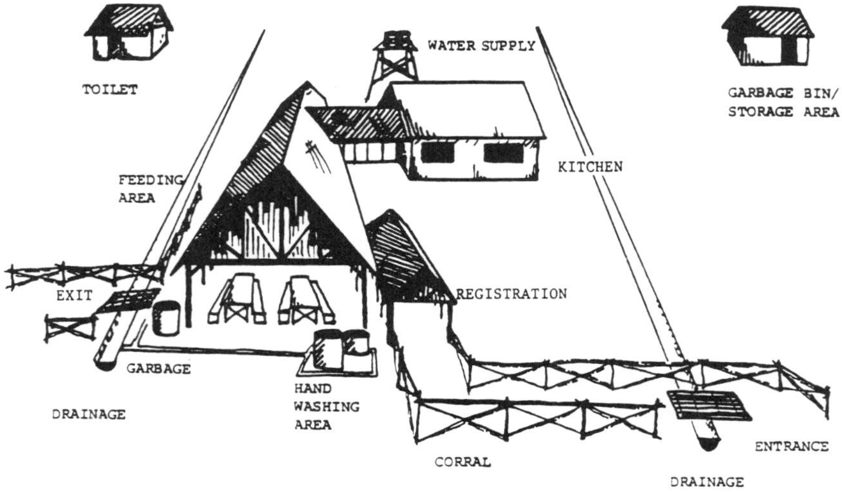

TOILET

WATER SUPPLY

GARBAGE BIN/ STORAGE AREA

FEEDING AREA

KITCHEN

EXIT

REGISTRATION

GARBAGE

HAND WASHING AREA

DRAINAGE

ENTRANCE

CORRAL

DRAINAGE

(Adapted from *Khmer food programme handbook*—WFP, 1980.)

Beneficiaries should, where possible, be required to bring their own cups/bowls/spoons each time. Where this is not possible, such utensils must be provided. Allow for many "disappearing".

Table 5/5

Utensils for an emergency SFP centre

Based on field experience, OXFAM supplies the following for an emergency centre to feed 250 children:

        1 cooking pot (100 litres) with lid
        1 cooking pot (50 litres) with lid
        2 wooden paddles for stirring food
    300 cups
    300 bowls
    100 teaspoons
        6 large spoons
        2 scoops
        2 measuring jugs
        2 ladles
        metal wisks
        2 tin openers
        1 scrubbing brush
        4 buckets with lids
        2 large jerry cans
    500 water sterilization tablets

Cleaning utensils, weighing scales, weight/height charts, MUAC tapes and reference books are also supplied: see ref. b. (The complete Oxfam kit (OFK2) costs about $825 excluding freight in 1985—$3.30/beneficiary.)

N.B. Empty 200 litre oil drums, cut in half and well cleaned have often made good, large pots. They may be available on the spot more quickly and cheaply than seeking "proper" pots.

Personnel

An organizer/manager should be appointed for each centre and given clear, written instructions concerning: storage of commodities—preparation and serving of meals—maintenance of hygiene—disposal of waste—registering beneficiaries—keeping records and preparing reports, etc.

Cooks and helpers should be found from within the community and given instructions in basic hygiene and the preparation of meals.

215

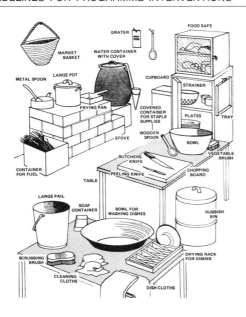

Figure 5/c
**Equipment for an
on-the-spot SFP centre**

for one preparing normal meals
for a small number of children

(Reproduced from ref. c)

All personnel should be strong and healthy. They should be medically screened at regular intervals. Noone with an infectious disease should be allowed to work in any centre.

Organization of feeding operations

Meals are served at fixed times each day which do not clash with normal family mealtimes or other important activities which mothers or older siblings may be involved in.

The best possible standards of hygiene are maintained. Cooks and other personnel should wash hands with soap, cover hair, avoid spitting, keep food and utensils covered when not in use.

Procedures ensure fair distribution and minimize the possibilities of cheating. See p. 211.

Sick children are coaxed to eat even if they have no appetite, are vomiting or have diarrhoea.

Beneficiaries do not take any food out of the centre. Siblings are discouraged from coming to the centre. Any food not eaten should be discarded into bins before beneficiaries leave the feeding eating area and be disposed of, e.g. as animal feed.

This is to ensure that those selected do in fact eat as much as they can of what is intended for them.

Food and meals

Meals should provide needed nutrients while being low in bulk. They should be:
- Based on local recipes to the extent possible;
- Palatable and acceptable, conforming to traditional local beliefs and practices;
- Prepared in ways to minimize nutrient losses; *and*
- Served hot, not reheated.

Type of meals is determined by what foods can be obtained and the facilities for preparation:
- In practice, meals are usually best prepared—initially—as porridges or thick soups which are easily digestible and suitable for all ages (based on cereals and legumes with edible oil added).
- If an SFP has to be continued for a long period, meals should be as similar as possible to normal family meals and weaning food be prepared separately for infants 5-12 months.

Table 5/6 shows some typical SFP rations based on a limited number of donated relief foods. More varied sample menus for preparing nutritious meals using items likely to be available locally and/or from donors are provided in the referenced publications. These should be adapted to local circumstances by field-experienced local nutritionists and instructions to cooks/demonstrators be issued in terms of local measures (see Table 3/4). Note that:
- Energy content of local recipes can often be increased by adding extra oil, or sugar. Protein (and vitamins) may be increased by extra legumes or adding small quantities of milk powder, fish meal, egg powder, etc.
- Fresh vegetables should be included whenever possible—available and affordable—to add vitamins (especially vitamin A from dark green leaves), flavour and variety.
- Small quantities of fresh, dried or canned fish or meat, and fruits should also be used whenever possible. Liver and orange/yellow fruits are also rich in vitamin-A.
- Vitamin-C content may be increased by sprouting (germinating) beans or, less satisfactorily, cereal grains *if* it is possible to maintain sufficient humidity under a glass/plastic enclosure.

Where such additions to the diet are not possible it will be necessary, in a long-running emergency, to seek donated commodities which are particularly rich/reinforced with the vitamins/minerals required.

217

Table 5/6

Composition of some typical SFP rations

Item	Daily ration			Quantity per month for 1,000 beneficiaries (metric tons)*
	Amount (g)	Energy (Kcal)	Protein (g)	
Maize meal porridge				
Maize meal	60	210	6	1.80
DSM	15	55	6	0.45
Oil	15	135	..	0.45
Sugar	5	20	..	0.15
Total	95	420	12	2.85

Plus 300 ml water: serving size approx. 400 ml.

CSM porridge				
CSM	55	210	11	1.65
Oil	10	90	..	0.30
Sugar	10	40	..	0.30
Total	75	340	11	2.25

Plus 220 ml water: serving size approx. 300 ml

WSB, rolled oats	100	360	20, 13	3.00

Milk drink (only if suitable cereals/blended foods are not obtainable)

DSM	40	140	14	1.20
Oil	10	90	..	0.30
Sugar	15	60	..	0.45
Total	65	290	14	1.95

Plus 330 ml water: serving size approx. 400 ml

The dry ingredients and oil are mixed first and a little cooled, boiled water stirred in to make a paste to which more water is then added before cooking (except the milk drink).

* The figures shown for tonnages required do *not* include any allowance for losses and wastage either in transportation or in feeding centres themselves. When planning requirements add 5 per cent or more: see p. 42.

Special biscuits may be useful initially in some circumstances: see p. 222. Milk drinks alone are of little value although requiring much effort in terms of the quantities of water to be boiled, then cooled, etc. If suitable cereal items are not obtainable, milk drinks may be considered *provided* oil and/or sugar is available to **218** increase the energy value.

Table 5/7

Blended foods

Corn-Soya-Milk (CSM), Wheat-Soy Blend (WSB) and other "blended" foods may be available through WFP or directly from some donors. They are nutritionally valuable, easy to transport and store, and can be very useful to initiate a supplementary feeding programme when appropriate local foods are lacking, *if*:

—They are available quickly; *and*

—The basic constituents of the blend are not unfamiliar to the local population.

Get a few bags and organize rapid acceptability trials before ordering/accepting large quantities of items which have not previously been used within the communities concerned.

Blended foods should be prepared and served in a manner as similar as possible to local dishes:

—They may usefully replace other cereals/flour in gruels, porridges, etc. and up to 40 per cent in bread.

—Used alone they are, in many countries, only palatable if sugar is added—but sugar is often not available or, if available, is expensive as well as difficult to store.

"Instant" varieties of such blends—e.g. ICSM—which are pre-cooked and need only to be mixed with clean water, can be very convenient, but are more expensive and less readily available than the raw blends.

Replace blends by locally familiar items as soon as feasible to increase the long-term educational benefit of the SFP.

Food preparation and cooking

Try to ensure that the loss of nutrients during preparation and cooking is minimized: see Table 5/8.

The availability of fuel (firewood) will often be a problem. Use fuel-efficient stoves if possible, also the fuel-less stove ("hay-box") method:

1. Boil the rice/soup etc. for a few minutes only;
2. Keeping lid tightly closed, remove the pot from the stove and immediately wrap it in straw, paper and/or blankets;
3. Leave it to sit for several hours.

Local cooks should experiment to determine actual cooking times needed for different recipes.

Table 5/8

Food handling procedures that reduce nutrient losses

Fresh fruit, vegetables, meat and fish are purchased daily.

No foods, except dry rations, are stored for more than a few days even in a refrigerator.

Liquid milk is kept covered and away from light.

Fresh vegetables are well washed, but not soaked, just before cooking. Beans are soaked in safe water.

Unnecessary slicing and peeling are avoided.

Leafy vegetables are placed in boiling liquid or gruel and cooked for the minimum time.

Soda is not used for cooking leafy vegetables.

Rice is washed only once or twice without rubbing.

Rice and vegetable water, and meat and fish juices, are used for stews, soups or as a drink.

Foods are cooked thoroughly, but are not overcooked.

Meals are eaten as soon as possible after preparation.

Reheating foods is avoided.

(Reproduced from ref. c)

Organizing a "take-home" SFP

Distributions must be made on a fixed schedule—normally weekly or fortnightly although perhaps at longer intervals for nomads—and at fixed locations where shelter and some temporary storage space is available. Drinking water should be available for beneficiaries.

Schedules and locations must be well publicized and carefully co-ordinated with those of any general food distributions. Corrals may be needed to facilitate orderly registration and distribution, see Figure 5/d.

Mothers collecting food for their young children should be required to bring those children with them to the distribution point each time, if possible. The children's condition can then be monitored on at least a spot-check basis.

Trained health workers should be present whenever possible to quickly identify any child (or mother) in need of medical treatment.

Figure 5/d
Possible arrangement for distribution of dry rations

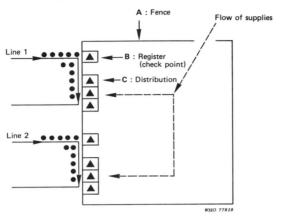

WHO 77818

A. Fence of mats, bamboo, wire, or rope depending on resources and needs. Narrowing aisles for line-ups might also be necessary.
B. Check point for cards. Sheltered by roof (or umbrella). The number of rations is called out clearly to distributors at C.
C. Distribution point. Several bags at a time can be emptied on to a tarpaulin for quicker distribution.

(Reproduced from ref. a)

Foods for "take-home" SFP distributions

Commodities must be ones which:
— Have high nutritional value;
— Carry and store easily; *and*
— Are easy to prepare/cook with the resources and facilities available to the recipients.

They should if possible be familiar to the population concerned, or at least be able to be prepared in a similar manner to local items, and have an acceptable taste. If the items are considered to be "children's food" they are less likely to be used for the family in general.

Rations should be determined on a basis similar to that for on-the-spot feeding, see Tables 5/2 and 5/3.

Milk powder should not be distributed as such. It has, however, successfully been pre-mixed with an appropriate cereal, e.g. rolled oats, before distribution, to be used in preparing porridges at home (e.g. in India in 1971).

221

Blended foods—see Table 5/7—can be very convenient provided they are locally acceptable, demonstrations are given beforehand to mothers on how to prepare them, and actual use at household level is monitored with further advice and demonstrations as necessary.

Special **biscuits** are available from some donors and can be useful to initiate supplementary feeding operations in situations where other commodities are not immediately available and cooking is difficult, but:

— Check the nutritional content: some are "high energy", others "high protein";

— Check the cost; *and*

— Get other foods (preferably locally familiar) as soon as feasible.

In some situations, biscuits have been produced locally—through contracts with bakeries—using wheat flour, CSM and DSM available within the emergency programme. This is also a way of using donated wheat flour which, in some countries, is not readily used in normal household cooking.

Using biscuits has no health/nutrition education value, but they may be more easily reserved for children than "normal" food items. Ask EOU for more information if required.

Possible UNICEF inputs

Depending on the assessemnt of actual needs and possibilities, some of the following inputs might be considered:

— Expertise: experienced feeding programme organizers and/or nutritionists to help plan and supervise the programme—possible finance for the participation of local nutrition institutes.

— Kitchen utensils (only if "on-the-spot"): see Figure 5/c and Table 5/5.

— Other equipment: hanging scales for infants—beam or bathroom scales for children/adults—weight-for-height charts—health/nutrition education materials

— Expendable supplies: soap and detergent—record ledgers and stationery.

— Food items, depending on the type of programme and unless/until WFP or others are able to supply.

— Operating costs. Financing as necessary for: local staff salaries and training—fuel for cooking and lighting—local purchases of expendables and food items—vehicle operating costs (for supply deliveries and supervision)—production, printing and distribution of programme instructions for centre personnel—health/nutrition education activities.

Further references

Practical guides:

a. *The management of nutritional emergencies in large populations*, C. de Ville de Goyet, J. Seaman & U. Geijer—WHO (1978)   E/F

b. *Oxfam's practical guide to selective feeding programmes*—OXFAM, Oxford (1984)   E

c. *Management of group feeding programmes*—FAO food and nutrition paper 23—FAO (1982)   E/F/S

Issues relating to supplementary feeding programmes:

d. *Supplementary feeding programmes for young children in developing countries*, G. Beaton & H. Ghassemi—report prepared for UNICEF and the ACC sub-committee on nutrition 1979, also published as supplement to *American Journal of Clinical Nutrition* vol. 35 No. 4 (1982)   E

ANNEX 6

THERAPEUTIC FEEDING
(NUTRITION REHABILITATION)

Objective

- **To save the lives and restore the nutritional health of severely malnourished children.**

Method and principles

Intensive special feeding is the essential treatment, but careful attention must also be given to correcting dehydration and controlling infections. Close medical supervision is essential.

At least 4—preferably 6—feeds must be given at regular intervals (every 2-3 hours) throughout the day and, if possible, one at night (especially for the most severe cases). Portions should be measured carefully each time to be sure that the child is taking sufficient food.

Feeds should be given slowly using a cup and spoon. In a few cases only, naso-gastric tube feeding may be needed initially (maximum 4 days), intra-venous drips as a last resort. Baby feeding bottles should *never* be used.

Recovery in all cases is best assured if the mother—or other mature relative—stays with the child all the time in a decentralized, community-level nutrition rehabilitation unit (NRU) or special Therapeutic Feeding Centre (TFC) and feeds the child under supervision. 3-5 weeks intensive feeding is typically required.

Often, especially with scattered populations, such residential treatment will not be feasible for many of those in need. If (a) facilities, personnel or other resources are not sufficient to provide residential care at community level for all severely malnourished children, or (b) mothers are unable/unwilling to reside at a TFC for 3-5 weeks due to other family responsibilities or other reasons:

—Children may be treated as out-patients being brought (by mothers) for feeding 5 times a day to a TFC; *or*
—Less satisfactorily, feeding might be given twice-a-day at a supplementary feeding programme (SFP) centre with special additional rations being given for feeding at home in between.

A TFC may provide both residential and outpatient treatment: e.g. facilities for 30 residents plus 70 outpatients.

Each TFC must be supervised by medically trained personnel (preferably be linked to an health clinic) and closely co-ordinated with a supplementary feeding programme to which every child discharged from the TFC is automatically admitted.

A balance must be maintained between TFC and other efforts to ensure that households have access to adequate quantities of appropriate foods (including any SFP activities). Inadequate attention to the latter may render any TFC efforts virtually useless!

Mobilize locally experienced medical-nutritionists at the outset to plan and organize any therapeutic feeding programme (TFP).

Planning a TFP—aspects to be defined

Needs and criteria

Obtain survey data and expert assessments. Thus estimate the numbers of severely malnourished children to be treated in particular areas and communities at the beginning of the programme and how the numbers are expected to evolve.

Decide the criteria and mechanisms to be used to identify the severely malnourished, and to enroll them in a particular treatment system appropriate to their needs and family possibilities (see p. 225)...

Resources/arrangements for providing treatment

Identify the organizational structures, premises, logistic facilities, and personnel through which therapeutic feeding might be organized:
  —Existing health units and PHC structures...
  —Other community services and facilities...
  —Womens groups and other organizations...

Thus determine the extent to which needs can be met in the various communities—taking into account population density and socio-cultural factors—by:
  —Increasing the capacity of existing community-level nutrition rehabilitation units (NRUs)...
  —Establishing additional such units within existing health centres/clinics...
  —Establishing special TFCs at community level...
  —Providing the necessary special foods and supervision at SFP centres...
[In practice, a combination of these mechanisms will often be necessary if treatment is to be accessible to all communities while facilities for intensive care are also available for the most severe cases.]

Define requirements for local contruction materials, equipment, utensils and other supplies to repair/expand any existing units and/or create new TFCs...

Determine whether any funds are already available and define the role and contribution the mothers and community in general...

Food and other supplies

Determine the types and quantities of suitable foods which are:
  —Able to be provided by the communities themselves...
  —Available from stocks held by government and others...
  —Available for purchase in local markets now and/or in the immediate future, and the prices...
  —Able to be delivered quickly by donors: when could they be delivered—what realistic ETAs?...

Thus decide:
  —From where the necessary milk, oil and sugar will be obtained...

226   —What other food items should be used to prepare semi-solid foods, what quantities will be required and from where they should be obtained (cf. weaning food and the SFP) . . .

Determine the quantities of drugs, cooking fuel and other supplies required, how and by whom they should be provided and transported . . .

Personnel

Define the types and numbers of personnel needed for each TFC—how and by whom they should be selected—what training should they be given, how, when and by whom—how, if at all, they should be remunerated (see p. 206): . . .

Supervision and reporting

Determine the type and number of personnel required to organize the setting up of TFCs and provide ongoing guidance and supervision:
  —Practical organizers . . .
  —Doctors, nurses and paramedical workers . . .

Determine what transport, equipment, facilities and funds they will need . . .

Define reporting arrangements—what reports should be submitted from each unit/TFC and to whom (see Figure 6/a): . . .

Overall plan and budget

See Annex 43

Admission and discharge arrangements

Criteria for admission

- **Clinically evident oedema or less than 70 per cent weight-for-height.**

If weight-for-height determinations are not immediately possible, admit those less than 75 per cent MUAC-for-height or MUAC less than 12.0 cm. See Annex 4.

The most severe cases (as judged by clinical examination) should receive residential care, at least initially, whenever possible.

227

Figure 6/a

Sample monthly report format for a TFC

Therapeutic Feeding Centre ....   Report for the month of: ....

Category	No. enrolled end last month a	New admissions this month b	Transfers to SFP: 80% wt/ht c	Drop-outs this month d	Deaths this month e	Total end this month =a+b−c−d−e	No. not gaining weight
Children 5–59 months { Less than 70% wt/ht (no oedema)..............							
With oedema..........							
Other children							
Medical referrals							
Totals							

	1	2	3	4	5	6	7	8	9	10	11	12	13	14	15	16	17	18	19	20	21	22	23	24	25	26	27	28	29	30	31
Number of children attending each day:																															

(Put slash / in boxes on days when SFP closed.)

Remarks

Signature:

(Adapted from ref. b)

Others should be enrolled as residents or out-patients depending on the avail-ability of facilities and the ability/willingess of mothers. A parent, or other responsible adult, should always agree (be persuaded) to allow the admission, and stay permanently with the child.

Any child with a communicable disease (e.g. confirmed TB or measles) should be kept and treated separately for the others to avoid cross-infection. New admissions should, if possible, be kept isolated from other residents for the first few days.

Criteria for discharge/transfer to SFP

- **No oedema, at least 80 per cent weight-for-height and gaining weight steadily.**

Patients should be clinically examined before being discharged from the therapeutic pro-gramme—transferred to the SFP. They should be active and free from infection.

Phasing out special TFCs

Special therapeutic feeding centres may be discontinued when the numbers of severely malnourished children has fallen to levels which can be adequately handled by regular health clinics and the ongoing SFP.

Establishing special TFCs

Special, temporary TFCs can be set up in schools, community centres, in impro-vised shelters or tents. 100 patients is a practical maximum for any one unit/TFC in order to assure adequate supervision and limit the danger of infections.

Community participation is essential. Involve mothers and community leaders. They must understand the objectives and methods of the programme and take as much responsibility as possible for running it. Involve traditional birth attendants and PHC workers.

Facilities required

The following will be required:
— A weather-proof shelter, sleeping mats and blankets adequate for the number of patients and the accompanying adults;

229

—Separate kitchen and latrines;
—A secure store for food, equipment and drugs;
—Sufficient clean water (ideally 20 litres/day/patient);
—Assured supplies of cooking fuel; *and*
—Night lighting.

Where feasible, space for the production of vegetables and keeping poultry, etc. can enable some of the TFC's own food requirements to be met by local efforts, particularly those of the patients' mothers, and also enhance the educational benefit of the operation.

Personnel

Each unit/TFC should be managed by an experienced public health nurse, paediatric nurse or medical intern. An additional nursing aide and two auxilliaries to train mothers and supervise actual feeding may be required for every 30 children under treatment. Other helpers will be needed for the kitchen, etc. Each should be given specific tasks/responsibilities. See Annex 5, p. 206 regarding remuneration.

A doctor or experienced public health nurse might supervise up to 10 TFCs if travelling distances are short.

Training

Provide written guidelines in an appropriate language and organize rapid orientation training for *all* personnel involved. Many doctors and nurses have little training in nutrition or in treating severe malnutrition.

If medical supervision will in fact be infrequent, train TFC workers to recognize and react to conditions which are likely to arise and could quickly prove fatal: e.g. fever, dehydration and hypothermia/hypoglycaemia.

Equipment and medical supplies

Table 6/1 suggests the utensils and other items which might be required to a TFC serving 100 severely malnourished children.

A limited number of non-expendable medical supplies will be needed in each TFC. Necessary drugs should normally be delivered from the responsible health centre/team.

Table 6/1

Feeding equipment for a TFC serving 100 severely malnourished children

Items provided by OXFAM on the basis of field experience. Nearest UNIPAC equivalent listed alongside.

2	Large cooking pots (50 litres) with lids	20-390-00
2	Wooden paddles for stirring food	
120	Cups	20-690-00
120	Bowls	20-514-00
300	Teaspoons (50 metal; 250 plastic)	20-867-00
2	Measuring jugs (2 litres)	02-610-00 + 20-225-00
2	Scoops	
2	Ladles	20-655-00
2	Whisks	
1	Food scale	05-500-00
1	Alarm clock	46-210-00
1	Scrubbing brush	
2	Large plastic jerry cans	50-071-00
4	Buckets with lids	02-638-00
2	Hurricane lamps	50-280-00
12	Candles with matches	
1	Torch + 4 batteries	06-300-00 + 18-022-12
500	Water purifying tablets	15-522-02
50	Naso-gastric tubes	03-730-00 + 03-735-00
5	Syringes	07-856-74
	Adhesive tape	05-010-50

Equipment for weighing and measuring children is also provided, including: hanging scales—weight-for-height charts—height stick—length board—tape measures—arm circumference tapes—stationery—pocket calculator. See also Annex 4.

Other items included are:plastic identity bracelets for identifying individual patients— medical record cards—"milk cards" to display the quantity of food each child should receive at each feed. See ref.c. The Oxfam kit (OFK3) costs about $600 excluding freight in 1985—$6/patient.

Measles vaccination should, if at all possible, be given to all children over 9 months before or within 2 days of admission—unless they are known to have just had the disease or to have been properly vaccinated already.

Vitamin-A injections or capsules should be given immediately to any children showing clear symptoms of the deficiency, and capsules to all others in areas where the deficiency is prevalent.

Ferrous sulphate and folate tablets should normally be given daily for at least 2 weeks to all except infants still also being breast-fed—whose mothers should receive instead.

Other drug needs should be covered by items in the WHO Emergency Health Kit, with the possible addition of anti-TB drugs *if* continuity of treatment can be assured.   **231**

Food and feeding procedures

Foods

K-Mix-II and oil can be useful to commence treatment (first 2-3 days after any necessary initial rehydration) and may also be needed in rare cases of lactose intolerance. Otherwise dried skim milk (DSM), sugar and oil make an adequate

Table 6/2

Preparation of feeding mixtures

K-Mix-II (UNIPAC 15-555-00)

Mix 100 gm K-Mix-II with 60 gm oil (stir well!), then make up to 1 litre by stirring in warm boiled water.

If weighing scales not available, measure by volume: 6 parts K-Mix-II with 2 parts oil and 23 parts water.

100 ml of the mix provides approximately 90 kcal and 3 g protein. 1 carton (20 kg) of K-Mix-II (plus 12 kg oil) is, on average, sufficient for each of 40 children for 3 days.

K-Mix-II is a specially formulated mixture of calcium caseinate, DSM and sucrose. Vegetable oil can be obtained from UNIPAC (15-550-20) but is often available locally from WFP or other sources.

"High energy milk"

Mix 420 gm DSM, 250 g sugar and 320 gm oil to make 1 kg of "premix". Stir in 4.4 litres of cold boiled water to make 5 litres (approximately 5 kg) of "HEM".

If weighing scales are not available, measure by volume: 10 parts DSM, 3 parts sugar plus 4 parts oil for the premix. 2 parts of freshly stirred premix plus 9 parts cooled boiled water for the prepared HEM.

For children with frequent diarrhoea or loosing oedema, 5.2 gm potassium chloride and 2.4 gm magnesium hydroxide should be added to each kg of premix. Alternatively, less satisfactorily, ORS may be given separately.

100 ml of HEM provides approximately 96 kcal and 3 g protein. 78 kg DSM plus 47 kg sugar and 55 kg oil makes sufficient "HEM" to feed, on average, 100 children for 1 week.

The premix can be kept for at least a week in clean, covered containers. Once made-up, the HEM must be used quickly.

and cheaper *"high energy milk"*. The oil must *never* be omitted. See Table 6/2 concerning the preparation of feeding mixtures.

Items as used in the weaning/supplementary feeding programme are required to prepare porridges to be introduced gradually once nutritional improvement starts (after 4-5 days for most patients) except for infants below 5 months. ICSM is excellent for this.

For all infants, breast-feeding should be continued in addition to the special food mixtures. The mothers' lactation must be re-established if necessary.

Feeding should initially provide provide about 100 kcal per kg of body weight per day using half-strength mixtures (i.e. 100 ml of the mixture diluted with a further 100 ml of water per kg body weight per day). This should be increased quickly to 150-200 kcal plus 3-4 g protein per kg per day (i.e. 150-200 ml of the full strength mixture per kg body weight per day).

In cases of extreme dehydration, rehydration with I-V fluids then ORS may be necessary for the first day before feeding starts.

Feeding arrangements

The gap between night and morning feeds must be kept to a minimum to reduce the risk of potentially fatal hypothermia or hypoglaecemia.

Unless refrigeration is available, food should be freshly prepared each time and prepared food not be stored for more than 2 hours.

The best possible standards of hygiene must be assured—hands well washed, utensils boiled before/after use and kept covered.

Children may have to be patiently coaxed to take food, and effort be devoted to overcoming initial distrust of families towards feeding methods which differ from traditional practices. Diarrhoea is common in the first few days, but feeding must be continued. Additional ORS drinks may be given.

Other practical aspects of TFC operations

Warmth

Patients must be kept warm, especially at night. They should sleep close to their mothers and blankets be provided even in apparently warm climates. (Metal foil and paper food sacks can also be used to wrap children.)

Records, monitoring and follow-up

Requirements are:
- —A TFC register with details of each child patient; and
- —Separate, individual record cards for each child recording: weight (every day or two)—the volume of feed to be given each meal and the volume actually consumed—drugs prescribed.

Weighing should be daily at first, twice-a-week later. If oedema is present, weight should actually be lost in the first few days as it is eliminated. Apart from this, weight gains of up to 10 g/day for each kg of body weight should be achieved.

Any child not able to take the prescribed quantities of feed and/or not gaining weight must be quickly referred to a medical officer.

TFC staff and members of the community should investigate (through home visits) cases of absenteeism to determine reasons and try to persuade/enable families to resume treatment of the child. Absentees may include:
- —In-patients who discharge themselves and do not return within 2-3 days.
- —Out-patients who stop attending.

Food for attendants

Attendants must not share the special, measured feeds provided for the patient!

Normally the mother or other adult staying with a child—and any siblings who cannot be left at home—should arrange to feed themselves. Meals may be sent from home, or food which the mothers present prepare collectively. In some cases food may have to be provided for the attendants also.

Possible UNICEF inputs

Depending on the assessment of actual needs and possibilities, some of the following inputs might be considered:
- —Expertise: experienced nutritionists and feeding programme organizers to plan and supervise the programme—finance to enable the participation of local nutrition institutes.

—Feeding equipment: see Table 6/1.

—Weighing/measuring equipment: see Annex 4.

—Other equipment: sleeping mats (including a few spares)—blankets (initial supply 2-3 per bed)

—Expendables: soap and detergent—disinfectant—growth charts—record ledgers and stationery.

—Food items: K-Mix-II (UNIPAC 15-550-00) and, unless/until WFP or others are able to supply: DSM (dry skim milk, vitamin-A fortified)—edible oil—sugar—cereal-based blended foods.

—Medicaments etc.

—Operating costs: financing as necessary for local staff salaries and training—fuel for cooking and lighting—local purchases of expendables and food items—vehicle operating costs (for supply deliveries and supervision)—production, printing and distribution of programme instructions for centre personnel.

Further references

a. *The management of nutritional emergencies in large populations*, C. de Ville de Goyet, J. Seaman and U. Geijer—WHO (1978) E/F

b. *The treatment and management of severe protein-energy malnutrition*—WHO (1981) E/F

c. *Oxfam's practical guide to selective feeding programmes*—OXFAM, Oxford (1984) E

MALNUTRITION, NUTRIENT REQUIREMENTS AND SOURCES*

Protein-energy malnutrition (PEM)

PEM results from low intake or poor absorption of food, usually due to inadequate availability or infection. It particularly affects children between 6 months and 5 years of age, especially at the time of weaning, and takes one of three forms:

Nutritional marasmus

The most frequent form of PEM in situations of long-term food shortage, resulting from prolonged inadequate food intake. Weight is lost, fat and muscle waste away:

— The child becomes very thin, may have sunken eyes, an "old man" face and loose folds of skin especially on the buttocks (like "baggy pants").
— The child may, however, appear relatively active and alert. See Figure 7/a.

---

* These notes and tables provide only a very brief summary. See referenced publications for details.

Kwashiorkor

Seen most commonly among infants recently taken off the mother's breast and in areas where tubers and roots (e.g. cassava) are the main staple foods, the main sign is *oedema*:

—Swelling of the feet and lower legs which may extend in advanced cases to the arms and face. Where there is gross oedema, the child may look "fat" and be regarded by parents as being well-fed.

Other signs, which do not always occur, include:

—Hair changes: colour becomes lighter—curly hair becomes straight—hair comes out easily with a gentle pull; and

—Skin changes: skin may become lighter in places—skin may peel off especially on the legs—ulceration may occur. See Figure 7/b.

Children with kwashiorkor are usually apathetic, miserable and withdrawn, and often refuse to eat. Profound anaemia is a common complication of kwashiorkor.

To check for oedema: Press with thumb or finger for 3 seconds on the top of the foot near the ankle. If a definite pit remains after the finger is removed, oedema is present. (Note: Oedema can also occur in other diseases.)

Marasmic-kwashiorkor

A common combination of the above two conditions. The child appears thin and wasted but with swollen lower limbs.

Vitamin and mineral deficiencies

Table 7/1 lists some of the deficiencies commonly encountered in situations of food shortage.

Acute deficiencies in individuals must be treated by providing concentrated doses of the particular vitamin/mineral.

If clinical signs of deficiencies are already widespread, or if evaluation of dietary intake indicates specific deficiencies:

—Try to improve the diet by including foods rich in the missing nutrients— especially by increasing, to the extent possible, the consumption of fresh vegetables and minimally processed cereals.

237

Figure 7/a

Child with marasmus

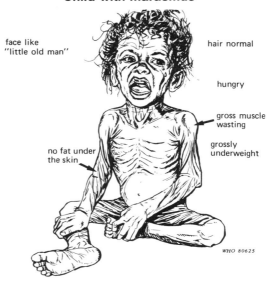

face like "little old man"

hair normal

hungry

gross muscle wasting

grossly underweight

no fat under the skin

WHO 80625

Figure 7/b

Child with kwashiorkor

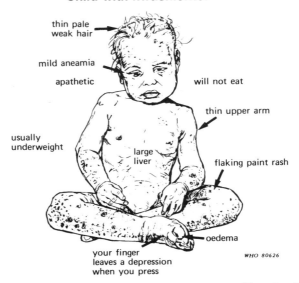

thin pale weak hair

mild aneamia

apathetic

will not eat

thin upper arm

usually underweight

large liver

flaking paint rash

oedema

your finger leaves a depression when you press

WHO 80626

(Reproduced from ref. d.)

—If diets cannot be improved sufficiently quickly, large-scale administration of the specific vitamin may be required.

Table 7/2 summarizes action in respect of vitamin-A deficiency.

The distribution of multi-vitamin tablets is usually a waste of time and money. Most contain only a small quantity of individual vitamins and may create a false sense of security.

Nutrient requirements

Indications of the energy and protein requirements of various categories of individual are provided in Table 7/4. The nature of the basic nutrients is summarized in Table 7/3.

In emergencies, food needs and provisions should be considered in a series of priorities/phases of increasing refinement:

1. Initially focus on ensuring sufficient dietary energy (kcal) for survival and maintenance.
2. Then assure the necessary general protein content.
3. Finally, try to assure appropriate intakes of particular amino-acids, vitamins and minerals.

Table 7/1

Likely vitamin/mineral deficiencies

Anaemia: caused by parasitic infections, low intake and/or poor absorption of iron and folic acid. Tongue, finger nails and inside of lower eyelids appear unusually pale.

Vitamin-A deficiency (xerophthalmia). Signs are poor vision in the dark, dryness or foamy material on the white of the eye and/or clouding of the cornea (the dark of the eye).

Vitamin-B1 deficiency (beri-beri). Loss of appetite, malaise and severe weakness expecially in the legs. May also lead to paralysis of the limbs or swelling of the body, heart failure and sudden death. Occurs when diet consists almost exclusively of white polished rice or starchy staples such as cassava.

Niacin deficiency (pellagra). Skin rash on parts of body exposed to sunlight. Occurs especially where maize and sorghum are the staples and other foods are lacking.

Vitamin-C deficiency (scurvy). Swollen gums which bleed easily; swollen painful joints. Occurs when fruits and vegetables are lacking.

For initial planning purposes in the absence of detailed demographic data:

— For short-term survival, 1,750 kcal may be taken as the average daily energy requirement for each individual over 10 years, and 1,250 kcal the average for each child under 10 years.

— For maintenance, average figures might be 2,100 kcal/day for individuals over 10 years and 1,500 kcal/day for children under 10.

Of these amounts, some 160 kcal should be in the form of protein (i.e. about 40 g protein).

Populations who are *already* malnourished will initially require more than the normal, average "required daily allowances" shown in Table 7/4 if their condition is to be restored and their children "catch-up" on lost growth. It is difficult to make precise recommendations concerning the increase required but 15% (i.e. multiplying the requirements shown by 1.15) may often be appropriate. The increased allowances should be maintained until the nutritional status improves.

Table 7/2

Prevention and treatment of vitamin-A deficiency

Prevention:
- Inclusion of dark green leafy vegetables, yellow fruits and vegetables, eggs, small dried fish and/or palm oil in the daily diets of all young children.

Treatment:
In all stages of active xerophthalmia, including night blindness and/or when changes can be seen in the eye itself:
- *Immediately:* one 200,000 IU capsule orally (UNIPAC 15-830-00/05 or equivalent) for children 1-6 years. Half the dose (100,000 IU) for infants below 12 months or children less than 8 kg.
- *The next day:* the same dose again.
- *1-4 weeks later:* the same dose yet again.

In the presence of persistent vomiting or very severe diarrhoea, a water-miscible injectable form of vitamin A (100,000 IU) may be substituted for the first dose. (Syringes and needles must be sterile.)

In cases where changes can be seen in the dark of the eye (corneal lesions), the patient should be referred, where possible, to a hospital, but without delaying initiation of the above treatment. Children with severe protein-energy malnutrition *and* xerophthalmia must be carefully monitored, and may require additional doses.

Chemoprophylaxis:
The occurrence of nightblindness in 1% of children 6 months-6 years—or of Bitot spots in 0.5%—indicates a public health problem justifying prophylactic distribution of vitamin-A:
- One capsule or equivalent for each child 1-6 years every 3-6 months. Half the dose to infants 6-12 months or children less than 8 kg.
- One capsule (once only) to women at the time of delivery or within 2 months of giving birth.

In communities in which vitamin A deficiency is a recognized problem (or the fatality rate of measles 1% or higher), all children diagnosed with *measles* should immediately be given the dose indicated above.

Food commodities and diets

A typical full daily emergency ration comprises:
  350-400 g of a staple (cereal)
  20-40 g of an energy-rich food (oil/fat)
  50 g of a protein-rich food (legumes)
Vegetables and other items (particularly to meet vitamin and mineral needs) should be added according to nutritional need, availability and custom. If the staple is a root crop, larger quantities of the other items are needed.

Table 7/5 indicates the energy and protein content of some common food items. The referenced publications provide further details and suggestions for various diets using items likely to be available and acceptable in various countries.

Not less than 20 per cent (but not more than 40 per cent) of the energy requirement should ideally be supplied from fats and oils. This greatly enhances the palatability of the diet and increases the energy density, and is particularly important for young children. Ideally, 10-15 per cent of protein should be of animal origin.

Table 7/3

Basic types of nutrients

All foods are made up of five basic types of nutrient in addition to variable amounts of water:

Carbohydrates are a source of energy, typically providing about 4 kcal/g. They are mostly starches and sugars of vegetable origin, and constitute the major component of cereals and tubers.

Fats and oils are the most concentrated sources of energy, some 9 kcal/g.

Proteins are body-building substances required for growth and tissue repair. They are found in varying quantities in foods of animal origin, in legumes and, to a lesser extent, in cereals. They also provide energy—about 4 kcal/g.

Requirements are usually specified in terms of "reference protein", equivalent to that of milk and eggs. The real value of the protein in any meal—the quantity actually absorbed—is obtained by adjusting (reducing) the nominal protein content of the constituent food items for "digestability" and "quality" which itself depends on the particular mix of amino acids in the meal.

A variety of **vitamins and minerals** are needed in small quantities for the adequate functioning of the body. Individual vitamins and minerals or combinations are found in all foods in very variable amounts.

Table 7/4

Average daily energy and protein requirements of individuals – planning guidelines

	Energy (kcal/day)[a]			Protein (g/day)[b]		Approximate proportions of a typical population[c]
	Recommended normal	Temporary maintenance	Emergency subsistence	Reference milk/egg	Mixed sources	
Infants 4-12 mths	110/kg body weight (average 820)			2/kg body weight (ave. 14)		3%
Children 1-3 years	1 250	1 200	1 100	15	18	9%
Children 4-6 years	1 750	1 600	1 300	20	24	9%
Children 7-9 years	2 000	1 800	1 500	27	32	8%
Children over 10 yrs and adults[d]	2 800	2 000	1 700	37-50	44-60	71%
Additional requirements for:						
Pregnant women	+250	+250	+250	+6	+7	1.5%
Lactating women	+500	+500	+500	+17	+20	1.5%

a Energy is sometimes expressed in "megajoules": 1 MJ = 239 kcals.

b The first column applies if the diet contains "high quality" proteins—a mixed diet including some animal protein. The second indicates the *minimum* quantities required if there is much fibre in the diet and protein is largely provided from cereals with some legumes (see Table 7/3).

c Figures indicate the rough proportions of the specified groups within the total population of a typical developing country. Specific estimates should be obtained for the proportions within the target population for any particular food programme. Actual proportions may be very different, especially among groups of displaced persons.

d Figures for energy requirements are averages for individuals who are sedentary or doing only light work. For individuals engaged in heavy work requirements may be 3000-3500 kcals/day. Protein requirements depend on body weight.

N.B.

(1) The above figures are only general planning guidelines. It is impossible to give exact figures in relation to individual requirements. People already malnourished need more than the amounts indicated above.

(2) Different requirements are frequently specified for boys and girls, men and women. Such differences are probably of little relevance for planning requirements in emergencies. The figures reflect the recommendations of the latest, 1981 joint FAO/WHO/UNU expert consultation. Some of the figures given for normal energy and protein requirements differ from earlier recommendations.

(Adapted from refs. a and d)

Table 7/5

Energy and protein content of some food items

Approximate values of nutrients provided by 100gms of the dry foods

Commodity	Energy (kcals)	Protein (g)	Notes
Cereals			Main source of energy and proteins in
Maize/maize meal	360	10	most diets. Milling reduces vit-
Rice	360	7	amins
Rolled oats	370	13	
Wheat, sorghum	330	13, 11	Sorghum lacks vitamin B
Roots/tubers			Very little protein; some vitamins and
Cassava fresh	149	1	minerals
Cassava flour	342	1	
Potato, yam	80-120	2	
Legumes/pulses			Useful sources of protein, some vita-
Dried beans/lentils	335	22	mins and minerals
Groundnuts, dry	549	23	
Soybeans	405	34	
Butter/Vegetable oil	850-900	—	Important concentrated source of energy: butter oil must be melted
Milk			
Whole cows milk	79	1	Must always be boiled before use
Dried whole milk	490	23	
Dried skim milk	360	36	See Table 3/2, p. 179
Fresh vegetables	20-30	1-5	Important sources of vitamins and mi-
Fruits	20-100	1	nerals: see also Table 5/8, p. 220
Fresh hens' eggs	140	12	
Meat/fish			Proteins readily utilized by body:
Pork (medium fat)	535	10	small quantities useful to improve
Goat (medium fat)	350	15	quality and palatability of diet.
Beef, mutton (med. fat.)	240	18, 15	
Chicken	139	19	
Fish, fresh	120	22	
Dried fish	300-380	63-66	
Fish protein concentrate (FPC)	330-390	75-82	Acceptability tests essential: can be added to soups/gruels in only very small quantities, if at all
Egg powder (dried)	575	45	
Blended foods			Valuable for SFPs when local foods
CSM/ICSM, WSB	380, 360	20	lacking: see Table 5/7, p. 219.
Soy-fortified bulgur	350	17	
Sugar	400	—	Difficult to store: gets wet quickly from humidity in air

243

(Extracted from ref. c)

Protein requirements

The large-scale use of specially formulated "high-protein" foods is very rarely justified. Most normal, mixed diets—of which sufficient is eaten to provide adequate energy—will also provide sufficient protein. A mixture of different foods is particularly important for children, and helps to ensure good absorption of protein.

Even a growing child, if heathly, requires no more than 10 per cent of total energy intake to be supplied in the form of protein. If energy intake is inadequate, protein will be burnt to provide energy—it will be used in the same way as carbohydrate or fat (which are usually much less expensive), not for growth and repair.

Further references

a. *Energy and protein requirements*, WHO Technical Reference Series 724-WHO (1985)   E/F/S

b. *Guide to food and health relief operations for disasters*, Protein-Calorie Advisory Group—UN (1977)   E/F/S

c. *Management of group feeding programmes*, FAO food and nutrition paper 23—FAO (1982)   E/F/S

d. *The management of nutritional emergencies in large populations*, C. de Ville de Goyet, J. Seaman & U. Geijer—WHO (1978)   E/F

e. *Manual on feeding infants and young children*, 3rd edition, M. Cameron & Y. Hofvander—Oxford University Press (1983)   E
(2nd edition, UN Protein Advisory Group, 1976, E/F/S)

f. *Control of vitamin-A deficiency and xerophthalmia*, WHO Technical Reference Series 672—WHO (1982)   E/F

ANNEX 8

MANAGEMENT AND STAFFING OF EMERGENCY HEALTH SERVICES

Objective

- To ensure the efficient organization and delivery of essential emergency health care at community level in the context of sustainable long-term services.

Overall management

Good organization—of both field services and supply operations—is the key to effective and efficient health care in emergencies. In a major emergency a (full-time) Co-ordinator for emergency health services should be designated by the government with appropriate authority and necessary administrative support.

Particular attention should be given to:
— Mobilizing and (re)assigning available medical and paramedical personnel— including any outside medical teams—according to priority needs.

— Redistributing and ensuring the controlled use of available stocks of drugs and other medical supplies. Ordering and receiving additional supplies (including control and co-ordination of donations).

— Establishing budgets for all aspects of health care operations, and ensuring the availability of operating funds to all field units.

— Systematically collecting and analysing data on the incidence of diseases (epidemiological surveillance) and ensuring prompt and appropriate reactions to any reports of outbreaks.

— Co-ordinating with other related operations—food, water supply, etc.

— Providing written guidelines to all personnel and teams engaged in health-related activities.

Guidelines should be in a language and style appropriate for the intended users and specify: standard treatment schedules to be applied using a limited number of essential drugs—what vaccination activities to undertake and how—how to requisition and take delivery of supplies—what reports to submit, and how.

Medical and paramedical personnel

Existing, trained health service personnel, community health workers and traditional birth attendants (TBAs) should be supported to provide necessary services to their communities. If, in a major disaster, the situation requires temporary special (additional) arrangements, these existing personnel must be fully involved and integrated in the operation.

Special medical teams sent to disaster areas should in general be small, mobile and very adaptable. In only a few instances will highly specialized teams be needed. Previous field experience and personal qualities are usually more important than advanced training and knowledge.

National personnel are to be preferred to expatriates—especially ones who do not speak the local language. (It has been recommended that any expatriate personnel should be ready to stay a minimum of 3 months in the field if they have relevant previous experience, 6 months if not.)

Adequate numbers of community health workers are essential to provide basic (primary) health care within all communities, and sufficient paramedical and auxilliary workers to ensure efficient use of the more highly trained medical personnel. Pharmacists and laboratory technicians will be needed to support curative services and the operations of medical teams.

Wherever there are major health problems or large population displacements, new health workers should be recruited from within the community and given rapid, initial training followed by regular supervision and in-service training:

— Carefully select candidates (from all sections and age-groups of the population if possible): ensure that they are accepted by the community—see also Table 27/2, p. 390;

— Establish clear policies for the remuneration of workers—see also Annex 5, p. 206.

— Prepare the training syllabus, methods and materials appropriate to the particular health problems being faced and the background of the trainees; *and*

— Give special attention to the selection and training of the trainers: involve existing trained nurses and other community workers.

The work—and therefore the training—of community health workers should normally focus on:

— Practical ways of improving hygiene and sanitation in the community including: preventing contamination of water supplies—sanitary disposal of excreta—arrangements for personal and food hygiene;

— Identifying malnourished children, arranging their enrolment in special feeding programmes, ensuring their attendance and advising/helping mothers to prepare weaning and supplementary foods;

— Immunization of children: registering children—organizing the community for vaccination sessions;

— Promoting home-based oral rehydration therapy for children suffering diarrhoea and ensuring treatment with ORS for cases of dehydration (see Annex 15);

— Bringing sick people and pregnant women to appropriate clinics, and ensuring assistance to women at child birth and with post-natal follow up wherever feasible.

Wherever health infrastructure is not extensive, promote the further training of village-level workers in the diagnosis and management of common disorders (e.g. dehydration, respiratory diseases, malaria, as well as the treatment of minor injuries). Provide them with simple, written guidelines.

Possible UNICEF inputs

Depending on the assessment of actual needs and possibilities, some of the following inputs might be considered:

— Funding for additional (preferably national) personnel to be mobilized for central and field level co-ordination and supervision of emergency health operations.

—Funding for the operation of special (national) medical teams, where needed, and the participation (travel costs, etc.) of appropriate personnel from national institutions who may not otherwise be able to be mobilized.

—Consultant missions to assist in assessments and the planning of rehabilitation assistance in areas of particular concern to UNICEF, e.g. paediatric care, MCH services, EPI programmes.

—Funding for the training of new paramedical and village health workers, including the preparation and production of training materials and guidelines.

—Materials, equipment, supplies and, possibly, some local costs to re-establish (in the rehabilitation phase) long-term training programmes for community health workers, nurses, midwives and paramedical workers.

Only in very exceptional circumstances does UNICEF provide or sponsor medical teams or individual medical field workers. The organizations of the Red Cross and Red Crescent and established voluntary agencies are normally able—and experienced—to provide and administer such teams/personnel when they are required. WHO may advise and assist the relevant authorities in overall management and co-ordination

Further references

Concerning health management in emergencies:

a. *Emergency health management after natural disaster*, PAHO scientific publication No. 407—PAHO (1981) E/S

b. *A guide to food and health relief operations for disasters*, Protein-Calorie advisory group—UN (1977) E/F/S

c. *Environmental health management after natural disaster*, PAHO scientific publication No. 430—PAHO (1982) E/S

Concerning health care in general in emergencies:

d. *Refugee community health care*, S. Simmonds, P. Vaughan & S. W. Gunn—Oxford University Press (1983) E

e. *Epidemiology of acute disasters*, J. Seaman—Kroger, Basel (1984) E

f. *Medical care in refugee camps*, Disasters, vol. 5 No. 3—International Disaster Institute, London (1981)

g. *Oxfam's practical guide to refugee health care*—OXFAM, Oxford (1983) E

h. *Assessment and surveillance of health problems: refugee populations*—Communicable Disease Centre, US Public Health Service (1983) E

Important basic health care references:

i. *Where there is no doctor*, D. Werner—MacMillan (1980) E/F/A

j. *Primary child care: Book 1—a manual for health workers*, M. & F. King, S. Martodipoero—Oxford University Press/WHO (1981) E

k. *Control of communicable diseases in man*, 14th edition, A. S. Benenson—American Public Health Association (1985) E

HEALTH FACILITIES AND EQUIPMENT

Objective

- **To ensure the restoration/provision of facilities and equipment essential for the delivery of basic health care services at community level.**

Premises

Where facilities (dispensaries, health centres, hospitals) have been damaged:

— Rapid provision of plastic sheeting/tarpaulins, locally available construction materials and/or limited funds should enable at least initial, temporary repairs to be made so that essential services can be continued/resumed.

— Detailed surveys and the preparation of quantity and cost estimates for any major reconstruction work (including of training institutions) should be undertaken later—but as soon as practicable—in order to plan and budget for the rehabilitation phase.

In cases of displaced populations:
- —Existing facilities in the area may need to be expanded, at least temporarily; *and/or*
- —New clinics be established from scratch.

Depending on local circumstances it may be appropriate to envisage a clinic for every 5-10,000 people plus a health centre for each main population concentration.

Tents may initially be necessary in a few situations where no premises exist but, where traditional structures can be erected quickly using locally available materials, this is generally a better solution. See also Annex 24.

Equipment

Where much equipment has been lost:
- —Provide standard sets of the most essential items for each type of unit as quickly as possible. (Take account of equipment which medical teams might be bringing with them).
- —Plan carefully, for the rehabilitation phase, any necessary re-equiping of larger institutions (including training units).

Ensure that provisions are appropriate to the levels of staffing and expertise which is and will, in the long term, be available at the various centres.

The WHO Emergency Health Kit list C (see Annex 11) suggests what might be appropriate to establish a clinic, including basic laboratory facilities, to serve a community of 10,000 persons. These kits are now being included in the UNIPAC emergency stockpile. Other standard UNIPAC kits may also be appropriate in rehabilitation operations, especially the midwifery, MCH-centre and public health nurse kits.

Emergency field hospitals are often offered by donors but are only rarely useful—although being very expensive especially when transported by air. They often arrive too late to be used in the first, casualty management phase, and contain many items which are not required for ongoing health care.

Vehicles

Where vehicles essential for mobile ("outreach") services have been lost or damaged, or services have to be developed/extended in new areas:

—Repair or, if necessary, replace vehicles to enable services to continue/be resumed;

—Ensure necessary supplies of fuel and lubricants; *and*

—Ensure arrangements/facilities for ongoing maintenance.

See also Annex 48 and Annex 33, pp. 437-8.

Possible UNICEF inputs

Depending on the assessment of actual needs and possibilities, some of the following inputs might be considered:

—Plastic sheeting, tarpaulins, large tents, locally available repair materials, funds—in the early phases.

—Other reconstruction materials (possibly including electric and water fittings) in the rehabilitation phase.

—Sets of basic equipment for clinics/dispensaries, MCH centres, hospitals, by diversion of stocks on hand or en route for regular programmes, local purchases or air deliveries from UNIPAC.

—Specific items for special units and training institutes in the rehabilitation phase.

—Spare parts/funds for the repair of damaged vehicles. Replacement vehicles where necessary.

During the first phase, any deliveries (especially by air) should normally be restricted to those items without which the necessary minimum level of service cannot be provided. Additional equipment might be provided later.

UNICEF inputs should normally be focused on the needs of the lower-level health care delivery facilities (dispensaries and health centres). Any equipment for hospitals should be for paediatric and maternity wards, outpatient and laboratory services.

ANNEX 10

DRUGS AND ESSENTIAL SUPPLIES

Objective

- **To ensure the availability of necessary essential drugs and other expendable supplies for community level health services, taking account of appropriate distribution policies and production possibilities.**

Delivering essential items

Immediate needs for drugs, dressings, soap, disinfectant, etc., will always have to be met from stocks already in-country held by the Ministry of Health, other agencies, producers and traders.

Additional inputs—to replenish government and agency stocks and to support the continuing emergency efforts—should, during the *initial* period, be restricted to:

—Items in the WHO Emergency Health Kit lists A and B (see Annex 11, p. 265); *and, where appropriate*

—Specific drugs needed for the continuation of pre-existing long-term treatment regimes (TB, leprosy).

Where there are virtually no stocks on hand and/or whenever the capacity to receive, sort and repack drugs is limited:

—Deliver drugs in *set-packed* kits ready for immediate distribution to user units;

—Quantities in each kit should be appropriate to the size of population served by the average medical team/health post.

Consider delivering drugs in bulk—or accepting donations of bulk-packed drugs—*only* where central pharmaceutical stores are well organized and operating efficiently.

The WHO Emergency Health Kit lists A and B suggest the types and quantities of essential drugs which might be appropriate initially, in most circumstances, to serve a population of 10,000 persons for 3 months. These kits are being included in the UNIPAC emergency stockpile.

Where significant stocks and organizational capacity do exist, and after the first 2-3 months in all instances:

—Tailor any ongoing inputs to the observed usage rates of different items in the basic list, to in-country stock levels and any ongoing local production.

Distribution of drugs

Policies for dispensing/distributing drugs should take account of established local practices and long-term policies as well as immediate needs. Try to avoid undermining any actual or proposed mechanisms of community self-reliance—e.g. village pharmacies selling at cost price—by large-scale (but short-term) free distribution of drugs. Consider augmenting the operational stocks of any such pharmacies where appropriate.

Local production

Where an indigenous pharmaceutical industry exists, use/restore its capacity where practicable, provided its production costs/delivery prices are not too unfavourable compared with the cost (including freight) of imports.

Where such local production has been disrupted and foreign exchange resources are limited, consider, for the rehabilitation phase, supplying spare parts and/or raw pharmaceuticals to enable the production *of essential items* to be restored.   **253**

Any continuing imports of drugs should then complement local production by supplying any essential items not able to be produced in sufficent quantity locally.

Practical aspects

Instructions for the use of available drugs should be issued in a locally-understood language. They must be carefully phrased—simple, unambiguous and fully comprehensible to the least trained of likely users.

Except when set-packed for immediate distribution, each different type of drug should be packed separately and outer packages be clearly marked to facilitate sorting and storage.

Both the inner and outer packaging of all drug consignments should be robust and weather-proof. All drugs supplied should have a remaining shelf life of *at least* 6 months and the expiry date be printed on the outer carton. (Deliveries from UNIPAC exceed these standards on all occasions.)

At all locations where drugs need to be stored, arrange:
—The best possible storage facilities;
—Prompt inspection and sorting of incoming consignments;
—Proper inventory control; *and*
—Systematic monitoring of requisitions.

Pharmacy students may be mobilized to operate temporary pharmacy stores in the field and to reinforce staff at central and regional stores. If available in-country expertise is limited/depleted, one or more experienced pharmacists may be brought in quickly to help (re-)establish central and/or regional medical stores.

Technicians to advise and assist in the rehabilitation and resumption of pharmaceutical production may also be needed during the rehabilitation phase.

Possible UNICEF inputs

Depending on the assessment of actual needs and possibilities, some of the following inputs might be considered:
—Sets of basic drugs (by diverting stocks on hand or en route for regular programmes, local purchases or air deliveries from UNIPAC).

—Quantities of specifically needed drugs and other supplies—soap, disinfectant, etc.

—Transport for the internal distribution of drugs.

—Local costs for the (re-)establishment and operation of necessary medical stores.

—Experienced pharmacists' services.

—Spare parts, raw materials and/or technical expertise for the rehabilitation and resumption of local production (in the rehabilitation phase).

Give priority to ensuring adequate supplies of drugs and other supplies relevant to the most basic, current health problems affecting children and mothers.

Co-ordinate closely with the WHO Programme Co-ordinator and other potential donors of drugs. The same basic list of requirements will often have been forwarded by the government to various potential donors.

For all requests:

—Check the numbers of people to be served and compare the quantities with those in the WHO emergency health kit lists.

—Seek specific explanations for any major discrepancies, and justification for any requests for items not in the WHO lists, or specific brand-name products.

The WHO Programme Co-ordinator should normally undertake or arrange such evaluation and furnish recommendations for action.

Evaluate offers of in-kind donations of drugs very carefully: see "unsolicited contributions" p. 154. "Doctors samples" and sophisticated non-essential drugs should normally be refused.

Further references

a.   *WHO emergency health kit*—WHO (1984)   E/F/S/A
       [Annex 11 reproduces these lists adapted to UNIPAC specifications]

b   *The use of essential drugs*, WHO Technical reference series No. 722—WHO (1985)   E/F

c   *Medical supply management after natural disaster*, PAHO scientific publication No. 438—PAHO (1983)   E/S

d   *The management of nutritional emergencies in large populations*, C. de Ville de Goyet, J. Seaman & U. Geijer—WHO (1978)   E/F

Other references to Annex 8 (p. 248)

WHO EMERGENCY HEALTH KIT

Explanatory notes

(Adapted from WHO emergency health kit — WHO, 1984.)

The WHO Emergency Health Kit is designed to establish a clinic and provide basic drugs to meet the essential needs for 10,000 persons for an initial 3 months.

The aims of this kit are to encourage standardization of the drugs and equipment used in an emergency, to permit swift initial supply from outside, to rationalize urgent requests and response, and to promote disaster preparedness by the provision of a kit that may be kept in readiness as a stock of essential items.

- **The current lists are expected to be thoroughly reviewed by WHO and other interested organizations in 1986. Check whether revised lists have been issued and/or the contents of the standard sets proposed by UNIPAC been modified.**

Lists A, B and C

The Kit is made up of two drug lists (List A and List B) and an equipment list (List C). Together the items on these lists and the re-order forms illustrated in the WHO booklet make up a complete prepackaged parcel ready for use. The component kits A, B and C may also be ordered separately depending on the needs of the situation.

List A drugs are for use by auxiliary and basically trained health workers. **List B** drugs are for use by doctors and senior health workers; they are additional to the drugs in List A.

With one exception, the drugs are those in the revised Model List of Essential Drugs published in the report of the WHO Expert Committee on the Use of Essential Drugs, 1983.

The lists below show the drugs actually supplied in the standard kits assembled by UNIPAC in 1986. The quantities are, in some cases, adjusted from the published WHO Lists to correspond to the unit package quantities stocked by UNIPAC.

In many instances various other drugs could serve as alternatives to those listed, which may be considered as examples of a therapeutic group; these are distinguished in Lists A and B by an asterisk (*). Choices must be made at the national level based on the availability and comparative cost of equivalent products.

List C in the 1984 WHO booklet includes basic clinic equipment, expendable clinic supplies for 3 months, and a set of laboratory equipment and supplies (no details prescribed for the latter). It is likely that, when the kit is revised (in 1986) these elements will be separated so that they can be ordered separately, e.g. clinic equipment with or without laboratory equipment, and additional sets of expendables if necessary.

The list below reproduces the existing WHO list, adapted to UNIPAC specifications and subdivided between basic clinic equipment and the expendable supplies. Appropriate standard sets of laboratory equipment and expendable supplies are being developed.

When defining needs and placing orders, consider carefully whether laboratory equipment is needed/can be properly used at all the locations, also whether and when additional quantities of the expendable supplies might need to be ordered (taking account of what is expected to be available locally/from other sources).

The basis of the kit

The composition of the kit is based on epidemiological data, population profiles and disease patterns typical of emergency situations, and certain assumptions borne out by experience as follows:

257

(a) An assumption that clinics will usually be staffed by health workers with only basic training, who will treat symptoms rather than diagnosed diseases and will refer patients who need more specialized treatment;

(b) An assumption that half the population is 0-14 years of age (5,000 persons) and half is 15 years old or more (5,000);

(c) For each half of the population, an estimate of the likely numbers of the more common symptoms or diseases presenting in a 3-month period at the early stage of an emergency, and an assumption that standardized schedules will be used to treat these: see Tables 1 and 2 in the WHO booklet.

Emergency needs

The drugs listed are *intended to cover initial needs only* pending a proper assessment of, among other things:

—The demographic pattern of the community;
—The physical condition of individuals;
—The incidence of symptoms and diseases as determined, for example, from clinic and health centre records and nutritional surveillance;
—The prevalence of symptoms as determined, for example, from household and nutrition surveys;
—The causes of mortality and morbidity;
—Likely seasonal variations of symptoms and diseases;
—The likely impact of improved public health measures;
—Local availability of drugs and equipment, taking account of national drug policies (see above);
—Drug resistance;
—The capabilities of the health workers;
—The referral system.

When this assessment has been made, a special list should be drawn up in the light of the situation and appropriate arrangements made to supply the necessary quantities.

Exclusions

Lists A and B do not include vaccines or drugs to control certain communicable diseases. To be sure of acting in accordance with national policies (e.g. for an EPI or tuberculosis or leprosy control programme), the vaccines and drugs needed and the best methods of supply should be discussed and agreed with the national health authorities. See also Annexes 13 and 14.

Delivery of kits

UNIPAC is able to deliver sets corresponding to lists A, B and C at short notice as well as the individual items which make up those lists. As with all standard kits, sets may be modified to meet specific local needs if necessary, but delivery will then be a little slower.

Cost and packed size of kits

For kits assembled by UNIPAC in 1986 the approximate costs (excluding freight), packed volume and weight of the kits are as follows:

	Cost (dollars)	Volume (cu m)	Weight (kg)
Kit list A	1,600	1.3	490
Kit list B . . . . :	650	0.15	36
Kit list C			
Basic clinic equipment	880		
Clinic expendables	530	1.35	203
Laboratory equipment and supplies . . .	1,060		
Total, one of each	4,720	2.8	730

List A—Basic drug requirement for 10,000 persons for 3 months

(List adapted to UNIPAC specifications—UNIPAC set 99-060-00: contents as of January 1986)

Item No.	UNIPAC stock No.	Drug	Form, strength, packaging	Quantity per set No.	Units
Analgesics					
01	15 060 02	Acetylsalicylic acid	Tablets 300 mg, scored, tin of 1000	17	tins
02	15 559 65	Paracetamol	Tablets BP, scored 500 mg, tin of 1000	5	tins
Antihelmintics					
03	15 553 55*	Mebedazole	Tablets 100 mg, bottle of 100	21	bottles
04	15 600 25	Piperazine citrate	Syrup USP, bottle of 30 ml	170	bottles
Antibacterials					
05	15 050 85*	Ampicillin	Powder for 60 ml oral suspension 125 mg/5ml	420	bottles
06	15 579 82	Penicillin G	Inj powder BP 1 mega unit without diluent	500	vials
07	15 438 02	Diluent (distilled water for injection)	BP, ampoule of 5 ml	500	amp.
08	15 590 80	Phenoxymethylpenicillin	Tablets 250 mg, tin of 1000	10	tins
09	15 590 25	Procaine benzylpenicillin	Injections 3 g (3 million IU)	375	vials
10	15 371 00*	Sulfamethoxazole + trimethoprim	Tablets BP 400 mg + 80 mg, tin of 500	15	tins
11	15 690 00*	Tetracycline	Capsules BP 250 mg, tin of 1000	9	tins
Antimalarials [a]					
12	15 320 00*	Chloroquine	Tablets 150 mg base BP, tin of 1000	8	tins
13	15 339 85*	Chloroquine	Syrup, 50 mg/50 ml, bottle of 1 litre	3	bottles
Antianaemia					
14	15 500 10	Ferrous sulfate + folic acid	Tablets 60 mg + 0.25 mg, tin of l000	15	tins
15	15 500 00	Ferrous salt	Tablets 60 mg, tin of 1000	30	tins

Dermatologicals

No.	Code	Name	Description	Quantity
16	15 150 20	Benzoic acid + salicylic acid	Ointment, tube of 40 g	100 tubes
17	15 051 20*	Antibiotic dermatological	Ointment, tube of 30 g	37 tubes
18	15 230 00*	Calamine	Lotion, bottle of 500 ml	10 bottles
19	15 200 00	Benzyl benzoate	Saponated concentrate, bottle of 1 litre	35 bottles
20	15 520 02	Gentian violet	Powder medicinal BP, bottle of 25 g	8 bottles

Disinfectants

| 21 | 15 315 00* | Chlorhexidine | Conc. solution 20%, bottle of 100 ml | 50 bottles |

Antacids

| 22 | 15 040 00 | Aluminium hydroxide | Tablets 500 mg, tin of 1,000 | 5 tins |

Cathartics

| 23 | 15 625 00* | Senna | Tablets 7.5 mg, pack of 100 | 4 packs |

Diarrhoea (replacement solution)

| 24 | 15 611 05 | Salts, oral rehydration | Powder, packet for 1 litre | 6000 packets |

Ophthalmologicals

| 25 | 15 100 00* | Tetracycline | Eye ointment 1%, tube of 5 g | 750 tubes |

Solutions

| 26 | 15 438 00 | Diluent (distilled water for injection) | BP, ampoule of 2 ml | 500 each |
| 27 | 15 438 04 | Diluent (distilled water for injection) | BP, ampoule of 10 ml | 500 each |

Vitamins

| 28 | 15 830 00 | Vitamin A (high potency) | Caps. 200,000 IU, bottle of 500 | 1 bottle |
| 29 | 15 830 10 | Vitamin A | Caps. 25,000 IU, bottle of 100 | 4 bottles |

[a] For treatment of chloroquin-resistant malaria, see List B item 09.

* Alternative drugs could be used.

Abbreviations: amp = ampoule; caps. = capsules; inj. = injection; IU = international units.

List B—Drugs for use by doctors and senior health workers

(in addition to List A)

(List adapted to UNIPAC specifications—UNIPAC set 99-061-00: contents as of January 1986)

Item No.	UNIPAC Stock No.	Drug	Form, strength, packaging	Quantity perset No.	Units
Local anaesthetics					
01	15 552 00*	Lidocaine hydrochloride	Injection BP 1%, vial of 50 ml	10	vials
Analgesics					
	*	(Pethidine—see note a)			
Antiallergics					
02	15 317 00*	Chloraphenamine maleate	Tablets, tin of 1000	1	tin
Antiepileptics					
03	15 436 25	Diazepam	Injection 5 mg/ml in 2 ml amp., box 10 amp.	1	box
Antiinfectives					
04	15 556 50*	Metronidazole	Tablets 250 mg, tin of 1000	2	tins
05	15 580 00	Benzylpenicillin	Injection 3.0 g	100	vial
06	15 310 00*	Chloramphenicol	Capules (or tablets) BP 250 mg, tin 1000	2	tins
07	15 373 00*	Cloxacillin	Capules 500 mg, bottle of 500	6	bottles
Antimalarials					
08	15 606 60	Quinine	Inj. 300 mg/ml in 2 ml amp., box of 10 amp.	2	boxes
09	15 680 45	Sulfadoxine + pyrimethamine	Tablets 500 mg + 25 mg, tin of 1000	1	tin
Plasma substitute					
10	15 432 00	Dextran-70	Intravenous infusion BP, bottle of 500 ml	10	bottles

Cardiovascular

11	15 515 00	Glyceryl trinitrate	Tablets 0.5 mg, bottle of 100	1 bottle
12	15 606 50*	Propranolol	Tablets 40 mg, bottle of 100	1 bottle
13	15 437 00	Digoxin	Tablets 0.25 mg, tin of 100	1 tin
14	15 437 20	Digoxin	Inj. 0.25 mg/ml in 2 ml amp., box of 10 amp.	1 box
15	15 010 00	Epinephrine (adrenaline)	Inj. 1 mg/ml in 1 ml amp., box of 10 amp.	1 box

Dermatologicals

| 16 | 15 559 00 | Nystatin | Cream 100,000 IU/g, tube of 30 g | 10 tubes |
| 17 | 15 525 00 | Hydrocortisone | Cream 1%, tube of 30 g | 10 tubes |

Diuretics

| 18 | 15 505 30* | Furosemide | Tablets, 40 mg, tin of 100 | 1 tin |
| 19 | 15 505 25* | Furosemide | Inj. 10 mg/ml in 2 ml amp., box of 10 amp. | 1 box |

Gastrointestinals

20	15 592 00*	Promethazine	Tablets BP 25 mg, bottle of 100	1 bottle
21	15 592 05*	Promethazine	Syrup, bottle of 250 ml	10 bottles
	*	(Codeine — see note a)		

Hormones

| 22 | 15 526 00 | Hydrocortisone | Powder for injection in 100 mg vial | 10 vials |

Opthalmologicals

| 23 | 15 660 00 | Sulfacetamide | Eye ointment 10%, tube of 5 g | 250 tubes |

Psychotherapeutics

| 24 | 15 436 30* | Diazepam | Tablets 5 mg, bottle of 100 | 1 bottle |

Respiratory

25	15 020 00*	Aminophylline	Inj. 25 mg/ml in 10 ml amp.	10 amp.
26	15 620 20	Salbutamol	Oral inhalation 0.1 mg per dose	5 aerosols
27	15 115 00	Beclomatasone	Oral inhalation 0.05 mg per dose	5 aerosols

263

List B *(continued)*

Item No.	UNIPAC stock No.	Drug	Form, strength, packaging	Quantity per set	
				No.	Units
Solutions					
28	15 608 00*	Compound sodium lactate (Ringer)	Inj. solution BP 500 ml with IV giving set	20	sets
29	15 435 15	Glucose	Inj. solution in 10 ml amp., box of 10 amp.	1	box
30	15 643 20	Sodium chloride	Inj. solution BP 500 ml with IV giving set	10	sets
31	15 438 04	Diluent (distilled water for injection)	BP in 10 ml ampoule	100	amp.
Oxytocics					
32	15 460 00*	Ergometrine maleate	Tablets BP 0.2 mg, vial of 10	10	vials
33	15 450 00*	Ergometrine maleate	Inj. BP 0.2 mg in 1 ml amp., box of 10 amp.	1	box

[a] Pethidine injections (50 mg in 1-ml ampoules, total 10 ampoules) and codeine tablets (30 mg, total 100 tablets) are recommended by WHO but are subject to international control under the Single Convention on Narcotic Drugs (1961) and the Convention on Psychotropic substances (1971). They are *not* included in kits assembled by UNIPAC or bought from other international sources but should be obtained locally in accordance with approved national procedures.

* Alternative drugs could be used.

Abbreviations: amp. = ampoule; inj. = injection; IU = international units; soln. = solution.

List C—Basic medical equipment and supplies for a clinic

(List adapted to UNIPAC specifications—UNIPAC set 99-062-00: contents as of January 1986)

N.B. Items listed with UNIPAC code beginning with 67 are not normally stocked by UNIPAC in 1985.

Item No.	UNIPAC Stock No.	Description	Quantity per set No.	Units
Basic clinic equipment				
001	07 835 00	Syringe hypo 2ml, Luer glass	5	each
002	7 845 00	Syringe hypo 10ml, Luer glass	5	each
003	7 490 00	Needle hypo 1.25x51mm / 18Gx2″, Luer, box of 12	2	boxes
004	7 520 00	Needle hypo 0.90x38mm / 20Gx1½″, Luer, box of 12	6	boxes
005	7 495 00	Needle hypo 0.90x51mm / 20Gx2″, Luer, box of 12	2	boxes
006	7 505 00	Needle hypo 0.70x32mm / 22Gx1¼″, Luer, box of 12	4	boxes
007	7 510 00	Needle hypo 0.55x19mm / 24Gx¾″, Luer, box of 12	6	boxes
008	7 515 02	Needle hypo 0.45x10mm / 26Gx⅜″, Luer, box of 12	4	boxes
009	5 220 00	Gauze-pad sterile 12-ply, 76x76mm square	5000	each
010	5 630 00	Suture catgut and needles	15	boxes
011	7 429 90	Holder, needle straight, Metzenbaum baby, 150mm SS	1	each
012	4 750 00	Knife handle, surgical for minor surgery No. 3	2	each
013	7 275 00	Forceps, hemostat straight, Rochestr-Pean, 160mm SS	2	each
014	7 205 00	Forceps, dissecting spring-type, curved fine points, 115mm SS	2	each
015	7 735 00	Scissors, surgical straight, 140mm sharp/blunt points SS	2	each
016	7 740 00	Scissors, surgical straight, 140mm sharp/sharp points SS	2	each
017	7 445 00	Scissors, surgical straight, 140mm blunt/blunt points SS	2	each
018	7 446 40	Scissors, suture baby, 114mm sharp points SS	1	each
019	4 810 50	Thermometer, clinical oral, dual celsius/fahrenheit scale	5	each
020	4 810 60	Thermometer, clinical rectal, dual celsius/fahrenheit scale	5	each

List C (*continued*)

Item No.	UNIPAC Stock No.	Description	Quantity per set	
			No.	Units
021	6 860 00	Stethoscope, binaural complete	2	each
022	6 865 00	Stethoscope, foetal, Pinard monaural	2	each
023	6 830 00	Sphygmomanometer, aneroid 300mm with cuff	1	each
024	6 610 00	Otoscope-ophthalmoscope set (without batteries)	1	set
025	7 775 00	Speculum, vaginal bi-valve, Graves medium SS	1	each
026	7 780 00	Speculum, vaginal bi-valve, Graves large SS	1	each
027	7 830 00	Syringe, irrigating, Kramer, 90ml metal	1	each
028	6 200 00	Tongue depressor, 165mm metal	1	each
029	3 730 00	Tube nasal-feeding, infant 8FR, 380mm polyethylene	10	each
030	3 750 00	Tube nasal-feeding, infant 16FR, 500mm soft rubber	5	each
031	7 445 00	Infusion-set, paediatric scalp-vein, sterile/disposable	50	each
032	3 280 00	Gloves, surgeon's, latex size 6½	100	pairs
033	3 285 00	Gloves, surgeon's, latex size 7	100	pairs
034	3 295 00	Gloves, surgeon's, latex size 8	100	pairs
035	2 765 00	Tray, instrument/dressing with cover, 310x195x63mm SS	4	each
036	2 100 00	Basin, kidney, 475ml (16oz) SS	2	each
037	2 560 00	Jar, needle or ointment, with cover and handle, 180ml	4	each
038	2 250 00	Bowl, sponge, 600ml SS	4	each
039	5 410 50	Plaster of Paris bandage BPC, 3 inches x 3 yards	12	rolls
040	3 610 00	Sheeting, plastic clear vinyl, 910mm wide	2	metres
041	3 050 00	Apron, utility, 900mm x 1m opaque plastic	2	each
042	6 900 00	Tape measure, 2m/6feet, calibrated cm/inches, steel	2	each
043	1 405 00	Scale, physician adult, metric, 140kgs x 100g	1	each
044	1 455 50	Scale, infant spring type, hanging, with trousers, 25kg x 500g	1	set
045	1 444 00	Height measuring instrument	1	each

046	1 560 00	Sterilizer, dressing, pressure cooker, 350x380mm (39 ltr), fuel	1 each
047	1 700 00	Stove, kerosene, single burner, pressure type	1 each
048	56 199 02	Filter, water, aluminium, with 4 Sterasyl candles	1 each
049	7 007 00	Airway, Guedel, rubber, infant size 54mm	1 each
050	7 008 00	Airway, Guedel, rubber, child size 67mm	1 each
051	7 009 00	Airway, Guedel, rubber, small adult size 82mm	1 each
052	67 005 48	Book "WHO Emergency Health Kit"	1 each

Clinic supplies which may need to be replaced every 3 months

101	7 822 00	Syringe hypo 2ml, Luer disposable	4000 each
102	67 003 78	Syringe hypo 10ml, Luer disposable	1000 each
103	7 474 30	Needle hypo 0.8x40mm / 21Gx1$\frac{1}{2}$", Luer disposable	2500 each
104	67 003 79	Needle hypo 0.5x16mm / 25Gx$\frac{5}{8}$", Luer disposable	2500 each
105	7 460 00	Knife blade, surgical for minor surgery No. 10, packet of 5	20 packets
106	18 022 12	Battery, alkaline dry cell "D" type, 1.5V	2 each
107	3 735 00	Tube nasal-feeding, premature 5FR, 380mm polyethylene	5 each
108	67 003 81	Gauze swabs, 5x5cm in packets of 100	10 packets
109	67 003 82	Gauze swabs, 10x10cm in packets of 100	10 packets
110	67 003 83	Sterile gauze swabs, 10x10cm in packets of 5	50 packets
111	67 003 84	Eye pads (sterile) in packets of 10	6 packets
112	67 003 85	Paraffin gauze dressing, 10x10cm in tins of 25	3 tins
113	67 003 86	Sanitary towels, packet of 20	10 packets
114	5 196 00	Cotton wool, absorbent, non-sterile, roll of 500g	2 rolls
115	5 010 50	Plaster, surgical adhesive tape, reel 25mm x 10m	120 reels
116	5 121 00	Bandage, gauze non-sterile 25mm x 9m	50 rolls
117	5 121 01	Bandage, gauze non-sterile 50mm x 9m	50 rolls
118	5 121 02	Bandage, gauze non-sterile 75mm x 9m	50 rolls
119	67 003 87	Pneumatic splint set, multipurpose	1 set
120	5 390 00	Pins, safety, medium size 40mm, bag of 12	40 bags

List C (*continued*)

Item No.	UNIPAC Stock No.	Description	Quantity per set No. Units
121	5 750 00	Towel, huck, 430x500mm	2 each
122	5 520 00	Soap, toilet, 113g bar unwrapped	60 bars
123	5 140 00	Brush, hand surgeon's, white nylon bristles	5 each
124	67 005 45	Health cards with plastic envelopes	10000 each
125	15 448 25	Envelopes for tablets, polythene, packet of 100	100 packets

Laboratory items

Sets of laboratory equipment and expendable supplies suitable to establish field diagnostic facilities in conjunction with an emergency clinic are being developed. The provisional list as of January 1986 includes 79 items and costs, ex UNIPAC, approximately $1,060. Definitive sets are expected to be established end 1986. Check with WHO, UNIPAC and/or EOU.

IMMUNIZATION PROGRAMMES

Objective

- **To protect children against measles and other preventable diseases which are — or could become — prevalent.**

This must be pursued within the limits of practical possibilities and in the framework of a national Expanded Programme of Immunization (EPI).

Priorities

Where an effective EPI programme served the population previously, top priority should be given to assuring its continued functioning and increasing its coverage if necessary.

Where previous immunization coverage was limited:

— The immunization of all children 9 months — 3 years old against *measles* will be a high priority in any temporary camps, crowded communities and areas where (seasonal) outbreaks are common. Immunization should there be undertaken just as soon as the necessary cold chain and other capacity can be mobilized.

— In similar conditions, *DPT, polio and BCG* vaccination of infants and young children is highly desirable but should be attempted only if the necessary operational capacity is assured, the population expected to remain relatively static for at least a month, and the operation can be integrated into a national programme within a short time.

Apart from measles, immunization operations should not be undertaken as immediate "emergency" measures but be planned as the first phase of an ongoing long-term programme. The general practices of the national EPI programme (if any) should be followed. Records must be kept.

Unless previous services are known to have had wide coverage, *all* children under 5 years may be vaccinated. First priority, however, is for children in the first year of life. Malnutrition, diarrhoea and/or minor illnesses are *not* contraindications to immunization.

Where neo-natal *tetanus* is a risk, immunize pregnant women with two doses of tetanus toxoid beginning as soon as pregnancy is recognized. This may be advisable in any situation were conditions of hygiene and general sanitation are poor.

With presently available vaccines, *mass* vaccination programmes (e.g. against cholera or typhoid) are generally *not* useful, but waste effort and resources which could better be used in implementing other, more effective control measures—especially environmental sanitation.

In certain areas, other specific preventable communicable diseases may be major—possibly seasonal—problems, e.g. meningococcal meningitis (in Sahelian Africa), yellow fever, Japanese encephalitis (in parts of Asia). It *may* in certain circumstances then be appropriate to give these vaccines, specific to the local strain, on a mass basis.

Organizing vaccination operations

General organization

Get experienced personnel to plan any immunization activities, especially any "crash" measles (or other) programme:

— Vaccines, personnel, equipment and the target children and women must all be brought together in the right place and at the right time!

— The expiry dates and storage conditions of *all* vaccine stocks must be closely monitored.

— Individual immunization cards (possibly combined with a growth chart) should be issued to each child immunized.

—National personnel should do the injecting.

Refer to the WHO EPI training guidelines (ref. a) for details on the organization of immunization programmes.

Advance preparation for vaccination sessions:
—Ensure that the purpose of vaccination is understood by mothers and community leaders.
—Plan actual sessions with the community a few days in advance.
—Ensure that sufficient health workers and community volunteers will be available—as well as the vaccines, equipment, vaccination cards and record books.
A typical set-up for vaccination sessions is shown in Figure 12/a.

The transportation and handling of vaccines requires *very* careful attention. All vaccines must be kept cool and shaded from sunlight at *all* times:
—Always keep cold boxes and vaccines carriers in the shade.
—Open cold boxes/vaccine carriers only at the last minute when vaccines are to be given: check the temperature on opening cold boxes.
—Keep prepared vaccines shaded during sessions: metal foil can be very useful for this.
Ensure close supervision of field operations and plan follow-up monitoring operations carefully.

Figure 12/a   Typical field vaccination session

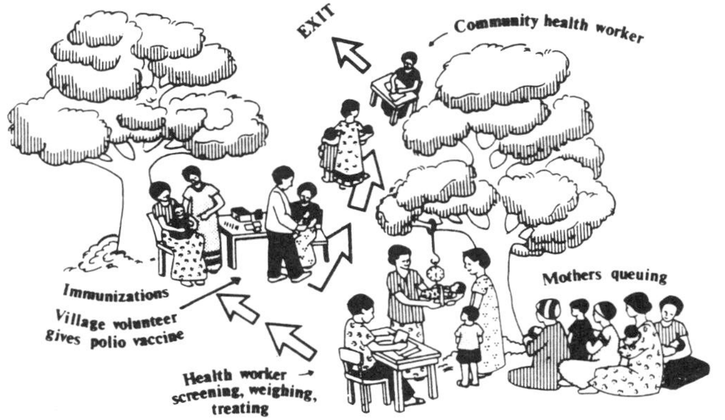

A rural immunization session with three stations, two health workers, a community health worker, and a village volunteer.

(Reproduced from ref. a, module 5)

271

Table 12/1

Dosage and storage of vaccines

Vaccine	Dose	Number and timing of doses	Diluent	Storage[b]	When ready for use
Measles	0.5ml (10,50)	1 dose at not less than 9 months	Special diluent. Must be cool. (Distilled water may be used in an emergency).	2 years at 0°C to +8°C	Destroyed by sunlight. Must be stored below +8°C. Will last for 3 hours after mixing, a full session if kept cold and well shaded
Polio (oral)	2 or 3 drops, depending on manufacturer[c] (20)	3 doses at 4-week intervals starting at 6 weeks. Add one extra dose at birth if feasible, especially in polio-endemic areas	None. (Droppers needed)	6-12 months at 0°C to +8°C 1-2 years at −20°C	Keep cool and shaded
DPT	0.5ml (20)	3 doses at 4-week intervals starting at not less than 6 weeks	None	18-24 months at 0°C to +8°C Do not freeze	Keep cool and shaded
BCG	0.1ml (50)	1 dose from birth	Normal saline. Must be cool	12 months at 0°C to +8°C	Destroyed by sunlight. Must be stored below +8°C.
Tetanus	0.5 ml (20)	2 doses at 4 week intervals beginning at first contact for pregnant women	None	2-3 years at 0°C to +8°C Do not freeze	As above for measles

[a] Figures in brackets indicate normal number of doses per vial.
[b] General indications of storage lives: check specification leaflets for manufacturers' recommendations for each individual lot of vaccine.
[c] Polio vaccines supplied by UNIPAC always require only 2 drops. Vaccines from other sources may require 3: check the manufacturer's specifications.
N.B. Technical opinion has changed over the years. The indications given above for the timing of doses and the storage life of vaccines correspond to the latest (1985) WHO recommendations.

Supplies and equipment needed

Vaccines

It will normally be possible to initiate any special/new immunization operations by *borrowing* supplies from the national programme. Any requirement for additional deliveries (by air) should thus be planned to replenish stocks as and when needed, and to cover any continuing increased level of demand. Specify whether diluent is required to be delivered or not.

Table 12/1 shows the dosages and storage properties of the various vaccines.

N.B. There is always a certain wastage of vaccine. Allow for this when ordering. If specific data on wastage rates in local operations is not available, multiply the number of doses of BCG planned to be administered by 2, and the number of doses of other vaccines by 1.3.

Cold chain

To keep vaccines cold all the way from delivery at the airport to use in a field vaccination session requires:
- —Cold room/freezers at airport and/or the capital;
- —Refrigerators at regional/area level;
- —Cold boxes for transfers between locations; *and*
- —Small vaccine carriers for field operations.

Table 12/2 provides details concerning the cold storage capacity required for particular quantities of vaccine. Table 12/3 lists the most important factors to be taken into account in selecting/specifying the particular cold chain elements to be supplied. *Supdir 55 Amendment 5* provides technical details of available items.

Vaccination supplies

In most cares, a plentiful supply of *needles and syringes* will be required:
- —Reusable plastic syringes are recommended: they last for approximately 200 sterilizations.
- —Needles may last, on average, only half as long: order twice as many needles as syringes.

273

—Sterilization equipment must be available: portable sterilizers and stoves will normally be appropriate for use in the field.

—Each needle and syringe should be used for only one injection between sterilizations.

Disposable needles and syringes should only be used if it is sure that they will be effectively destroyed after having been used once only.

Table 12/4 summarizes the kinds of equipment needed.

When very large groups of children are to be vaccinated (say 500 or more per session), the use of *jet injectors* (e.g. Ped-o-jets, UNIPAC 07-447-00) greatly increases speed and decreases the risk of infection. They are appropriate for "mass" vaccination operations conducted by small numbers of well-trained vaccination teams:

—Specific training (at least 1 day) must be provided to vaccination team members in the operation and maintenance of the equipment;

—For each team, a separate injector will be required for each antigen plus one spare;

—Spare parts must be on hand, also operation and maintenance manuals;

Table 12/2

Cold storage space needed by vaccines
(in cc per dose / litres per 1,000 doses)

| | | Actual space required in cold chain elements | | |
Vaccine	Packed volume	Freezers and cold boxes	Refrigerators	Cold rooms
Measles	3.0	3.6	6	12
DPT	2.5	3.0	5	10
BCG	1.0	1.2	2	4
Polio	1.5	1.8	3	6
Tetanus	2.5	3.0	5	10

Notes:

1. The above figures include space for the packaging and the diluent necessary for the respective vaccines.

2. As a rule of thumb for full EPI operations, the vaccines necessary to fully immunize a single child represent a packed volume of 30 cc, requiring an actual space of 36 cc in freezers and cold boxes plus 60 cc in refrigerators and 120 cc in cold rooms.

—Vaccines must be delivered in multi-dose bottles (usually 50-dose although 10 and 20-dose bottles can also be used).

A team undertaking mass measles vaccination alone would need 2 injectors. Full EPI operations would normally be undertaken through community health workers but, if a limited number of teams are to implement a mass campaign injectors might then be used: 1 for measles, 1 for DPT, possibly 1 for tetanus, plus 1 spare = 4 per team.

Ped-o-jets require the seals to be replaced after 10,000 injections, and major parts after 50,000. Some other injectors have to be returned to the manufacturer for maintenance!

Table 12/3

Choosing cold chain equipment

Aspects to be considered for cold boxes and vaccine carriers:

☐ Volume capacity—How much vaccine will be carried?

☐ Cold life (quality of insulation)—How long will the vaccine be in transit and in what ambient temperatures?

☐ Weight—How will the box be carried?

☐ Durability—What conditions will the box be exposed to?

☐ Price—Which box meets the above needs for the lowest price?

Aspects to be considered for refrigerators and freezers:

☐ Volume capacity—How much vaccine must be stored (a) at 4°C? and (b) at -20°C?

☐ Icemaking performance—How much ice/icepacks must be frozen per 24 hours?

☐ Refrigerator performance—What are local temperatures, day and night?

☐ Power source—What reliable sources are available: electricity (voltage, frequency); bottled gas (type); kerosene?

☐ Cold life—For how many hours may contents need to be kept below 8°C in case of power source failure?

☐ Reliability—What facilities and parts are available locally for different types of equipment?

☐ Price—What model meets the above requirements for the lowest cost?

See *Supdir 55 Amendment 5* for technical details of available equipment. Note that the length of time for which the vaccines will be kept cold without power ("cold live") varies enormously between different items.

Emergency immunization kit

A standard kit of supplies to enable an emergency immunization operation to be mounted in the absence of any existing vaccination supplies or cold chain is being

Table 12/4

Vaccination supplies

In most situations:

For BCG:

Syringe 0.1 ml sterilizable plastic, Luer	(07-822-15)
Needle, hypo, 10 mm, 26G, Luer	(07-515-02)

For all other vaccines:

Syringe 1.0 ml sterilizable plastic, Luer	(07-822-22)
Needle, hypo, 32 mm, 22G, Luer	(07-505-00)

For reconstituting vaccines

Syringe 5.0 ml sterilizable plastic	(07-819-05)
Needle, hypo, 76 mm, 18G, Luer	(07-488-00)

If there are no existing supplies, complete *syringe kits* may be appropriate: 99-070-00 for sessions of up to 40 injections; 99-071-00 for up to 80 injections. A spares kit, 99-072-00 might then be appropriate for a field base servicing 10 field units/teams.[a]

In certain circumstances where it is absolutely certain that the material will be effectively destroyed after having been used once only:

Syringe, immun 2 ml with needle, disposable	(07-822-25)

For vaccination of very large groups of children:

Ped-o-jets (UNIPAC 07-447-00) with spares (07-447-05).

Sterilization equipment

If needles and syringes are being used, portable steam (pressure) sterilizers will probably be needed for field operations: 01-571-10 for 42 syringes and 50 needles; 01-571-00 for 84 syringes and 100 needles. Stoves will be needed, e.g. 01-700-00 (kerosene pressure type). Complete sterilization kits (including sterilizer, forceps, timer, sharpening stone and soap box) may be useful: 99-080-00 for 42 syringes; 99-081-00 for 84 syringes.

Sterilization takes 20 minutes. Five minutes venting plus 15 minutes actual sterilization.

---

[a] Details of these kits are being finalized. They will be available from UNIPAC in 1986.

developed jointly by WHO, UNHCR and OXFAM. It will include a refrigerator (capacity for 5,000 doses of vaccine), cold box, vaccine carriers, syringes, needles sterilization equipment, small generator, fuel containers, record cards and also instruction manuals on how to set up and run an emergency measles (or other) vaccination operation.

Necessary vaccines and fuel will have to be provided separately, but the kit should provide everything else that would be required to undertake a crash immunization operation in an isolated camp of displaced persons—or other situation where there is no existing EPI stracture/capability. 5,000 children will be able to be immunized against measles between replenishment deliveries of vaccine from national cold chain facilities elsewhere. If other vaccines are to be included, the number will be correspondingly less. The equipment can afterwards be used— with additional items—in a subsequent, ongoing EPI operation.

Details of the kits should be available from WHO, UNHCR and OXFAM—and EOU/UNIPAC—during 1986. Each kit will cost about $2,500 and weigh about 200 kg.

Possible UNICEF inputs

Depending on the assessment of actual needs and possibilities, some of the following inputs might be considered:

—Vaccines (against a carefully planned delivery schedule).

—Ped-o-jets (with spares kits) or syringes, needles and sterilizers—see Table 12/4.

—Cold chain components: refrigerators, cold boxes, vaccine carriers, ice packs, thermometers, spare parts for refrigerators; etc.

—Transport.

—Local operating costs (including kerosene for fridges).

Further references

a. *Immunization in practice*—WHO (1984) E/F
    [Set of seven simple training modules and a trainers guide on practical aspects of vaccinating in the field.]
b. *Logistics and cold chain for primary health care*, volumes 9 and 12-21—WHO (1983) E/F
    [Simple guidelines on estimating vaccine requirements and looking after cold chain equipment.]

277

EPIDEMIOLOGICAL SURVEILLANCE

Objective

- **To detect any signs of particular health problems and enable early action to be taken to contain any outbreak of communicable disease.**

Method and principles

Reports from health facilities and medical teams must be received, analysed and evaluated regularly. Any reports of specific outbreaks of disease must be rapidly investigated. Sample surveys may be undertaken to determine the prevalence of particular conditions. Note that clinic attendance rates and the incidence of symptoms/diseases observed there are not necessarily representative of the health situation on the community as a whole. The appearance of new diseases or sudden changes in observed rate of incidence are, however, often significant.

The restoration and reinforcement of pre-existing reporting and surveillance systems is a high priority in any emergency. A thorough understanding of how those systems operated previously is essential.

In the absence of any effective, pre-existing arrangements—and especially if laboratory facilities are lacking and diagnostic criteria not well standardized:

— Request regular reports from all health posts/medical teams on the occurrence of a *limited number of symptom complexes* suggestive of specific diseases which are (a) likely to arise in the particular circumstances, and (b) amenable to control measures.

— Don't try to establish a sophisticated system from scratch, or request reports on the number cases of specific diseases actually diagnosed.

This minimizes the administrative demands on hard-pressed medical workers while providing enough information to prompt more specific investigations by epidemiological personnel when particular symptom complexes become prevalent.

A sample report form is provided in Figure 13/a. Such a report might be integrated with summary reports of nutrition status data and special (supplementary and therapeutic) feeding operations.

The central surveillance unit should:

— Present the appropriate decision-makers with a summary of the data, conclusions and specific recommendations for action; *and*

— Feed back summary data and conclusions to all reporting units.

In all situations, reports and information from *informal sources* should also be taken note of and be investigated to reassure the population (by defusing any unjustified rumours) and avoid other resources being diverted/expended unnecessarily.

Practical aspects

All health workers and medical teams must understand the importance of surveillance and therefore of submitting their own reports regularly—including zero returns when necessary rather than no report.

Give clear guidelines to health workers at each location on how and to whom (as well as when) to send their *reports*:

— Telephone, telex or radio may be used where available.

— Otherwise reports may be sent by hand of previously identified personnel (e.g. those involved in food distribution) who are touring.

— The schedule and deadlines established for the submission of reports must be enforced.

Ensure *staffing* of the central epidemiological unit by appropriately trained and experienced, national epidemiologists. Mobilize international assistance where needed to expedite the establishment of an appropriate system.

Figure 13/a

Sample form for epidemiological surveillance reporting

Health unit,
camp or   Report for
medical team: ....   the period: ....

Mortality data

	Less than 1 month	1-12 months	1-4 years	5-14 years	Adult	Total
Respiratory disease						
Diarrhoeal disease						
Malaria						
Measles						
Neonatal						
Maternal						
Other						
Total						

Morbidity data   [Number of new cases seen with the following as the major presenting condition: count each new case once only.]

Symptoms/clearly recognizable diseases	Number of new cases	Percentage of total
Fever, no cough		
Fever + cough (possible respiratory infections)		
Fever + chill (possibly malaria/dengue)		
Diarrhoea with blood		
Diarrhoea, no blood		
Malnutrition		
Dehydration		
Measles		
Eye infections		
Other significant medical problems:		
....		
....		
Total		100

Significant developments/changes affecting health conditions:

Signature: ....   Date: ....

(Adapted from PAHO ref. a, *UNHCR handbook for emergencies* and *Oxfam practical guide to refugee health care*.)

The epidemiological unit must have ready access to *transport and laboratory facilities* (possibly including WHO collaborating centres) in order to be able to respond promptly to any indications of disease outbreaks and to obtain definitive diagnoses.

Medical personnel specifically assigned to surveying and surveillance functions should, if at all possible, be able to refer cases requiring treatment to others and not be required to take responsibility for individual patients.

Possible UNICEF inputs

Depending on the assessment of actual needs and possibilities, some of the following inputs might be considered:

—Financing of expert epidemiological services (only if WHO, Red Cross or other medical assistance agencies are not able to do so).

—Transport.

—Laboratory equipment and supplies.

—Office supplies and local operating costs.

Further references

a. *Epidemiological surveillance after natural disaster*, K. Western, PAHO scientific publication No. 420—PAHO (1982) E/S
b. *Guide on emergency measures for the control of outbreaks of communicable disease*—WHO (1985) E (F/S/A to follow)
c. *Safety measures for use in outbreaks of communicable disease*—WHO (1985) E (F/S/A to follow)
    (Companion volume to "*Guide* ...", ref. b, above)

CONTAINING OUTBREAKS OF COMMUNICABLE DISEASE

Objective

- **To contain any epidemic outbreaks of communicable diseases as quickly as possible, and offer treatment to those infected.**

For measures to prevent outbreaks of communicable disease see Annexes 16-22 on water and sanitation aspects and Annex 23 on vector control.

When an outbreak has occured in a neighborouring country and can be expected to spread, measures should be taken in anticipation to deal with it.

Priorities

Actions required:
- —Epidemiological investigations;
- —Public health measures; *and*
- —Treatment for individual cases.

Any reports of epidemics must be quickly investigated to check diagnoses (through laboratory analyses and detailed examination of clinical descriptions and associated epidemiological factors) and the actual rates of incidence.

In outbreaks of exceptional magnitude/severity, special response measures may be needed including the assignment of additional medical and sanitation personnel and, possibly, the creation of a special task force responsible for containing the outbreak (if an appropriate inter-ministerial disease control body does not already exist).

Note: Epidemics of communicable disease can be precipitated by a variety of factors not necessarily connected with any other form of "disaster". However, disasters *may* create conditions favourable for the rapid spread of diseases which are already endemic in the areas.

Cholera

Preparedness

When outbreaks have occured in the region and can be expected to spread to a nearby country/area not yet affected—or in anticipation of the usual cholera season in areas where is it endemic—action should be taken to:

1. Strengthen surveillance, particularly along the routes of possible disease introduction and in cholera-receptive areas (characterized by overcrowding and unhygienic environments);
2. Improve water supply, excreta disposal and food safety measures, supported by health education;
3. (Re)Train health workers in clinical management of acute diarrhoeas including cholera;
4. (Re)Train laboratory workers in the detection of cholera vibrios; *and*
5. Assemble modest stockpiles of ORS, IV fluids, antibiotics, laboratory supplies and sanitation supplies, see Table 14/1.

Close co-ordination between the ministry of health, WHO, UNICEF, bilateral assistance, NGOs and other concerned agencies is essential.

During an outbreak

Priority must be given to:
—The prompt identification and treatment of individual cases;

283

Treatment supplies required during a cholera outbreak
*Requirements for 200 cases, typical for an outbreak in
a total population of 100,000.*

Rehydration supplies

240	litres Lactated Ringer with giving sets	(UNIPAC)
	= 480 sets of 0.5 litre each	(15-608-00)
10	disposable syringes 5-10 ml	(07-824-00)
10	needles 18G for adults	(07-490-00)
20	needles 22-24G for children	(07-505-00)
10	scalp-vein sets	(07-445-00)
10	naso-gastric tubes	(5 each 03-730-00 and 03-750-00)
1,300	pkts ORS (15-611-05 or locally produced), *or* bulk-packed ORS to make up 1,300 litres: see calculation Table 15/2.	

Antibiotics

For the treatment of cases:

3,200 caps Tetracycline, 250 mg (15-690-00) (16 caps/case)
and, for young children:
20 x 60ml btls Erythromycin syrup (15-463-00) *or* Sulfamethoxazole
+ trimethoprim syrup (15-371-05).

If chemoprophylaxis is planned, additional requirements for 5 close contacts per case (= 1,000 contacts) are: *either*

16,000 caps Tetracycline, 250 mg (16 caps/person) *and*
100 x 60 ml btls Erythromycin syrup *or* Sulfamethoxazole + trimethoprim syrup (for young children);
or 3,000 caps Doxycycline, 100 mg (3 caps/person) *and*
10 x 60 ml btls Doxycycline syrup.

Other treatment supplies

A field treatment facility treating 200 cases should also have:

2	large water dispensers with taps (marked at 5, 8, 10 litre intervals) for making ORS solution in bulk	
20	bottles (1 litre) ⎫ for ORS solution	(empty I.V. bottles
20	bottles (0.5 litre) ⎭	may be used)
40	tumblers, 200 ml	(20-950-00)
20	teaspoons	(20-867-00)
20	tablespoons	(20-865-00)
10	tubeclamps	(09-305-00)
3	kidney dishes	(02-110-00)
3	forceps	(07-210-00)
5	spirit lamps	(05-300-00)

plus: flashlights (2)—strong twine (1 reel)—cotton (5 kg)—alcohol (250ml)—adhesive tape (3 reels).

[The list has been agreed with WHO. It differs slightly from that in ref. e which is in the process of revision.]

—Public health measures—the improvement of water supplies, personal hygiene, sanitary disposal of excreta and food safety, supported by intensive health education; *and*

—Ensuring rapid in-country transport and distribution to community level of all needed supplies.

Mass vaccination is *not* useful with presently available vaccines. Chemoprophylaxis is recommended *only* for very close contacts of cholera patients and only if community health care is well developed and drug administration can be closely supervised. Distributing soap and organizing home visiting to ensure its frequent use and the best possible personal and domestic hygiene will be more beneficial and should have a higher priority than distributing drugs, especially when resources are not plentiful.

Cases should be treated near their homes to decrease spread of the disease. For this, appropriate training and supervision of community-level health workers and adequate (but not exaggerated) quantities of ORS should be assured. Intravenous rehydration may be required initially for about 20 per cent of cases.

Table 14/1 suggests the quantities of supplies which may be required to treat 200 cases, of which 40 (20 per cent) may intially require intravenous fluid. (ORS is required to follow on and also for the other 160 cases.) 200 is the number of cases which may be expected during an outbreak in a population of 100,000 in a cholera-receptive area.

Table 14/2 lists the other, complementary items which will be needed for diagnostic and public health purposes.

An attack rate of 0.2 per cent is typical in outbreaks in Asia. In Africa the rate may reach 1 per cent or more in some local situations, but 0.2 per cent remains valid for the wider population and as a basis for calculating requirements in the absence of any definite data to the contrary.

Other diseases

Shigellosis

Epidemics of shigellosis (bacterial dysentery) due to *Shigella dysenteriae 1* are increasing, particularly in Asia and Africa. Treatment of cases and public health measures, particularly personal and food hygiene, are the essential control measures. Hand washing with soap before handling food and after visits to the toilet is particularly important.

Treatment consists of oral rehydration plus appropriate antibiotics. Thorough laboratory tests are essential to determine which drugs should be used as certain **285**

Table 14/2

**Laboratory and public health supplies
required during a cholera outbreak**

Laboratory diagnostic supplies

1,000 rectal swabs (where not able to be produced locally);
500 g Cary-Blair medium;
3 x 300 g TCBS medium;
5 x 2ml Polyvalent cholera diagnostic antiserum.

Necessary nutrient agar (500 g), bacto-peptone (1 kg), glassware (500 petri dishes, 1,000 disposable bijou bottles) should already be available in a competent bacteriological laboratory.

Public health requirements

Sufficient disinfectant (e.g. cresol/lysol);
Sufficient chlorine chemicals for water treatment, see Tables 18/5 and 18/6, pp. 339, 340;
Water testing kits (5), orthotlidine with reserve solution.
Megaphones/portable loudspeakers (3), e.g. UNIPAC 18-450-00.

---

strains of shigella organisms are resistant to many antibiotics. The preferred drugs, if the local strain is not resistant to them are ampicillin (UNIPAC 15-050-75) and sulfamethoxazole + trimethoprim (15-371-00). Nalidixic acid has had to be used in some instances.)

Typhoid

Priority should be placed on public health measures especially food sanitation. Mass vaccination with currently available vaccine has not been found to be useful on account of reactions and consequent inacceptability. Drugs generally used for treatment are chloramphenicol (15-310-00) and sulfamethoxazole + trimethoprim (15-371-00).

Malaria

The need is for:

—Mosquito control;
—Individual treatment of fever cases (including access to referral centres for severe cases and treatment failures); *and*

—Laboratory facilities to confirm diagnoses and determine any drug resistances.

Mosquito control requires indoor and space spraying (see Annex 23) and, where possible, careful selection of camp sites and protection/screening of shelters.

Quinine perfusions may be needed to treat the most severe cases in referral centres with proper medical facilities.

The prophylactic use of drugs should normally be limited to pregnant women. However, more general prophylaxis *may* be considered for an initial period for non-immune populations displaced into malarial areas.

The likelihood of widespread malaria is reduced if people live 1km or more away from the breeding places of anopheles mosquitoes, especially surface water. The draining off of stagnant water is desirable but unlikely to be possible in the very short term.

Meningitis

In outbreaks of meningitis it is essential to determine the particular strain of the disease. Treatment of meningococcal meningitis is by a single injection of an oily suspension of chloramphenicol. (Treatment of pneumococcal meningitis which is endemic in many areas is with penicillin.)

Vaccination is effective in containing outbreaks of meningococcal A and C, but is very expensive and may be restricted to children (not less than 2 years) and young adults, with priority to those in the immediate contact groups of diagnosed cases. Prophylaxis of case contacts—using sulfonamides or other drugs depending on the strain—is much cheaper but may be less effective.

Vaccine should be given appropriate to the particular serogroup of the index case (frequently A in developing countries). If the particular serogroup has not yet been determined, group A + group C — or, better, A+C+Y+W135 — vaccine should be given provided one of these subgroups is known to have been prevalent in the community.

Measles and other common diseases

Mass vaccinations of children should be undertaken if at all possible in instances of epidemic measles and, possibly, yellow fever, polio, Japanese encephalitis.

Also ensure that parents are advised of the need to provide adequate food and water—and especially to continue breast-feeding—for sick and recovering children. These illnesses increase requirements and the practice of withholding food and fluid, traditional in many cultures, can prove lethal. **287**

For **measles,** all children 9-36 months should be vaccinated. Within this age range, a child may be excluded only if it is absolutely sure that he/she has already been *effectively* vaccinated. To be sure that any previous vaccination was indeed effective is it necessary to check the records/cards, cross-check the history with the mother (or other responsible adult), and be satisfied that (a) the vaccination was not given before 9 months and (b) the cold chain was operating efficiently at that time. Revaccination has no harmful side effects. Children diagnosed with measles may require vitamin A supplements, see Table 7/2, p. 240.

See Annex 15 concerning diarrhoeal diseases, and the referenced publications for other diseases.

Possible UNICEF inputs

The expertise and resources of WHO should normally be swiftly mobilized by the government. Where the health of children is directly at risk, some complementary inputs from UNICEF may be necessary. Depending on the assessment of actual needs and possibilities, some of the following inputs might be considered:

For cholera and shigellosis:
— Support to sanitary surveys and hygiene and sanitation measures (especially disposal of human excreta, provision of soap, disinfectant, etc.): see Annexes 20-22.
— Support to water supply improvement measures including chlorination: see Annexes 16-18.
— Support to rehydration therapy and provision of antibiotics: see Annex 15.
— Preparedness measures in areas into which current outbreaks elsewhere may spread.

For measles: (also yellow fever, polio, Japanese encephalitis where outbreaks are severe)
— Support to the immunization of young children. See Annex 12. In general, immediate needs will be able to be met by diverting supplies intended for the national EPI programme, but emergency immunization kits may be useful in situations where existing cold chain and other equipment is not immediately adequate.

For meningitis
— Vaccination and/or prophylactic drugs for children/young adults in close contact with cases.

For typhoid:
— Support for measures to improve water supply (including chlorination) and sanitation: see Annexes 16-22.

For malaria and typhus:
—Support to appropriate vector control measures: see Annex 23.

Plus, in most epidemics:
—Support for special "crash" training for health workers.
—Support for in-country transport and distribution of priority supplies, and personnel. Transport may be temporarily diverted from other programme purposes.
—Specifically focused health education programmes among the most vulnerable communities.
—Laboratory diagnostic supplies.
—Specific drugs required for treatment.

Where specific epidemics are common—virtually annual events—in particular localities, provision to respond to the predictable needs for assistance should be included in the regular UNICEF health programme budget and recourse be made to "emergency" assistance processes only if the epidemic takes on unusally major proportions or generates extraordinary needs.

Further references

General

a. *Guide on emergency measures for the control of outbreaks of communicable disease*— WHO (1986) E (F/S/A to follow)

b. *Safety measures for use in outbreaks of communicable disease*—WHO (1986) E (F/S/A to follow)
[Companion volume to "*Guide . . .* ", ref. a, above]

c. *Control of communicable diseases in man*, 14th edition, A. S. Benenson—American Public Health Association (1985) E/F

Enteric diseases

d. *Guide to simple sanitary measures for the control of enteric diseases*, S. Rajagopalan and M. Shiffman—WHO (1974) E/F/A

e. *Guidelines for cholera control*, WHO/CDD/SER/80.4—WHO (1984 being revised 1985) E/F

f. *Manual for laboratory investigators of acute enteric infections*—WHO (CDD 83.3) (1983) E/F

g. *Guidelines for co-operation in cholera control*, PRO/1985-007— UNICEF/PDPD Sept. 1985 E/F/S

Malaria

h. *Basic principles for the control of malaria and general guidelines for UNICEF/WHO support*—UNICEF/WHO joint statement—JC25/UNICEF-WHO/85.6 (1985) E (F expected 1986)

Meningitis

i. Report of the WHO working group on strategies for the control of epidemics of meningococcal infections, March 1983—WHO (BAC/CSM/84.3) E

289

PREVENTION AND TREATMENT OF DIARRHOEAL DISEASES

Objective

- **To reduce diarrhoeal disease morbidity and mortality in children.**

This is particularly important when water and/or food supplies have been disrupted, or people displaced and in crowded conditions. For response to outbreaks (epidemics) of cholera, see Annex 14.

Methods and principles

Prevention of diarrhoea

General communal measures which can reduce the incidence and spread of diarrhoeal diseases are summarized in Table 15/1. Specific water and sanitation measures are described in Annexes 16-22.

Treatment of diarrhoea and prevention of dehydration

During an attack of acute diarrhoea, dehydration can be prevented by an appropriate, immediate response by the parents to:
- —Maintain breast-feeding;
- —Maintain or increase the intake of normal fluids; *and*
- —Give the child additional home-prepared fluids: rice water—thin gruels of available cereals (e.g. sorghum)—vegetable soups—sugar and salt solutions (if sugar is available).

Anti-diarrhoeal drugs are entirely inappropriate. Antibiotics should be used only in cases of bloody dysenteries—shigellosis (see p. 285) and amoebiasis (for which metronidazole is required)—and cholera.

Treatment of dehydration

If a child becomes dehydrated, adequate rehydration can prevent death. In the vast majority of cases, *oral rehydration*—using Oral Rehydration Salts (ORS) disolved in clean water and administered using a cup, or cup and spoon—is possible and sufficient. Solutions must be prepared fresh each day.

Table 15/1

Communal measure to reduce morbidity due to diarrhoeal diseases

- ☐ Promotion of breast-feeding (which has a specific and considerable protective effect);
- ☐ Sound feeding practices, especially at weaning;
- ☐ Timely vaccination against measles (but not cholera);
- ☐ Clean drinking water supplies;
- ☐ Environmental sanitation, especially disposal of faeces;
- ☐ Personal hygiene, especially hand-washing with soap after using latrine and before preparing food;
- ☐ Hygienic food preparation and storage;
- ☐ Eating cooked food while it is still hot; *and*
- ☐ Relevant health and nutrition education.

Figure 15/a **A severely dehydrated child**

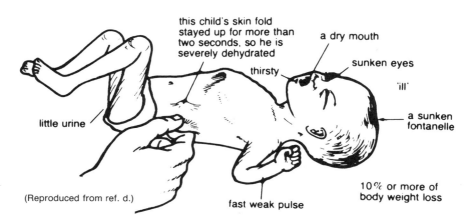

this child's skin fold stayed up for more than two seconds, so he is severely dehydrated

a dry mouth

sunken eyes

thirsty

'ill'

little urine

a sunken fontanelle

(Reproduced from ref. d.)

fast weak pulse

10% or more of body weight loss

If the child is vomiting, ORS should still be given (slowly in sips) either by cup and spoon or by naso-gastric tube. The child will normally retain more fluid than is vomitted out.

In only a very small number (less than 5 per cent) of cases, *severe* dehydration leads to shock and the child is unable to drink. The *intravenous* administration of fluids is then the surest treatment but ORS can, as an emergency measure, also be administered—under medical supervision—using a naso-gastric tube.

If a child has collapsed, is vomiting very severely and persistently and/or there are other serious complications, the administration of I.V. fluids is necessary. Adequate skilled nursing care and inpatient facilities must be available.

N.B. The above applies to cases of cholera as well as other cases of acute diarrhoeas: see Annex 14. The provision and administration of I.V. fluids costs more than 50 times as much as treatment by ORS.

A dropper may be used to introduce oral solution into the mouths of very small babies. If an infant is habituated to bottle feeding and rejects a spoon, it may be necessary to give ORS solution using a feeding bottle initially—to save the child's life without resorting to naso-gastric tubes or I.V. fluids. Education of the mother and replacement of the bottle should follow.

Estimating ORS requirements

Obtain local estimates for:

292   —The percentage of children under 5 years in the total population;

—The average number of episodes requiring ORS per child every 3 months;
—The proportion of cases expected to receive ORS from health services; *and*
—Probable wastage rates for packets.

Table 15/2 provides examples of calculations of the quantities of ORS which might be required.

1 episode every 3 months and 20 per cent of cases receiving ORS are typical in many endemic situations, but higher or lower figures may be appropriate in some communities. Requirements are likely to be very much higher in camp situations, especially due to higher coverage.

For outbreaks of cholera, only a small, additional quantity of ORS is required to treat cholera patients over and above the "normal" requirement for diarrhoea in the community.

Table 14/1 indicates the supplies necessary for intravenous rehydration. In cases of severe dehydration not involving cholera, antibiotics are not required; the other quantities remain applicable for 40 cases initially requiring I.V. fluids.

Practical and policy aspects

A definite policy must be agreed (nationally if possible) concerning the level of health services to receive ORS packets. In general it is appropriate to:

—Promote the use of home-made solutions by mothers to prevent dehydration and treat cases which remain mild at home using ingredients available in the household;
—Provide ORS for use in treating dehydration by trained community health workers and in health centres and in hospitals.

(The use of ORS packets in the home is neither necessary nor feasible in most countries.)

Train all levels of health workers in the use of both home-prepared solutions and ORS: include doctors as well as all levels of nurses and para-medical workers who have not already had such training.

Educate mothers to:

—Prepare and use home-prepared fluids as soon as diarrhoea starts;
—Recognize a few signs of dehydration; *and*
—Seek the help of a community health worker when the signs appear or if diarrhoea continues.

Identify a local container (of 1 litre or another appropriate size) for measuring the volume of water and provide instructions for the preparation of ORS in those **293**

Table 15/2

Examples of calculations of ORS requirements

In a "normal" community situation

The need is mainly for children under 5 years. On average, 2 packets of ORS are needed to treat a child. ORS requirements *for a 3-month period* can therefore be roughly estimated as follows—assuming there is a good programme to use the packets:

Total population (e.g. 100,000)
x Percentage of children under 5 in the total (say 17 per cent)
x Number of episodes per child every 3 months requiring ORS (say 1)
x Percentage of cases expected to receive packets (say 20 per cent)
x 2 packets per episode
x 1.10 (= +10 per cent) for wastage
= Total number of packets needed every 3 months.
100,000 x 0.17 x 1 x 0.20 x 2 x 1.10) = 7,480
say 7,500

In camps of displaced persons

Proportion of children under 5 in the total population may be abnormal (say 25 per cent).
Number of episodes per child every 3 months is often higher than "normal" (say 2).
Percentage of cases expected to receive packets may be high (say 75 per cent).
2 packets per episode.
Wastage less than "normal" (say 5 per cent thus multiply by 1.05).

For such a camp population totalling 100,000 the requirement for 3 months may then be:

(100,000 x 0.25 x 2 x 0.75 x 2 x 1.05) = 78,750 packets
say 80,000

In outbreaks of cholera (*see Table 14/1*)

0.2 per cent of the total population in an area is typically afflicted in a severe outbreak.
Coverage of cases may be very high (say 100 per cent) in a camp situation but very much lower among a scattered population.
On average, 6 packets of ORS are required to treat each case.

Thus for a (camp) population of 100,000 the *additional* requirement for dealing with the outbreak (assuming 10 per cent wastage) may be:

(100,000 x 0.002 x 1.00 x 6 x 1.10) = 1,320 packets
say 1,300

terms. Ensure the use of the best available drinking water in both home-prepared and ORS solutions.

To the extent possible, arrange for daily checks by health workers of children being treated at home.

Organize public education on diarrhoea prevention as part of overall health and nutrition education. Use community structures, media, religious and women's organizations, etc. in addition to the person-to-person efforts by doctors and nurses when providing treatment.

Possible UNICEF inputs

Depending on the assessment of actual needs and possibilities, some of the following inputs might be considered:

For oral rehydration therapy:

—ORS (UNIPAC 15-611-05 or locally produced)

—Naso-gastric tubes (UNIPAC 03-730-00 and 03-750-00)

—Measuring jugs, water containers, cups, spoons, stirrers, cleaning materials, etc.

—Support for (a) training of health workers and (b) health/nutrition education of mothers and the community in general.

N.B. Avoid overestimating the material requirements—e.g. the number of ORS packets (see Table 15/2)—and underestimating the training, education and logistic needs.

For intravenous rehydration:

—Small quantities of fluids and complementary supplies as indicated in Table 14/1 may be supplied to meet the needs of those cases which cannot be treated using ORS and for which there are facilities and staff able to properly administer I.V. fluids.

Further references

a. *Treatment and prevention of acute diarrhoea — Guidelines for the trainers of health workers*—WHO (1985)   E/F

b. *A manual for the treatment of acute diarrhoea — for physicians and other senior health workers*, WHO/CDD/SER/80.2 Rev.1—WHO (1984)   E/F

c. The treatment of diarrhoea and the use of oral rehydration therapy—Joint WHO/UNICEF statement (1983)   E/F/S

d. *Primary child care: Book 1—a manual for health workers,* M. & F. King, S. Martodipoero—Oxford University Press/WHO (1981)   E

295

DISTRIBUTION AND STORAGE OF WATER

Objective

- **To conserve and protect available supplies, and make reasonably safe water accessible to community services and all population groups.**

Table 14, p. 85 provides guidelines for estimating the quantities of water required.

Priorities

- **Restoring/providing supplies to and within hospitals, other health facilities and premises being used for special feeding programmes has the highest priority.**

- **Access to other available supplies must be shared as equitably as possible between all community groups and households.**

Special attention to the distribution and storage of water is necessary whenever:

—Existing piped distribution systems have been damaged and/or contaminated;

—Traditional sources are no longer usable and supplies are available only at some distance from the people; *or*

—Displaced persons are concentrated in small areas.

Action is then required to:

—Inventory available sources of supply, storage and distribution capacities—their location, quantity and quality—and estimate requirements in each area;

—Minimize waste and possibilities for contamination of available supplies;

—Make at least minimum quantities of reasonably safe water accessible to people where they live; *and*

—Warn people of the dangers of using particular sources and supplies which are known to be unsafe.

Wherever water supplies cannot be assumed to be safe, immediate action to provide adequate capacity to store water and therefore improve its quality—at distribution points and/or in households—is a logical first step.

If large numbers of people have to be served from a small number of sources:

—Feed/deliver water into storage tanks;

—Provide appropriate means for users to draw off water—probably through rows of taps; *and*

—Prevent access to the sources themselves by individual consumers.

The larger the number of people using a single source or outlet, the greater the risk of pollution and damage. Table 16/1 provides guidelines for setting up temporary storage and distribution points.

Consider delivering water by truck only as a very short-term, temporary measure.

Waste water

To reduce health hazards and maximise the benefit in situations where supplies are short, repair/construct channels or pipes to drain waste water away from distribution points, household and communal services to soakage pits or tanks (or lined pits) from which it can be recycled—e.g. for watering livestock, irrigating crops/vegetable gardens (if not soapy), or use in flush latrines.

Municipal (piped) systems

If piped systems have been *damaged,* ensure rapid action to:

— Isolate the damaged sections to minimize losses/waste and prevent pollution seeping into the whole system;

— Provide sufficient supplies for all communities through standpipes wherever possible;

— In localities where a piped system has been totally disrupted, deliver necessary minimum/survival supplies by truck for a few days until sufficient stand pipes can be restored/established;

— Make whatever immediate/temporary repairs are possible with the materials and expertise on hand; *and then*

— Organize detailed surveys to prepare plans and estimates for complete rehabilitation.

Remember that communities on high ground will always get less water than those lower down, especially if pumping in the system is intermittent.

If the system has been *contaminated,* and also after any repairs (temporary or permanent) have been made, ensure disinfection of the sections concerned by:

— Increasing the pressure in the system as a whole (if possible); *and*

— Increasing the residual chlorine content in the water (assuming a chlorination treatment facility exists).

In all cases, ensure the availability and the effective organization of necessary equipment and personnel (including a functioning public health laboratory) to:

— Monitor the water quality at delivery points; *and*

— Respond quickly when any breakdowns, leaks or contamination are discovered.

Locations lacking infrastructure

If previous sources are usable or able to be rehabilitated quickly and demands have not increased, restore *pre-existing* arrangements for distribution. During the emergency phase, changes/improvements should only be attempted if the necessary materials and manpower are readily available and the restoration of supplies—of a quality not worse than that to which the population was previously accustomed—will not be further delayed.

298 *New* arrangements for distribution and storage may be necessary when output from existing sources has to be substantially increased and/or new sources be developed (see Annex 17) because:

—Some previously used sources are no longer available or not yielding sufficient water; *or*

—An enlarged population has to be served.

Table 16/1

Temporary water storage and distribution points

The storage *capacity* required at each distribution point depends on the number of people to be served and the frequency of deliveries. Assuming 20 litres/person/day, 1,000 litres provides for 50 people if filled once a day; 100 people if filled twice daily, etc.

3-4,000 litres (3-4 cubic metres) galvanized steel tanks are often suitable and available locally. Otherwise it may be necessary to obtain collapsible rubber/PVC tanks (by flying them in if absolutely necessary).

Tanks should be mounted on raised platforms or mounds so that water can be drawn off from the bottom. Collapsible tanks must be on level surfaces free of glass or sharp stones and surrounded by a barrier to prevent rolling.

Users' containers must *never* be dipped into tanks. Tanks should be covered and taps be installed either directly in the tank or on pipes leading from it. There should, if possible, be one tap for every 200-250 users, and an ample stock of replacement taps. As a last resort only, a single, clean "captive" container may be provided to be dipped into a tank (as for an open well).

Screw-type and push taps are frequently broken or jammed. Self-closing valve taps have proved reliable: those made in India are inexpensive— $3.40 excluding freight in 1985. Ask UNIPAC for details, delivery possibilities and current prices.

Collapsible tanks are available from UNIPAC—5,000 litres UNIPAC 56-750-00; 1,500 litres UNIPAC 56-750-01. They can sometimes be obtained as donations in-kind from governments. OXFAM can supply tanks complete with distribution systems. Ask EOU and UNIPAC for further advice.

To disinfect a tank:
1. Half fill the tank with water;
2. Pour in 1 litre of 1 percentage chlorine solution for every 100 litres of tank capacity: see Table 18/5, p. 331.
3. Fill the tank up with water.
4. Leave for 12 hours.
5. Drain off and discard the water.

If the water is of good quality at source but needs to be brought closer to the population: deliver it through watertight pipes into storage tanks at suitable distribution points, if possible. Table 16/2 provides some guidelines concerning pipes.

If water is of poor quality or moved in open channels: store, filter and/or chemically treat it at the distribution point to make it safe for domestic use (see Annex 18).

In areas liable to flooding during the rainy season, or where the source is a river of which the level may vary markedly during the expected period of use, ensure that

Table 16/2

Pipes for small-scale distribution systems

Bamboo may be able to be used for short-term/temporary installations. Otherwise plastic pipes are usually the cheapest, light to transport and easiest to lay. They are available in lengths of coiled, flexible pipe up to a diameter of 100mm, or in rigid lengths.

The *diameter* of pipes needed depends on the required flow rates, the length of the pipeline, any rise and fall on the route, and whether gravity-fed or pumped. It should be calculated by experts. The figures below, extracted from ref. a, provide only a general indication for a gravity-fed system:

Pipe diameters in mm.

Flow rate (ltr/sec)	Steel		Bamboo		Plastic (PVC)	
	Flat	Steep	Flat	Steep	Flat	Steep
0.10	19	19	25	19	19	12
0.20	25	19	32	25	19	19
0.40	32	25	37	32	25	25
0.60	37	32	50	32	32	25
0.80	50	32	50	37	37	32
1.00	50	37	62	50	37	32
2.00	62	50	76	62	50	37
3.00	62	50	76	62	62	50

"Flat" = pipes sloping at less than 1:15 (7 %) but more than 1:50 (2 %).
"Steep" = pipes sloping at more than 1:15 (7%) but less than 1:5 (20%).

If the system is expected to be used for an extended period, pipes should be buried for protection, and sections of the system should have isolating valves. If pipes cannot be buried, galvanized iron pipes must be used.

Joints must be watertight. If there are leaks, pollution will be sucked in when pressure drops or the system is turned off.

See p. 339 and *Guide list OLGA* for further details.

all pumps, storage and treatment systems are located above the highest water level which might be anticipated.

Consider deliveries by truck only as a last resort, and only for as long as it takes to pipe water in, develop other sources, or move the population.

A typical water tanker of capacity 8,000 litres carries sufficient water to meet the normal minimum requirements—15 l/day/person—of only 530 people for just one day, or the survival requirements for drinking alone—3 l/day/person—of 2,700 people for one day. Attempts to truck in water for large numbers of people are likely to be extremely expensive, or quite impracticable.

Delivering water by truck

Where there is no alternative to *temporary* truck deliveries:
- —Mobilize suitable tankers;
- —Establish temporary storage/distribution tanks at strategic locations;
- —Chlorinate water in the tankers; *and*
- —Schedule deliveries according to carefully determined priorities.

Water tankers may be available with the military, fire services, dairies or bottled drink factories including breweries. It is difficult to adequately clean petrol and oil tankers. If suitable tanker trucks cannot be found, place steel or collapsible tanks on ordinary trucks. Secure them firmly: for collapsible tanks use strong webbing or nets. 1 cubic metre (1,000 litres) of water weighs 1 metric ton.

Static tanks should be set up at the selected distribution points so that trucks do not have to wait while individuals collect their needs/rations: see Table 16/1.

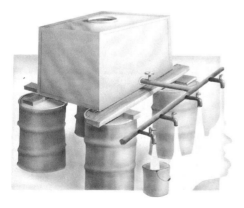

Figure 16/a

A temporary water distribution point

Trucks must carry pumps to deliver water into the static tanks (unless the trucks can deliver from a higher level than the tanks so that gravity feed is possible).

After community services, priority must be given to delivering supplies to public distribution points. No deliveries to private/domestic tanks should be permitted until the demand for water at public distribution points is fully satisfied.

People with their own transport should be encouraged to collect water from the more distant sources so that quantities delivered to local distribution points remain for the less priviledged members of the community.

Water for such operations may be drawn from: usual municipal sources if still usable and quantities are sufficient—tubewells belonging to industrial establishments or other institutions—surface water as a last resort while other sources are being developed.

Providing for institutions

Ensure adequate, safe supplies from:
- —Any existing municipal system;
- —The institution's own well—pre-existing or newly constructed; *and/or*
- —The pumping and careful treatment of river water.

Deliveries by truck may be necessary on an emergency basis while other arrangements are made.

Arrange for the rapid repair of internal, piped water distribution systems within hospitals and health centres, including necessary pumps and the power sources for them. Generators may be needed until normal electric power supplies are resumed.

Possible UNICEF inputs

Depending on the assessment of actual needs and possibilities, some of the following inputs might be considered:
- —Expertise to help to plan and implement appropriate arrangements: sanitarians and practical water supply engineers.
- —Spare parts and other materials for emergency repairs to piped water distribution systems serving hospitals, other health facilities and special feeding centres.

—Water tanks, pumps, pipes, pipe fittings, solvents for plastic pipe joints, pipe cutting and other tools, etc. to establish emergency storage and distribution arrangements for communities.

—Funds for the operations of trucks for emergency deliveries to community services and particularly needy communities (where there is no immediate alternative).

—Supplies and other support for water testing and treatment operations: see Annex 19.

Further references

a.   *Small water supplies,* S. Cairncross and R. Feachem, Ross Bulletin No. 10—Ross Institute, London (1978).   E

b.   *Guide to simple sanitary measures for the control of enteric diseases,* S. Rajagopalan and M. Shiffman—WHO (1974).   E/F/A

c.   *Guide list OLGA*—UNICEF (1975).   E

d.   Manufacturers' catalogues (available from UNIPAC: see catalogue).

ANNEX 17

WATER SOURCES
(EXPLOITATION AND REHABILITATION)

Objectives

- **To ensure the availability on a continuous basis of (a) sufficient safe water for hygiene and domestic use, and (b) adequate water for livestock and community level food production.**

This includes the operation and maintenance of the systems installed to raise/ deliver the water as well as the development of sources themselves.

N.B. Insufficient water can be more detrimental to health than slight contamination. Apart from potentially fatal dehydration when daily intake is insufficient to replace moisture lost from the body, parasitic, fungal and other skin diseases, eye infections and diarrhoeal diseases all increase when bodies, clothes and cooking utensils cannot be properly cleaned, and food not be adequately prepared.

Choosing sources

Table 17/1 (next page) lists possible sources and some of the main considerations regarding their use:

- Rain and ground water from natural springs or deep wells—when adequately protected—is usually microbiologically safe.
- Surface water is unlikely to be safe: water in ponds and lakes (i.e. not flowing) is often grossly polluted.

Shallow wells often deliver filtered surface water; sometimes they tap ground-water sources.

Rehabilitate and increase the yield of previously established sources if possible before seeking new ones. Remove any sources of pollution (especially latrines) that may be within 30 m.

If new sources are necessary:

- Thorough surveys and/or reliable existing data are essential before resources (time and funds) are committed to digging or drilling for ground water.
- If new sources are needed and ground water is known to be available, the choice of method of exploiting it depends on the depth of the water table, yield, soil conditions and the availability of expertise and equipment.
- If new wells are to be sunk, they should be at least 30 m away—preferably uphill—from any sanitation facilities or other obvious sources of possible pollution. (Very deep borewells may be excepted.)

Figure 17/a suggests the main criteria involved in determining how available sources may be exploited. Table 17/2 lists the aspects to consider in choosing between alternative sources and means of exploitation.

Table 17/2

Criteria for choosing between alternative sources

- ☐ Speed with which sources can be made operational;
- ☐ Potential yields;
- ☐ Reliability of supply (taking into account seasonal variations and, if necessary, logistics);
- ☐ Water purity, risk of pollution and ease of treatment if necessary;
- ☐ Simplicity of technology and ease of maintenance;
- ☐ Costs; *and*
- ☐ In the case of displaced populations, the rights and welfare of the local, indigenous population.

Table 17/1

Water sources and their utilization

Source	Treatment	Extraction	Distribution	Remarks
Rain	Unnecessary if catchment and receptacles clean.	Channelling off suitable roofs and/or hard ground.	Collection directly at household or institutional level	Useful as supplementary source of safe water in certain seasons.
Ground water				
Natural spring	Unnecessary if properly protected.	Simple gravity flow; preferably piped from a protective "box".	Individual collection directly, via storage tanks or gravity-fed distribution system.	Source must be protected; yield may vary seasonally.
Deep well (low water table)	Unnecessary if properly located, constructed and maintained.	Handpump possible if water table less than 60 m deep and output required is low, otherwise motor pumps necessary.	Individually pumped by hand, or motor pumped to storage tanks, possibly linked to distribution systems.	Yield unlikely to vary much with seasons unless prolonged drought. Special construction equipment and expertise required. High yields often possible.
Shallow well (high water table)	Unnecessary if properly located, constructed and maintained.	Hand pump or hand drawn container.	Pumped or drawn directly from wells by individuals.	Yield may vary seasonally; can be dug/drilled by local skilled labour. Care needed to avoid pollution.
Surface water				
Flowing (stream, river)	Often necessary: sedimentation, filtration and/or chlorination.	Preferably pumped to storage and treatment tanks.	Individual collection preferably from storage/treatment tanks.	Yield may vary seasonally; access to source should be controlled.
Standing (lake, pond)	Always necessary, as above.	As above.	As above.	As above.

(Adapted from the UNHCR *Handbook for Emergencies*)

Sea water can be used for almost everything but drinking and irrigation, thus reducing fresh water requirements. Desalination is not a feasible means of providing fresh water in an emergency. If there are no fresh water sources, the population may have to be moved.

Rain water

If other sources of safe water are limited, organize the collection of as much rain water as possible. Reasonably pure rain water can be collected if:

— The roofs of buildings (not thatch) or tents are clean and guttering in place; *and*

— Appropriate collection and storage containers (e.g. plastic, glass or earthenware pots but preferably not metal) are available to households and institutions.

Allow the first rain after a long dry spell to run off, thus cleaning the catchment of loose dirt.

In some situations it may be possible to collect and store rain water which runs off hard ground during heavy storms:

— Dig pits (or build small dams) in suitable locations and line them with polythene.

— Keep them covered if possible when not directly receiving rain.

Rain water can be a major source only in areas and during periods when there is adequate and reliable rainfall, but it can be:

— A useful source of safe water, for both household and institutional use, during

Table 17/3

Estimating potential for rainwater collection

One millimetre of rainfall on one square metre of roofed area gives 0.8 litres on average, after allowing for evaporation.

Thus, if the roofed area measures 3 m x 4 m and the rainfall which might, on average, be expected during a particular month is 120 mm, the amount of rain water which might be collected in that month is:

$$3 \times 4 \times 120 \times 0.8 = 1,152 \text{ litres}$$

i.e. an average of about 38 litres per day—sufficient to meet the survival needs of 8 people, or the normal minimum requirements of 2-3 people.

(The rainfall may, of course, not be spread evenly throughout the month and, if the rains fail, there could be none).

the rainy season when surface water is particularly likely to be contaminated (i.e. at a time when other water is plentiful but unsafe).

—A useful supplement to general needs at any time: e.g. through special collection for community services—such as health and feeding centres—where the safety of water is most important.

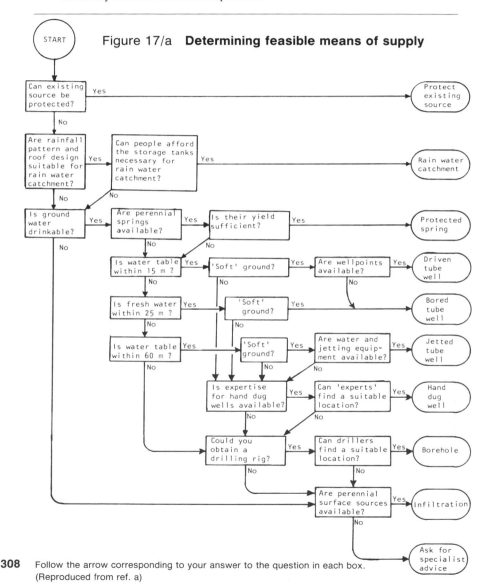

Figure 17/a **Determining feasible means of supply**

308 Follow the arrow corresponding to your answer to the question in each box. (Reproduced from ref. a)

Natural springs

Spring water is usually pure at the source and can be piped—often by gravity feed—to storage and distribution points. The locations of springs are normally known to the local population: they are typically indicated by a concentration of vegetation greener than most of the surroundings.

Protecting and exploiting springs

Check the true source: some apparent springs may really be surface water which has seeped or flowed into the ground a short distance away.

Draw water off at the source itself, if possible. Otherwise prevent any human activity or animal grazing between the source and the take-off point.

Protect the source itself against pollution:

—Construct a simple "box"—of bricks, stones or concrete—dug into the ground which encloses and covers the source, and from which the water flows directly through a pipe to a tank or collection point nearby: see Figure 17/b. See refs. a, d, f, for further, practical details.

—Fence off the source wherever possible and place the delivery point outside the fence.

Disinfect any source which has been polluted and any "box" which has been repaired or constructed:

—Scrub the box with 2-3 bucketsful of a strong chlorine solution: see Table 17/7, p. 318; *then*

Figure 17/b **Protection of a natural spring source by a "box"**

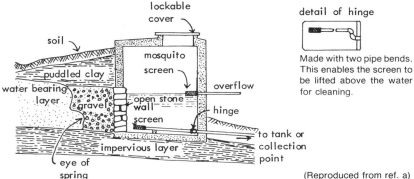

detail of hinge

Made with two pipe bends. This enables the screen to be lifted above the water for cleaning.

Table 17/4

Characteristics of different types of well constructions

Type of well	Approximate maximum depth	Technique	Comments	
Driven tube well	10-15 m	Pipe with special tip is hammered into ground. Can be sunk in 1-2 days.	Small. Cannot be sunk in heavy clay soil or rock. Needs special filter "well point" at tip of pipe.	Driven tube well / well point
Auger-bored tube well	25 m	Hole bored by hand using a suitable auger (different augers for different soils). Can be sunk in 2-3 days.	Larger than driven tube well. Augers may need to be imported but locally available boring tools can often be used.	Bored hole well / auger
Hand dug well	30-40 m	Requires skilled workers otherwise dangerous. Speed depends on soil conditions: 2-10 metres per week for a team of 4-8 men	Needs no pump, but easily contaminated by mis-use or if workmanship is poor. Convenient where such wells are traditional and other equipment/materials lacking.	Hand dug well
Jetted tube	80 m	Water is pumped down the well pipe to loosen and carry solid back up out of the hole thus enabling the pipe to be driven further down.	Process of sinking requires much water. Can be done by hand in delta areas with little equipment but skilled labour; otherwise special drilling equipment needed.	Jetted tube well
Drilled tube well (borehole)	Over 100 m	Large mechanized drilling rig. Several days depending on soil/rock conditions.	Expensive equipment requiring skilled operators, good maintenance, sufficient tools and fuel, and efficient logistic support.	Borehole

The yield potential of a well depends on the geological formation in which it is sunk, the contours and gradients of the land, the well construction. Actual output up to that maximum depends on the pump. If wells are sited too close together, yields will be reduced.

(Table adapted from UNHCR *Handbook for Emergencies*, sketches from ref. a.)

—Let it flow until the residual chlorine level drops and the water is acceptable to taste.

Estimating yield of a spring source

If water is delivered from the source through a pipe, simply use a watch to determine how long it takes to fill a calibrated container (e.g. a 1-litre jug or 10-litre bucket). See ref. a for alternative methods.

N.B. The yield may vary widely with the seasons. It will be at its minimum at the end of the dry season.

Tube wells

Methods for sinking tube wells depend on the depth of the water table and the soil conditions above it: see Figure 17/a and Table 17/4.

In all cases, a concrete apron at least 2 metres in diameter and sloping down towards the outside all round is necessary to prevent any waste or other surface water seeping into and contaminating the well. See Figure 17/c. A gutter (shallow trench) should drain waste water away to a gravel/stone-filled soakage pit, or animal trough.

Equipment and materials required

The construction of tube wells requires:
- —Drilling equipment appropriate to the soil conditions, depth of water table, and technical expertise available;
- —Pipes and well screens of appropriate sizes;
- —Pumps: see Annex 19; *and*
- —Construction materials: adequate quantities of cement—sand—gravel—bricks/stones—reinforcing rods—shuttering—etc. to make the well head.

Pipes are normally of steel (with treaded joints between sections) or PVC (with either threaded or glued joints). Bamboo may be able to be used, on a temporary basis, in some situations.

Well screens are commonly made of brass or PVC but improvisation with bamboo may be possible—plug the bottom and cut many narrow slots into the sides.

Figure 17/c **Typical tube-well (with a driven point)**

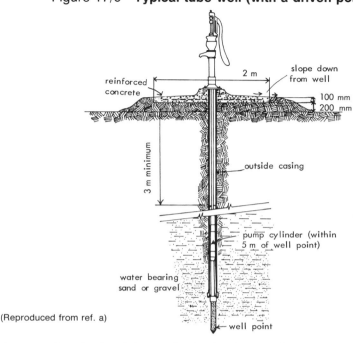

reinforced concrete

2 m

slope down from well

100 mm
200 mm

3 m minimum

outside casing

pump cylinder (within 5 m of well point)

water bearing sand or gravel

(Reproduced from ref. a)

well point

Any new tubewell or borehole must first be "developed" to full yield by an initial period of pumping at a fast rate. This has the effect of pumping out finer soil particles, thus allowing water to pass more easily into the well.

If the site is liable to flooding in the rainy season, design the installation accordingly—e.g. provide a raised platform or a flexible connection from a raft to a sealed well head and install a submersible electric pump.

Rehabilitation of tube wells

Tube wells may be damaged/polluted by: physical damage to the well head and pumping installation—and/or contamination by polluted water entering through a damaged well head or an inadequate apron. They may also dry up, partially or completely, if ground-water conditions change.

For the repair/replacement of **pumps**, ensure sufficient, appropriate spare parts, tools, transport and mechanics.

If the tube well itself has been **damaged** or **blocked** with debris:

312   —It is sometimes possible to withdraw the pipe and screen and intall replacements in the same hole: an appropriate hoist is needed as well as replacement pipes, joints and screens, and materials to reconstruct the apron.

—Frequently, however, a new well will have to be sunk nearby, or an alternative source be found.

If water has become **contaminated**:

—This can sometimes be cleared by rapid pumping over an extended period and washing out the pump itself with a strong chlorine solution: see Table 17/7, p. 318.

—Alternatively, 3 buckets of strong chlorine solution may be poured into the well tube, left for some hours and then pumped out.

—Repair/replace the concrete apron around the well head and improve the drainage to a soakage pit as necessary.

—Thoroughly wash out and disinfect any storage and distribution system connected to the well.

Test the water to see if the pumping/disinfection has succeeded. If not, try to determine and remove the cause of the pollution.

Deepening/enlargement of tube-wells

If the yield from a well has fallen, try to redevelop the well by fast pumping. If this fails—or if contamination has not been cleared by other efforts—try to deepen the well. If the existing pipes can be withdrawn, the same hole may be deepened by whatever means/equipment is available and appropriate to the soil conditions. Otherwise construct a new well nearby.

If more water is needed than is presently able to be pumped, and if test pumping shows greater yield to be possible:- withdraw the existing pipes, if possible, then rebore, sink a larger diameter pipe and install a larger capacity pump or additional handpumps.

Construction of new tube wells

Before investing hope or resources in any drilling operations:- check existing hydrogeological data or organize necessary surveys to confirm whether water of acceptable quality is likely to be present with worthwhile yields in the localities concerned.

When drilling *is* to be undertaken, ensure all necessary inputs including: technical expertise—skilled labour—tools—equipment—pipes—screens—pumps—transport—funds for operating expenses.

Where deep ground water is being sought: organize rapid test drilling (using rotary rigs) where survey data is encouraging—immediately develop those "exploratory" holes which yield adequate water into production wells (by enlarging the hole and installing the necessary lining, well pipes and pumping mechanisms).

Hand-dug wells

Hand dug wells can satisfactorily meet the requirements of very large populations in some circumstances, e.g. more than a million Afghan refugees in Pakistan 1982/3.

Depending on the soil conditions, wells may be dug to as much as 40 metres in depth. Experienced, skilled labour must be mobilized, especially for operations below 5 m depth: see also Table 17/5.

Table 17/5

Precautions when digging/deepening hand-dug wells

For depths greater than 5 m, ensure:
— The provision and use of safety ropes, and the capability at all times to evacuate workers from the bottom of the well;
— Sufficient light using mirrors and flashlights; *and*
— Adequate aeration/ventilation of the well before workers descend and while they work.

Where it is necessary to continuously pump water out of a well ("de-watering"), use an electric or preferably compressed-air-operated pump, with the generator or compressor well away from the well. Never use a petrol or diesel motor inside a well.

Raising and lowering a large bunch of leaves inside the well for some time may be sufficient to purge the air within many wells.

For very deep wells and any where there is a risk of toxic fumes entering the well (and accumulating at the bottom):
— Lower a lighted candle first: if it goes out there is excessive carbon dioxide in the well which must therefore be ventilated before anyone descends; *and*
— Ensure continuous aeration using a fan or suitable compressor (with a oil filter fitted on the air supply) to pump fresh air down to the bottom of the well.

Wells should be *lined*—with stone, bricks or reinforced concrete—for at least the first 3 m below ground level to prevent surface water entering the well and to prevent the sides caving in. In sand/gravel soils the lining should extend to 6 m depth.

Water may be raised by various mechanical devices, but most commonly it is hand-drawn using buckets or similar containers on the end of a rope. Figure 17/d and Table 17/6 suggest measures to minimize risks of pollution.

If large numbers of people need to use a single well, it is best to cover it and install a pump: see Figure 17/e.

The final deepening of any dug well should take place at the end of the dry season when the water table is at its lowest level. A 20-cm layer of coarse sand/gravel placed at the bottom of a well helps to filter out sediment.

Rehabilitation of dug wells

Open, dug wells may be damaged/polluted by: collapse of the lining and/or headwall—contamination by flood water or other surface water seeping in through a damaged well head or lining—contamination by debris (and possibly bodies) falling in. They may also dry up, partially or completely, if ground-water conditions change.

Figure 17/d   Typical dug well intallation

HOIST ARRANGEMENTS SHOULD AVOID DRAWERS LEANING OVER WELL (E.G PULLEY OR ROLLERS).

HEADWALL HIGH ENOUGH TO PREVENT CONTAMINATION, NARROW ENOUGH NOT TO BE STOOD ON.

SIMPLE WOODEN WINDLASS CLOSE TO HEADWALL MAY BE USEFUL — CHECK LOCAL PRACTICE.

SURFACE WATER RUN-OFF IN RAINY AREAS.

WIDE AND IMPERVIOUS SLOPING APRON TO AVOID MUD, & STAGNANT WATER (DRAINING TO SOAKAWAY OR DITCH).

SIDES SEALED FOR 3 M BELOW GROUND.

SINGLE PUBLIC TETHERED CONTAINER : USE OF INDIVIDUAL CONTAINERS PROHIBITED.

Figure 17/e **An improved dug well**

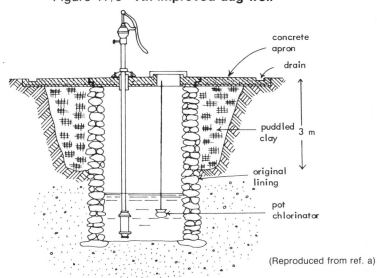

concrete apron

drain

puddled clay — 3 m

original lining

pot chlorinator

(Reproduced from ref. a)

"Puddled" clay is clay which has been thoroughly mixed with a little water and sand to the consistency of a thick paste and well compacted into position.

Table 17/6

Preventing pollution of a dug well

Users' own containers must *never* be lowered into a well. One or two special containers must be fixed in place and be used by everyone.

The captive bucket/container should be lowered either from a pulley suspended above the well or across a roller/bar fixed across the headwall. The bucket must not scrape the side of the well.

A solid concrete *apron* should be constructed at least 1m wide and sloping away from the well in all directions to a gutter which leads to a soakage pit, preferably filled with stones or gravel, 10 m away.

A *headwall* about 50 cm high should be sealed into the apron: it should not be so wide that people can stand on it.

Prevent anything falling or being thrown into the well. Cover it, if possible, when no one is using it.

If heavy rains are expected, dig a drainage ditch around the well about 10 m away with a channel to lead excess surface water away, possibly to the soakage pit.

If a well has become contaminated, been blocked with debris or the side-walls have collapsed:

—Lower the water level as much as possible by rapid, continuous pumping (a suitable, not directly-coupled motorized pump is needed, see Table 17/5); *then*

—Take out any solid debris, inspect and clean/repair the inside of the lining.

If water is seeping into the well through the lining (within 3-6 m of the surface):

—The lining must be renewed or improved: patching is rarely successful.

—As an alternative to replacing the lining, the soil around it may be dug out to a depth of about 3m and filled in with puddled clay: see Figure 17/e.

—A layer of concrete reinforced with wire mesh should, if possible, be placed between the old lining and the clay.

In all cases:

—Inspect the headwall and protective apron; repair or replace as necessary, including the pulley or rollers for lowering the bucket; *then*

—Thoroughly wash down and, if possible disinfect the well.

A pot chlorinator may afterwards be suspended in the well to continuously disinfect the water if necessary. See Annex 18, p. 332.

Especially if the well has been seriously contaminated, scrub the lining and inside wall with a strong chlorine solution (see Table 17/7)—particularly between the current, low water level and the highest point to which water is expected to rise. Then pour a quantity of the same solution into the well and agitate the water by raising and lowering a bucket in it. Leave for 12 hours if possible. (If possible: estimate the quantity of water in the well—pour in 5 litres of the strong chlorine solution for every 100 litres of water in the well—add more if the residual chlorine concentration is less than 0.3 mg/l after an hour.)

Deepening dug wells

If a well has run dry or the yield is inadequate, seek water at a greater depth by:

—Deepening the well itself; *or*

—Sinking a tube well into the bottom of the well and mounting one or several handpumps on a concrete slab (with a manhole) sealed over the well head: see Figure 17/e.

Alternatively, yield *may* be able to be increased by driving perforated pipes radially outward from the bottom of the well into the surrounding soil across the direction of flow of the ground water, but this may be less cost-effective.

Table 17/7

Preparation of a "strong" chlorine solution

To make 10 litres (1 bucketful) of a strong solution for disinfecting pumps, wells, spring boxes, etc., mix the quantity shown of one of the following chemical sources with 10 litres of water in a plastic bucket:

Chemical source	Percentage available chlorine	Quantity required	Approximate measures
Bleaching powder	35	6 g	1 dessertspoon
Stabilized/tropical bleach	25	8 g	1 tablespoon
High test hypochlorite solution	70	3 ml	1 teaspoon
Liquid laundry bleach	5	40 ml	3 tablespoons or 5 dessertspoons
Liquid laundry bleach	7	30 ml	2 tablespoons
Javelle water	1	200 ml	1 teacup or 6oz milk tin

This "strong" solution contains 0.02% chlorine = 0.2 g of chlorine/litre = 200 mg/litre = 200 ppm ("parts per million").

Avoid skin contact with any of the chemical sources or the strong chlorine solution. Avoid inhaling the chlorine fumes.

Digging a new well

The requirements for digging a new well are similar to those of rehabilitating an old one, although more time and larger quantities of materials (especially concrete) are required:

- Choose the site carefully, where water is known to be available at not-too-great a depth and well away from sanitation facilities; *and*
- Disinfect the well before use as for a rehabilitated well.

Water will often be found at shallow depths close to river banks and lakes, also in low-lying places where the vegetation is rich.

Sub-surface dams

Where rivers have dried up and the river bed is of sand, gravel or shale, water *may* still be flowing in the river bed itself. If so, it may be possible to access this water by constructing sub-surface dams across the flow and then leading the retained water off to wells in the river bank. Such operations, organized by OXFAM, were successful in helping to meet the needs of 40,000 refugees in northern Somalia in 1982/3.

First determine whether sub-surface water is present by digging in the river bed until hard rock or impervious clay is reached. If water is present:

1. Dig a trench right across the bed down to the impervious layer;
2. Construct a dam using rocks (and concrete if necessary and available) to a level below that of the river bed itself;
3. Construct an infiltration gallery (stone-filled trench) across the river bed a short distance upstream of the dam and extending some metres into the dry river bank;
4. Dig/sink a well in the bank to intersect with the infiltration gallery to extract the water: see Figure 17/f.

Water obtained in this way is often of good quality unless it is flowing close to the soil surface. See ref. h.

Figure 17/f Sub-surface dam and infiltration gallery

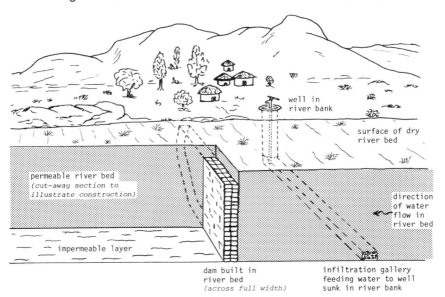

(Adapted from *Ground-water dams for rural water supply in developing countries,* A. Nilsson—Royal Institute of Technology, Stockholm, 1984)

319

Surface water

Water in streams, rivers, ponds, lakes and reservoirs is rarely safe, it needs to be improved in quality and if possible treated before it is used for drinking.

If the source holds water all-year-round:
- Dig/sink shallow wells near the banks if these are porous (the water table can be expected to be near the surface); *or*
- Intall a river bed filter, if the bed of the lake or river is sandy; see below.

If this is not feasible—if, for instance, the ground is not sufficiently porous—the surface water may have to be drawn directly. The quality and safety of the water can then be improved by one or a combination of: storage and sedimentation—slow sand filtration—chemical treatment. See Annex 18.

Regardless of how the water is to be extracted and treated:
- Draw water as far away as possible from and in the case of a river upstream of any other human or animal use;
- Fence off the area of the bank where drinking water is to be drawn off and, if necessary, organize guards to prevent pollution by keeping people and animals away; *and*
- Designate other areas, downstream, for washing and watering animals.

Lake/river bed filters

If the bed of the lake or river source is permeable, dig a filter box into the bed as shown in Figure 17/g and pump water out directly to storage tanks. This method

Figure 17/g   **Lake/river bed filter**

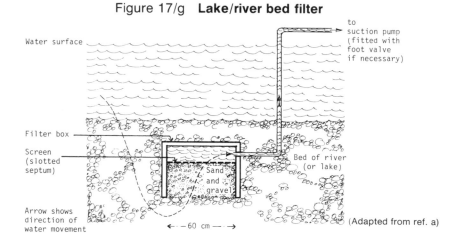

to
suction pump
(fitted with
foot valve
if necessary)

Water surface

Filter box

Screen
(slotted
septum)

Bed of river
(or lake)

Sand
and
gravel

Arrow shows
direction of
water movement

←– 60 cm —·→

(Adapted from ref. a)

has been used successfully in lakes and slow-flowing rivers, but is difficult to construct and operate in fast-flowing rivers.

The watertight box is open at the bottom and has a filter plate sealed into it about ⅓ from the top. The fine slots in this plate ("septum") should, if possible, taper outwards towards the top so that sand particles do not clog it. The box itself is normally made of reinforced steel but it is possible to improvise with other local materials.

Initial rapid pumping will build up a graded layer of soil below the filter plate after which normal pumping will deliver properly filtered supplies.

Maintenance of systems

The breakdown of a pump or any other component of an extraction and delivery system can have disastrous consequences for the population. Ensure arrangements for regular maintenance and prompt repairs, including:

— Defined responsibilities for maintenance (if possible by designated community members);

— Training and tools for local operators and mechanics;

— Availability of sufficient, appropriate spare parts; *and*

— Availability of spare/stand-by pumps (which can be used while one which has broken down is being repaired).

Establish systems by which spares and expert mechanics can be mobilized very quickly whenever needed.

Possible UNICEF inputs

Depending on the assessment of actual needs and possibilities, some of the following inputs might be considered:

General

— Expertise to help plan and implement appropriate programmes: hydrogeologists, hydrologists, water engineers, sanitarians, drillers, mechanics, including mobilizing locally available technical expertise.

— Laboratory equipment and/or small field test kits ("portable water analysis" kits) for water quality testing.

— Chlorine chemicals for disinfecting wells and associated installations.

— Local costs for operations including maintenance of installations (preferably by motivation and training of local populations).

321

Rain water collection

—Materials for the rapid repair/construction of guttering.

—Containers—jerry cans or buckets with lids—for households to collect and store water.

—Local costs for the establishment of collection systems at feeding centres, health centres and hospitals.

Natural springs

—Materials and, possibly, local costs for the repair/construction of spring "boxes" and associated storage and distribution arrangements.

Tube wells and hand-dug wells

—Expertise and/or local costs for expert surveys of wells and, if needed, the ground-water potential.

—Tools: spades—buckets—block-and-tackle—pliers—trowels—levels—cutlasses—measuring tapes—rope—hard hats, etc.

—Pipes, screens, cement, reinforcing bars, etc. for the (re)construction of wells: see guide list OLGA.

—Spare parts and/or new pumps.

—Local operating costs for repair and construction work.

Surface water

—Tools and materials for the construction of storage tanks, filter units, etc.

—Pumps for raising/moving water.

Further references

a. *Small water supplies,* S. Cairncross & R. Feachem, Ross Bulletin No.10—Ross Institute, London (1978).   E

b. *Self-help wells,* R. G. Keogel, FAO irrigation and drainage paper No.3—FAO (1977).   E

c. *Hand-pump maintenance in the context of community well projects,* A. Pacey—OXFAM/Intermediate Technology Publications (1980).   E

d. *Water supply for rural areas and small communities,* E. Wagner & J. Lacroix—WHO (1959)   E/F/S

e. *Small community water supplies,* Technical series paper 18—International reference centre for community water supplies and sanitation, The Hague (1981)   E

f. *Environmental health engineering in the tropics (an introductory text),* S. Cairncross & R. Feachem—J. Wiley (1983)   E

g. *Appropriate technology for water supply and sanitation,* vol.12 (of 12 volume series)—World Bank (1980)   E

h. *Field Engineering,* P. Stern et al—Intermediate Technology Publications, London (1983)   E

i. *Guide List OLGA*—UNICEF (1975)   E
    [lists and specifications of supplies and equipment likely to be needed]

ANNEX 18

WATER QUALITY AND TREATMENT

Objective

- To ensure that water is safe for human consumption.

Methods and priorities

- Avoid the need for any treatment by finding good quality sources, if possible, and give high priority to preventing contamination.

- Improvement/treatment, where necessary, should be the minimum required to ensure acceptably safe water, using appropriate technology and a method that is reliable.

323

If water needs to be improved/treated on a large scale:- mobilize sanitary engineers to determine how it should best be done, and to organize the operation and maintenance of appropriate systems.

In all cases give high priority to domestic hygiene and measures to protect the water between collection and use.

Dangers and sources of contamination

The greatest risk associated with polluted drinking water is the spread of diarrhoeas, dysentries—caused by a variety of viruses, bacteria and protozoa—and infectious hepatitis. The pathogens (disease-causing organisms) are largely transmitted in faeces:

—Contamination by *human faeces* is the major concern, although animal (and bird) faeces in water may also cause disease transmission;

—Children's faeces are more dangerous than those of adults;

—Contamination by urine is a significant threat only in areas where urinary schistosomiasis is endemic.

Table 18/1 lists the priorities for testing water quality and the possibilities for improving it when necessary.

Table 18/1

Testing and improving water quality

If possible, test the quality of water at source, in storage tanks and tanker trucks:

—Before any new source is used;

—At regular intervals during use; *and*

—Whenever any contamination—especially by faeces—is suspected.

It *must* be tested immediately any outbreak of a typically water-borne disease is reported.

Water may be improved/treated by:

—Covered storage for 1-2 days (during which many viruses, protozoa and bacteria die off and solid particles settle out).

—Slow sand filtration in specially constructed filter units, which effectively removes protozoa, most bacteria and solid particles.

—Chemical treatment, normally with a chlorine-based compound, which kills bacteria, viruses and protozoa.

—Boiling which kills bacteria, viruses and protozoa.

Improvement/treatment methods

Chemical treatment is the surest way of making water safe for drinking, but such treatment must be properly controlled and supervised on a continuous basis. Except in the context of well-established municipal systems, or situations where adequate numbers of competent sanitation personnel are on the spot, this may be difficult to assure. Chemical treatment may, however, be appropriate for supplies for hospitals, feeding centres, etc.

Storage plus **slow sand filtration** requires considerable effort—and materials—at the outset to establish the systems (tanks, etc.) but, once set-up, should be able to be operated by suitably instructed members of the community with only oc-casional inspection/supervision by professional sanitarians. (Where a system serves a large community, those responsible for its day-to-day operation may need to be remunerated.)

Water purification tablets and boiling are rarely appropriate for water treatment on a large-scale, but may be used in hospitals, feeding centres, etc. In many situations, storage/sedimentation followed by slow sand filtration or chemical treatment in separate storage tanks is the best approach.

Testing water quality

Samples should, if feasible, be sent to a public health laboratory for expert analy-sis. Otherwise they may be tested on the spot by trained sanitarians using field test kits.

Taking samples requires no particular expertise, but considerable care: see Table 18/2. Samples should, to the extent possible, be kept cool and in the dark. They must reach the laboratory—or be analysed in the field—within 24 hours of col-lection.

The actual test done will depend on the normal practice of local water laboratories and the experience of the local sanitarians. The most widely used tests are those that detect and enumerate faecal coliforms: see Table 18/3. Membrane filters will probably be required for field testing.

In cases where the water is already being disinfected by chlorination it is easier and more appropriate to test for the presence of chlorine than for bacteria directly. If chlorine is present at concentrations of 0.2-0.5 mg/litre at the distribution point, the water can be considered safe. Residual chlorine test kits will be required.

Table 18/2

Taking water samples

Collection bottles

Bottles should be sterile and have an air-tight seal.

Don't fill them completely. Tie a piece of greaseproof paper or aluminium foil over each cap after closing it.

Ideally, 100-200 ml glass bottles with ground glass stoppers or rubber-lined screw tops should be used. They should preferably be autoclaved—e.g. in a pressure cooker for 40 mins.—after first tying a piece of brown paper securely over the open mouth and wrapping the cap in similar paper. In practice, Coca-Cola or similar fizzy drink bottles can be used if new caps and a manual capping machine are available (e.g. UNIPAC 20-515-20 + 20-525-00). The caps must also be wrapped and autoclaved.

If sampling from a chlorinated supply, put a few drops of 10 per cent sodium thiosulphate solution in each bottle first.

Sampling from surface water

Take samples at least one metre from the bank and 20-30 cm below the water surface: see Figure 18/a.

If schistosomiasis is prevalent, protective boots and gauntlets should be worn if risks of contracting the disease are to be avoided.

Sampling from a dug well

Lower a weighted sampling bottle into the well without touching the sides: see Figure 18/b; *and*

Take samples separately from water raised in the captive communal bucket (to check whether the bucket itself is contaminated).

Sampling from a tubewell pump

1. Wipe the mouth of the pump with a clean rag;
2. Operate the pump for long enough to clean out the water standing in the well tube;
3. Sterilize the mouth of the pump with a gas or alcohol flame, if possible; *then*
4. Take a sample holding the bottle in the middle of the stream of water.

Sampling from a tap

1. Wipe the mouth of the tap with a clean rag;
2. Run the water fast for at least 1 minute;
3. Sterilize the mouth of the tap with a gas or alcohol flame, if possible;
4. Run the water for 1 minute; *then*
5. Take the sample.

Figure 18/a
Sampling from a stream

Waterproof
gauntlet

FLOW

20 cm

Bottle or
sample cup

(Reproduced from ref. b)

Figure 18/b
Sampling from a dug well

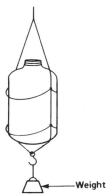

Weight

Table 18/3

Faecal coliform levels

The presence of faecal coliforms indicates that the water has been contaminated by faeces of humans or other warm-blooded animals. Concentrations are usually expressed per 100 ml of water. As a rough guide:

0-10	faecal coliforms/100 ml = reasonable quality
10-100	faecal coliforms/100 ml = polluted
100-1,000	faecal coliforms/100 ml = dangerous
over 1,000	faecal coliforms/100 ml = very dangerous

Storage/sedimentation

Leaving water undisturbed in large tanks—or household containers—improves its
quality as many pathogens die off and any heavy matter in suspension settles out
(sedimentation):

—Storage of untreated surface water for 12 to 24 hours brings about an ap-
preciable improvement in its quality.

—The longer the period of storage and the higher the temperature, the greater
the improvement.

—48 hours storage helps to prevent transmission of bilharzia, provided snails do not enter the tank.

Storage tanks should be covered: the dangers of contamination of open tanks more than offset the advantages of direct sunlight.

The storage area should be fenced off, and if necessary guarded, to prevent children playing in the water.

Storage capacity should, if possible, be equivalent to at least 24 hours requirements for the population to be served.

A two tank system is often used:

— The first tank is the settling tank in which water is left undisturbed for at least 48 hours, more if possible.
— The clarified water is then transferred to the second tank from which it can be used. The sludge at the bottom of the first tank is discarded.

If treatment is still required, the water can be chlorinated in the second tank before it is used. If the bottom of the first tank is above the top of the second, the clarified water can simply be drained or siphoned from the first into the second.

The numbers of viruses and protozoa in stored water decreases with time. They decrease most rapidly at warm temperatures. Bacteria generally behave similarly but, in exceptional circumstances, may multiply in polluted water. The dose of bacteria needed to establish an infection in the intestine may be large, however, whereas the infectious dose of viruses and protozoa is typically very low. Prolonged storage therefore greatly reduces the dangers.

Schistosomiasis (bilharzia) parasites die if they do not reach the fresh water snail within 24 hours of excretion by an infected person, or a human or animal host within 48 hours of leaving infected snails.

The stirring in of some dissolved alum (aluminium sulphate) crystals accelerates the sedimentation process but *not* the dying off of pathogens. 50-500 gms of crushed alum is required for every 1.000 litres of stored water, depending in the alkalinity of the water. Dissolve it in a bucket of water first.

Slow sand filtration

As water passes through fine sand, solid particles are filtered out and, more important, the thin layer of micro-organisms which develops on the surface of the sand bed breaks down any organic matter in the water.

Table 18/4 and Figure 18/c provide brief details of the "packed-drum" filter which can provide 40-60 litres of good quality water per hour for health and feeding centres, or drinking water for small groups of households.

Table 18/4

Packed drum filters

Requirements

—A suitable drum with a cover (e.g. an empty 200 litre vegetable oil drum; empty fuel drums can be used but not drums which have contained chemicals).

—Pipes; pipe fittings; taps; sand; gravel; tools.

Preparation

1. Thoroughly clean the drum; drill holes and fit pipes; then disinfect the drum with a strong chlorine solution.
2. Put large gravel in the bottom to a level 5 cm above the bottom (outlet) hole.
3. Fill with washed sand (grain size in the range 0.2-0.5 cm) to a depth of 75 cm.
4. Disinfect by filling with a strong chlorine solution (see Table 17/7) and leaving for 12 hours.
5. Flush out with water until there is no longer a strong smell of chlorine.

Operation/use

The rate of drawing water must never exceed 60 litres/hour:

—If possible, establish a continuous, slow flow: feed water into the filter from another tank at a higher level through a valve adjusted to allow a flow of not more than 1 litre/minute—collect the filtered water in another storage container.

—Otherwise, simply draw water off from a tap at the bottom and immediately add a similar quantity of unfiltered water to the top.

Cleaning

Clean the filter occasionally but not too often—when the rate of flow has fallen significantly:

1. Drain off the top water.
2. Scrape off and discard the top 1-2 cm (¾") of sand.
3. Loosen the new surface of sand, then restart the filtration.

Top up with fresh, washed sand occasionally.

The filter must never be allowed to run dry. There must always be a layer of water above the surface of the sand.

The referenced publications provide details for the construction of larger systems which can deliver 100 litres/hour for every square metre of filter surface area. They may, however, not be practicable in many emergency situations.

Figure 18/c **Packed drum filter**

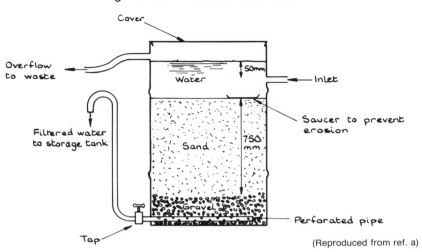

(Reproduced from ref. a)

Chemical disinfection

Chemical treatment of water on a large scale is, as a rule, recommended only in situations where storage and/or filtration cannot meet the need. All disinfection systems require close control and supervision. They are of little value unless fully reliable. Get expert advice.

Chemical disinfection of new and rehabilitated wells, sand filters, pumps and piped water systems is, however, essential.

Chemicals

The most generally available chemical suitable for use in emergencies is bleaching powder (calcium hypochlorite). "High Test Hypochlorite" solution, if available, has advantages. Liquid bleach and javel water can also be used. Note that:

— Each of these products contain a different amount of usable chlorine, hence different quantities of each are required for the same purpose. All lose active chlorine over time.

— All chemicals and made-up solutions should be stored in tightly closed containers made of dark coloured glass, ceramic or plastic (not metal), and kept in a cool dark place.

330

—For small-scale operations it is best if chemicals are delivered in small-sized containers (e.g. 1 kg plastic bags).

Chlorination in storage tanks

Chlorination should normally be undertaken after an initial sedimentation or filtration process. The quantity of chlorine required depends on the degree of pollution and the amount of sediment in the water.

1. Prepare a 1% chlorine solution: see Table 18/5;
2. Pour sufficient of the 1% solution into the tank to produce an initial chlorine concentration of 5-7 mg/litre: see Table 18/6;
3. Leave for at least 30 minutes (1-2 hours if protozoa or helminths are likely to be present); then
4. Test the water to determine the residual chlorine content, add more chlorine solution or neutralize excess chlorine as necessary: see Table 18/6.

Table 18/5

Preparation of 1 per cent chlorine stock solution

To make 1 litre of the stock solution, mix the quantity shown of one of the following chemical sources with 1 litre of water in a glass, plastic or wooden container:

Chemical source	Percentage available chlorine	Quantity required	Approximate measures
Bleaching powder	35	30 g	2 heaped tablespoons
Stabilized/tropical bleach	25	40 g	3 heaped tablespoons
High test hypochlorite solution	70	14 ml	1 tablespoon = 4 teaspoons
Liquid laundry bleach	5	200 ml	1 teacup or 6 oz milk tin
Liquid laundry bleach	7	145 ml	10 tablespoons
Javelle water	1	Is itself a 1 per cent stock solution.	

A 1 per cent solution contains 10 g of chlorine/litre = 10,000 mg/litre or 10,000 ppm (parts per million.)

Avoid skin contact with any of the chemical sources or the stock solution. Avoid inhaling chlorine fumes.

Table 18/6

Disinfecting water using 1 per cent stock solution

To produce an initial chlorine concentration of 5-7 mg/litre in the water to be treated, stir in 0.5-0.7 ml of the 1 per cent stock solution for every litre of water. Quantities required for particular volumes of water are:

Volume of water to be disinfected	Quantity of 1 per cent solution (ml)	Approximate measures
10 litres	5-7	1½ teaspoons
50 litres	25-35	2 tablespoons
100 litres	50-70	4 tablespoons
1,000 litres	500-700	3 teacups or 6oz milk tins

Leave the water to stand for at least 30 minutes, then test it to determine the residual chlorine content:

—If concentration is 0.2-0.5 mg/litre (or more), all harmful organisms will have been killed and the water can be used.

—If concentration is less than 0.2 mg/litre, add more 1% solution, wait 30 minutes and test again.

—If concentration is greater than 0.5 mg/litre, the water may taste unpleasant: neutralize the excess chlorine (see below) and add less of the 1% solution to the next batch of water.

Field "residual chlorine test kits" are available: only basic laboratory experience is required to use them. After treatment excess chlorine may, if necessary, be neutralized by adding a little sodium thiosulphate ("Hypo"): 1 crystal to a litre of water, 4-5 crystals to a bucketful.

Chlorination in dug wells

If it is necessary to chlorinate water in a dug well, and little equipment or technical expertise is available, a *pot chlorinator* may be suspended in the well—1 metre below the water level. This requires some expertise but, as a general indication:

—A single pot chlorinator—see Figure 18/d—may be sufficient to treat a well or tank being drawn on at a rate of about 1,200 litres/day (say 60 people). It would need to be replaced every 1-2 weeks.

—A double pot chlorinator—see Figure 18/e—would be sufficient to treat a well being drawn on at about 400 litres/day (say 20 people). It should be replaced every 2-3 weeks.

332 For larger wells, two or more pots may be used.

Figure 18/d **Single pot chlorinator**

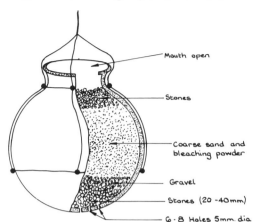

Mouth open

Stones

Coarse sand and bleaching powder

Gravel

Stones (20 -40mm)

6 - 8 Holes 5mm. dia

The pot should have a total capacity of 12-15 litres and contain 1 kg of bleaching powder mixed with 2 kg coarse sand.

(Reproduced from ref. c)

Figure 18/e **Double pot chlorinator**

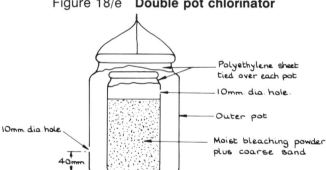

Polyethylene sheet tied over each pot

10mm. dia. hole.

Outer pot

Moist bleaching powder plus coarse sand

10mm. dia hole

40mm

The outer pot should be about 25 cm diameter and 30 cm high; the inner pot about 16 cm in diameter and 28 cm high. It should contain 1.5 kg bleaching powder mixed with 3 kg coarse sand, then moistened. The hole in the inner pot should be about 3 cm above the level of the mixture.

(Reproduced from ref. c)

Drip chlorinators

Various types of drip chlorinators can be constructed to feed a chlorine solution very slowly into a water supply which is being used (flowing) continuously: see referenced publications.

Boiling

Boiling is the surest method of water sterilization, but is not practical for the needs of large populations especially when fuel is short. It should be relied on to purify domestic water supplies only if the people have traditionally boiled their water *and* have sufficient fuel to continue to do so.

At low altitudes simply bringing water to the boil will destroy all pathogens that may be transmitted by drinking water. As a rule of thumb, boiling should be continued for one minute for every 1,000 metres of altitude above sea level, as the boiling temperature reduces with altitude.

Prolonged vigorous boiling is often recommended but is not necessary to destroy the faecal-orally transmitted pathogens. It is wasteful of fuel—boiling requires about about 0.5 kg of wood per litre of water—and evaporation of the water will increase the concentration of nitrates which could then be dangerous for very young babies.

Mobile drinking water units

Trailer-mounted drinking water units—comprising a motorized pump, hypo-chlorinator and filter—are available which are said to be capable of delivering up to 50,000 litres of good quality water per hour. Where local infrastructure is well developed and expertise exists to operate such units, they have been valuable for short-term use after certain high-impact disasters: e.g. in Lebanon and Peru.

Units may be available from the local military or rescue services. They might be obtainable as in-kind contributions from major donors. UNIPAC can provide information on purchase possibilities.

Possible UNICEF inputs

Depending on the assessment of actual needs and possibilities, some of the following inputs might be considered:

- Expertise—experienced sanitarians—to help in planning, organizing and supervising operations (in conjuntion with WHO).
- Bleaching powder or other chemicals.
- Local costs for establishment of storage, filtration and/or treatment units.

Further references

Concerning water testing:

a.   *Guidelines for drinking water quality,* vol.1 (recommendations) and vol.3 (drinking water quality control in small community supplies) —WHO (1985)   E/F

b.   *Field testing of water in developing countries,* L. Hutton—Water Research Centre, England (1983)   E

Concerning water treatment:

c.   *Small water supplies,* S. Cairncross & R. Feachem—Ross Bulletin no. 10—Ross Institute, London (1978)   E

d.   *Safe drinking water,* J. Howard—OXFAM, Oxford (1979)   E

e.   *Guide to simple sanitary measures for the control of enteric diseases,* S. Rajagopalan & M. Shiffman—WHO (1974)   E/F/A

WATER PUMPS, PIPES AND FITTINGS

Pumps

Pumps may need to be repaired, replaced or newly provided to raise water for direct distribution at a well and/or to move it through pipelines to storage tanks or other distribution points.

In most areas, *hand-operated pumps* are to be preferred, especially where they are already familiar locally and fuel supplies cannot be guaranteed. They are relatively easy to install and maintain, generally more reliable than motorized pumps and less dependent on supplies of spare parts as well as fuel from outside the community.

Motorized pumps—which can raise water much faster and from greater depths—may however be indispensable if the needs of large number of people have to be met from only a few sources, and those sources have high yield potentials. Regular maintenance and prompt repair/replacement in case of breakdown must be assured, as well as regular fuel/power supplies.

Handpumps

Handpumps can be used to raise the water if the water table is not more than 50-60m deep, the available yield and/or required output is low. If the water table is less than 7 m deep, suction pumps with the operating cylinder at the top (ground level) can be used. Otherwise the cylinder must be "down the well," not more than 5 m above the water level.

Yields of 750-900 litres/hour can be possible—about 10 cubic metres per day assuming continuous pumping for 12 hours. This could be sufficient, in theory, for 1,000 people. In practice, actual performance may be less than half of this.

The type of handpump already familiar in the area should normally be provided. "Experiments" should generally be avoided in the emergency phase. (Alternatives and refinements may be considered in the context of any long-term rehabilitation-cum-development programme when close, continuous supervision of all pump installations by a competent technician can be assured.)

Motorized pumps

Get advice from professionals, local technicians and community leaders regarding the selection and siting of pumps. The major considerations in pump selection are: local familiarity—fuel supplies—availability of spares—ease of maintenance—and, above all, reliability.

Alternative types are submersible electric pumps fitted "down the well" or mechanical shaft-drive pumps. Self-priming centrifugal pumps are usually recommended when water has to be lifted a considerable height (up to 100 metres) or pumped over a long distance. Low-speed pumps generally cause fewer operational problems and have a longer life than high-speed units.

Table 19/1 lists some of the main aspects to be considered and specified when ordering pumps. Any requirements for an initial stock of spare parts must also be stated at the time of ordering.

If spare parts are required to repair an existing pump, quote the make, model number *and* serial number of the pump.

Provided tank storage capacity is sufficient to meet peaks in demands during the day, the **delivery capacity** required of the pump is determined by dividing the total daily output needed by the number of hours the pump will be run each day. It must not be greater than the yield of the source concerned. Provide for some spare capacity to cover breakdowns, any possible increases in population, etc.

Pumps should generally not be run at night, and must be left idle for a sufficient period each day to allow the water in the source to recover to its original level. If the pump output is **337** greater than the yield of the well, the latter may be pumped dry and the pump itself then burn out.

Table 19/1

Specification of motorized pumpsets

The following characteristics must be considered and specified when pumps are being requested/ordered:

☐ Delivery capacity (litres or cu.ft. per minute).

☐ Inlet pipe diameter.

☐ Outlet pipe diameter.

☐ Whether diesel, petrol or electric. If electric, the voltage and number of phases and whether a stand-by generator also required. If diesel/petrol, whether hand or battery starter.

☐ The situation in which the pump is to be used: location and altitude of the site—depth and/or distance over which water is to be pumped.

☐ Any special considerations: e.g. salts in water which might affect certain materials in the pump.

☐ How the pump and motor should be mounted.

Pumps coupled to an engine mounted on the same base plate are generally the most convenient. The whole assembly may be mounted on skids—if light enough to be carried—or on a trailer.

See *Guide List OLGA* (p. 255) for further details.

Solar (photovoltaic) pumps

In some circumstances pumps powered by solar panels may be suitable. The present generation are still expensive for their output but very reliable and involve no direct running costs.

Such pumps naturally work best in direct sunlight but will still work with light cloud cover. As a rough indication, a solar pump powered by panels rated at 450W would lift 1-2 litres/second through 6 metres on a sunny day. Thus a solar pump might be a solution when the output of a hand pump would be insufficient but the high output of large mechanized pumps are not necessary.

Solar pumps performed well in refugee camps in Somalia delivering 55-75 cubic metres per day on an 8 m head.

Windmills

Windmills may be considered where wind speeds of at least 8 kms/hour (5 miles/hr.) can be expected for 60% of the time throughout the year. Some windmills can be connected to handpumps which can be operated by hand when necessary.

Pipes and fittings

Requirements for pipes and pipe fittings must be specified by experienced, practical technicians, but note that:

— Plastic pipes are usually cheaper and easier to install than other types.
— Plastic pipes can usually be glued together, but different solvents (glues) may be required for different pipe sizes.
— If used for transmission pipelines in camps, etc., plastic pipes must be buried—otherwise galvanized iron pipes should be used instead.
— If threaded (screw) joints are being used with metal and/or plastic pipes, it is often best—and delivery quickest—to order pipe in unthreaded lengths and to provide thread-cutting tools (dies) to enable threads to be cut on the spot.
— Order ample quantities of joints and other fittings: avoid special/unusual fittings as much as possible.
— When ordering lengths of rigid pipe, take account of possible problems in transporting long lengths to the field sites: 6-metre (or 20-ft) lengths are best in most situations.

Further references

a.   *Appropriate Technology Sourcebook,* K. Darrow & R. Pem—Volunteers in Asia publication (1976)   E
b.   *Guide list OLGA*—UNICEF (1975)   E

ANNEX 20

DISPOSING OF EXCRETA*

Objective

- **To ensure arrangements and facilities for the disposal of human excreta which minimize the risks of disease spreading due to contamination of the environment, especially water supplies, or the proliferation of vectors.**

Social as well as technical factors must be taken into account.

Priorities and methods

The sanitary disposal of excreta is likely to pose particular and urgent problems in two kinds of situation:

---

* The guidelines provided in this annex are largely derived from the *UNHCR handbook for emergencies* with additional details from the listed "further references".

a. Municipal sewerage systems or other arrangements in urban areas damaged/disrupted.
b. Displaced persons in crowded conditions in rural or urban areas.

In most cases, temporary arrangements will have to be made very rapidly to reduce immediate health hazards. Table 20/1 suggests the phases of action which might be appropriate. Table 20/2 summarizes some of the dangers of inadequate arrangements.

Weeks cannot be allowed to pass while waiting for expert advice, construction to be completed or material to arrive! Interim, emergency arrangements should be made, and these then be improved or replaced by better arrangements later—as soon as possible—based on thorough technical and sociological investigations.

Table 20/1

Phased actions to reduce health hazards

Where municipal systems are disrupted/inadequate:

1. Immediately establish temporary, alternative arrangements—probably communal trench latrines, and/or chemical toilets.
2. Disinfect the immediate environment of any damaged facilities.
3. Repair/replace facilities as quickly as possible.

Arrangements in non-urban areas:

1. Consult with community leaders, local health and sanitation personnel and social anthropologists to determine what arrangements to reduce health hazards would be feasible.
2. Immediately establish arrangements to control/localize defecation—probably in designated, enclosed areas of land or sea (unless sufficient latrines already exist).
3. Organize the establishment and maintenance of appropriate latrines:
    —Trench latrines may be needed initially but, where feasible, individual family latrines are usually much better.
    —Ensure that latrines are suitable for children, can be used at night, and that appropriate anal cleaning materials and hand washing facilities are available.
    —Organize necessary public education and arrangements for cleaning and regular inspection/supervision.

N.B. Latrines will not be used or themselves become a health hazard unless kept clean and properly maintained.

341

Uncontrolled surface defecation—or in the sea—is a major health hazard, but risks are significantly reduced if defecation is controlled/localized.

Possibilities for the successful establishment and operation of different **latrine systems** depend on:

—The physical characteristics of the area including geology, rainfall, drainage and the availability of water;

—Cultural considerations, including previous habits; *and*

—The space, materials, equipment and expertise immediately available.

Cost, ease of installation and maintenance will also be major considerations.

Failure to take proper account of any of these aspects can easily result in the system itself not being used and/or breaking down and rapidly becoming a health hazard.

N.B. What can be done during the emergency phase depends on the previous levels of services and facilities, and local habits. It is not realistic to expect that habits will be suddenly improved in the middle of an emergency. Modifications or adjustments of traditional practices can, however, be sought through simultaneous practical measures and public education.

Table 20/2

The dangers of insanitary excreta disposal

- The agents of most important infectious diseases are passed from the body in excreta and may reach other people.

- Excreta can, unless properly isolated, provide a breeding ground for insects which then act as direct or indirect transmitters of disease.

Note: Persons acting as carriers and transmitting an infection may in fact show little or no sign of disease. Conversely, persons in an advanced state of disease may have little or no importance in transmission.

The safe disposal of *human* excreta is more important than disposal of animal waste, because more diseases affecting humans are transmitted by human waste than animal. Human *faeces* are much more dangerous than urine. *Children's* faeces are more dangerous than adults'.

Diseases which can be transmitted through faeces include: typhoid, cholera, bacillary and amoebic dysentry, infectious hepatitis, polio, bilharzia, roundworm, hookworm, miscellaneous diarrhoeas and gastro-enteritis.

The disposal of *urine* also requires special attention in those areas of Africa and the Middle East where the *Schistosoma haematobium* species of bilharzia occurs, and wherever typhoid is common and endemic. Elsewhere it is probably sufficient in an emergency just to prevent contamination of the water.

Controlled surface defecation

In hot, dry climates where sufficient space is available, localized surface defecation in areas away from the dwellings and water supplies may be an adequate arrangement, particularly where this has been the normal practice. Table 20/3 lists actions to be taken if surface defecation is necessary, at least on an interim, emergency basis.

In time, the heat and sunlight render the faeces harmless, but watch out for increased numbers of rats in the area and keep the potential health hazards under review. Black rock is the best surface. Covering excreta with a little earth lessens risks.

Table 20/3

Controlling surface defecation

If space allows:

- Designate areas which are away and down-wind from dwellings but sufficiently close to be used and not in the path of any surface run-off during rain.
- Fence off the areas and dig cut-off ditches to protect them against any flooding;
- Provide privacy (screens), dig shallow trenches and provide spades if appropriate and possible;
- Publicize the arrangements and encourage people to use these areas and not defecate near dwellings; *and*
- Prevent defecation or urination in or near water supplies.

If the ground is flooded or marshy, or there is a high water table, the risks to public health are very high and arrangements to physically contain excreta (in an area away from dwellings and water sources) are even more vital, but also more difficult. Pending a proper latrine containment system:

—Construct simple raised platforms, about 50 cm high, to avoid people immediately being contaminated by excreta.

—Alternatively: cut one end out of empty 200-litre (45-gallon) oil drums, insert them open-end-down into the ground, after digging holes as deep as the water allows; leave the last half metre of each drum standing out of the ground and cut a small hole in its end to transform it into a squatting plate.

Figure 20/a

Considerations in excreta disposal in refugee camps

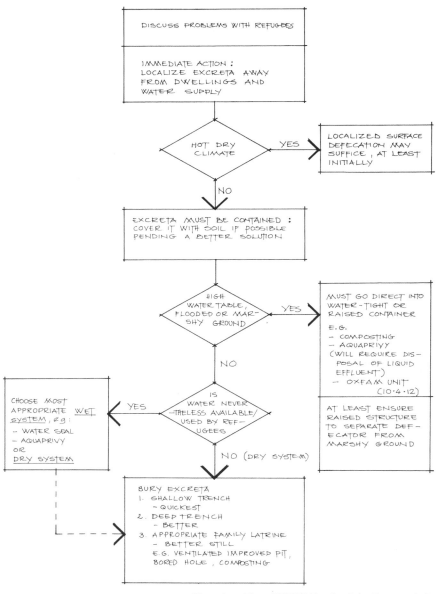

(Reproduced from UNHCR *Handbook for Emergencies*)

Defecation in the sea

Defecation in the sea is less harmful than indiscriminate defecation on land but should be discouraged unless there is no other option. The dangers increase greatly with population density. Where it is unavoidable:

— Localize it by fencing off a designated area, *and*
— Build structures out into the sea that permit defecation away from the immediate shore line.

Check the effects of tides, currents and prevailing winds and plan/locate these arrangements to minimize risks of direct contamination of the foreshore, especially areas used for washing and bathing. Pumping untreated excreta far enough out to sea so that it is carried away from the coastline is a longer term possibility.

Defecation in bays, estuaries or lagoons where fish or shellfish are caught should be avoided since this may spread infection.

Latrines

Types of latrine

There are "dry" latrines—trenches, pits (simple holes in the ground)—and "wet" or water-dependent latrines, which are flushed. Some of the different types are described in Annex 21. Some systems also incorporate composting or the cartage of excreta for use in agriculture or fish farming.

Latrines may be designed and allocated as:

— Individual family units.
— Centralized units with each latrine allocated to an individual family.
— Communal systems.

Choosing a system

● **Any system should be cheap, simple, easy to install and maintain: the latrines must be accessible and kept clean.**

345

- **Individual family units are, in most circumstances, to be preferred but emergency conditions often dictate the use — at least initially — of communal trench latrines.**

Population density will affect the *space* available and thus the types of system possible. Space must be available for replacement latrines when necessary.

Other physical considerations are outlined in table 20/4 and summarized in Figure 20/a. Cultural factors are listed in Table 20/5: they determine what types of system may be acceptable.

Once these factors have been taken into account, the cleanliness of latrines and their ease of access will determine whether or not they are used. Communal latrines are usually a problem. The best guarantee of proper maintenance is the individual family allocation of latrines.

Where space and soil conditions allow, the simplest and most common individual family unit is the **pit** or **bored-hole** latrine. They are most suitable in conditions of low to medium population density — up to 300 persons/hectare — but have been used satisfactorily in areas with twice this density.

Table 20/4

Physical considerations regarding latrines

The **nature of the soil** may impose certain constraints:

—Digging pit-type systems is difficult in rocky ground.

—Sandy soil demands special measures to prevent the side walls of pits collapsing.

—Impervious clay soils may exclude any system dependent upon seepage.

Note that soil conditions can vary over a short distance: a thorough survey is necessary. Take account of any difference between dry and wet season soil conditions.

Where the water-table is high, or flooding likely, excreta must be contained using water-tight or raised container systems. Simple dry systems cannot be used: if flood water entered such latrines, large areas could be contaminated.

If **water sources** are not adequate and reliable, "wet" systems should not be used. (Such systems are anyway generally more expensive than those which do not need water.)

Whatever the system, many communities will require at least a little water for anal cleaning.

Space should be available not only for the construction of one pit latrine per family, but also for the digging of new pits when the old ones are full. This is especially important when pit latrines are used as communal facilities.

Trench latrines can be dug quickly and need less space than a large number of individual family units. While shallow trenches may be a quick-action solution for a short initial period, deep trench latrines are incomparably more effective.

Siting of latrines

As a rule, at least one latrine seat/position should be provided for every 20 people. Latrines should normally be:

—At least 6 m from dwellings: 10 m or more away from feeding and health centres;

—Over 30 m and downhill from wells or other drinking water sources;

—Not more than 50 m from users' dwellings and easy of access. (If people have to walk far to a latrine they may defecate in a more convenient location regardless of the health hazard.)

If rains are likely to be heavy, anticipate where surface run-off will flow and keep latrines away from such flows—or dig drainage ditches to divert the flows.

Table 20/5

Cultural considerations relating to latrines

☐ Previous sanitation arrangements and practices: for adults—for children;

☐ Method of anal cleaning;

☐ Preferred position—sitting or squatting;

☐ Need for privacy;

☐ Segregation of sexes and/or of different groups or individuals with whom it is culturally unacceptable to share a latrine;

☐ Cultural taboos—e.g. against contact with anything that may have touched excreta of others;

☐ Social factors, including likelihood of community action to ensure proper use of proposed system; *and*

☐ Need for special orientation (direction) of latrines in some cultures.

N.B. Over half the world's population is not accustomed to using latrines.

Design and construction

A latrine must be easy to clean. The surfaces round the hole should be washable: avoid uncovered wood if possible.

People not used to latrines will generally prefer a large enclosure with no *roof* but—at least during wet seasons—it is preferable to cover latrines in order to prevent rain water filling the latrine, causing contamination around it, or weakening the surrounds. Make sure proper drainage off the roof is provided, away from any soakage pit.

The structure should be made of local materials which should also be used for reinforcing the pit where necessary. Ensure the availability of necessary tools, nails, etc.

In all **"dry" systems**, keep the squatting holes as small as possible (say 18 cm diameter) and ensure that close-fitting covers are provided and used—except with VIP latrines (see Annex 21, p. 354).

For **"wet" systems**, ensure the supply of sufficient squatting or sitting slabs and U-pipes—perhaps by organizing local manufacture (e.g. on-site casting of concrete slabs). See referenced publications for more details and get advice on local methods.

Where there is an established method of covering latrines, for example with a wooden lattice, it may be best to continue to use this during the emergency phase even if it is less easy to clean (thus less sanitary) than a special plate. Improved slabs/plates might be introduced in the rehabilitation phase.

Practical aspects of latrine operations

Use by children

Ensure that the latrines are safe and physically suitable for children and that all children are shown and encouraged to use them properly.

Children are both the main sufferers from excreta-related diseases and also the main excreters of many of the pathogens that cause diarrhoea. They may not easily be persuaded of the need to use latrines and are often frightened by unfamiliar arrangements.

Night lighting

Latrines must also be able to be used at night. For individual units, families may be able to arrange their own lamps, but for communal units some form of lighting should be provided.

Anal cleaning and hand washing

Assure the availability of appropriate anal cleaning materials at or near all latrines, and facilities for hand washing. This is essential to the maintenance of hygiene.

Control of insects and smells

Disinfectants should *not* be poured into the pits or tanks of latrines (as they dispose of excreta by biological degradation). The regular addition to trench or pit latrines of a little soil, ashes or diesel oil, if available, may help control insect breeding and reduce odour.

Communal latrines

Where communal latrines are unavoidable, ensure arrangements to keep them clean. Give particular attention to the maintenance and cleanliness of latrines serving community facilities such as health and feeding centres. They must be cleaned daily. Cleaners must be appointed/designated and close supervision be assured.

If maintenance is inadequate, even properly designed and installed systems will break-down—leading to contamination of the environment and a high risk of infection and disease.

Health education

The public health education programme must emphasize the importance of sound environmental sanitation practices. The link between disease and contamination by excreta must be clearly understood by all.

Possible uses of excrement

Biogas can be produced from excreta, with fertilizer as a by-product. While rarely likely to be a priority in an emergency, this possibility should be considered where fuel is short and effective local biogas systems already exist. The gas is generally best used in communal services. (There is a minimum effective plant size and conversion of a family's excreta to biogas only yields up to a quarter of their needs in cooking fuel.)

More simply, the contents of dry (e.g. pit) latrines may be **composted** and used on fields. Raw sewage or liquid effluent may be poured (in a controlled manner) into **fish** farm tanks/ponds.

Unless such usage was already practised before the emergency, it would not normally be appropriate to try to introduce any of them in the immediate emergency phase but, subject to proper advice and consultation, they might be considered in the context of rehabilitation (leading into development). **349**

Possible UNICEF inputs

Depending on the assessment of actual needs and possibilities, some of the following inputs might be considered:

—Expert sanitarians (in conjunction with WHO).

—Tools, construction materials and local costs for the repair/construction of latrines.

—Disinfectants and materials for the initial, temporary repair of sewerage systems to prevent pollution.

Further references

a. *Small excreta disposal systems*, R. Feachem and S. Cairncross, Ross Bulletin No.8 — Ross Institute, London (1978)   E

b. *Excreta disposal for rural areas and small communities*, E. Wagner and J. Lanoix — WHO (1958)   E/F/S

c. *Guide to simple sanitary measures for the control of enteric diseases*, S. Rajagopalan and M. Shiffman — WHO (1974)   E/F/A

d. *Guide to sanitation in natural disasters*, M. Assar — WHO (1971)   E/F/A

e. *Disaster prevention and mitigation*, vol. 8, *Sanitation aspects* — UNDRO (1982)   E/F/S

f. *Appropriate technology for water supply and sanitation,* vol. 11, *A sanitation field manual* — World Bank (1980)   E

TYPES OF LATRINE*

This annex provides brief descriptions of different types of latrine. The circumstances in which it might be necessary and appropriate to provide latrines are reviewed in Annex 20. More details of the various types can be found in the publications listed on p. 350.

Shallow/straddle trench latrines

These are very cheap and can, in many locations, be quickly dug with picks and shovels, but each trench will normally last for only a few days before needing to be

---

* The descriptions provided in this annex are adapted from the *UNHCR handbook for emergencies* with additional details from the "further references" listed on p. 350.

replaced. They can be valuable as immediate, emergency measures while other, better arrangements are being organized.

—The trench is usually 30 cm wide and 90-150 cm deep.
—For every 100 people, 3-5 m of length is recommended.
—Soil from the digging of the trench should be piled at the side and users throw/shovel a little in each time to cover their excreta.
—Boards should be placed along the sides of the trench to provide a sure footing and prevent the sides caving in.
—When the trench is filled to within 30 cm of the top, it should be filled in with soil and compacted, the site be marked, and a new trench (or improved system) be brought into use.

Privacy may be secured with brush, canvas, wood or sheet metal fencing. Anal cleaning materials should be provided. It may be necessary for special sanitation squads to inspect trenches daily and organize the filling in and replacement of them. Where possible, simple platforms might be placed over each trench: they should be easy to clean and to move on to the next, replacement trench.

Figure 21/a Shallow trench latrine

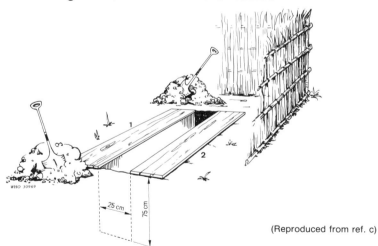

(Reproduced from ref. c)

Deep trench latrines

These are much superior to shallow trenches, can also be dug by hand, but digging takes much longer unless mechanical excavators can be quickly mobilized. Each trench can be used for several weeks and the system be operated for long periods if necessary—and if space is available for new trenches to be dug as old ones fill up.

—Trenches should be 1.8-2.5 m deep and 75-90 cm wide.

—For every 100 people, 3.5 m of length is recommended.

—Soil should be piled up and used as for shallow trenches.

—The sides of the trench should be shored up if there is any danger of collapse.

—Some sort of platform *must* cover the trench, with seats/squatting holes as appropriate and, if possible, lids to cover each one: see Figure 21/b.

The trench should be fly-proofed to the extent possible. Adding earth, ashes or oil will reduce flies. Privacy and inspection may be needed as for shallow trenches.

Figure 21/b Cover for deep trench latrine

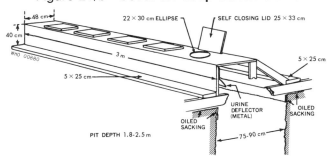

Trench revetted at sides. Anti-fly oiled sacking laid down for width of 1.25 m all round trench; wooden fly-proof cover of tongued and grooved wood on strong base.

Adapted from: O'Hara, A. S. (1967) *Environmental health in disaster,* Ottawa, Department of National Health and Welfare, Canada, p. 85.

(Reproduced from ref. d)

Pit latrines

The most common excreta disposal system around the world is the individual family pit latrine. It consists of a squatting plate (or seat) above a hole in the ground with a superstructure for privacy: see Figure 21/c.

Individual families can dig the pit and build the superstructure. If used by only one family these latrines are usually well maintained. Pit latrines can also be used in clusters as communal facilities.

—The pit should be about 1 m across and 2 m deep.

—The rim of the pit should be raised about 15 cm and cut-off ditches dug to divert any rainwater surface run-off.

—The sides of the pit should be reinforced, perhaps to a depth of one metre below ground level to prevent collapse.

—A light wooden squatting plate or wooden lattice, although harder to clean, may be more practical than a heavy concrete slab.

—When a pit is three-quarters full, it should be filled with soil and the superstructure and squatting plate moved to a new pit.

The danger of collapse may be further reduced by digging the pit as a trench only 50-60 cm wide or as a round pit. Oil drums can then be used for the lining.

The use of lids and the occasional addition of a little diesel oil can reduce odour and insect problems. If layers of ashes are applied as the pit fills, the excreta will decompose and in time the site can be used again.

Figure 21/c   Pit latrines

Simple pit latrine
(example with squatting slab)

Ventilated improved pit (VIP) latrine
(example with a seat)

(Reproduced from UNHCR *Handbook for Emergencies*)

"VIP" latrines

The ventilated improved version (VIP)—see Figure 21/c—should be built whenever possible:

—The vent pipe should be at least 15 cm in diameter, about 2 m high, painted black and placed on the sunny side of the latrine for maximum odour and insect control. It must be fitted with an insectproof gauze screen, when it will work as an excellent fly trap.

—The hole should not be covered by a lid as this impedes the air flow.

Bored-hole latrines

These are bored/drilled using a hand auger or mechanical drill and require a smaller slab than a pit. They can quickly be constructed as family units if augers are available. However, the side walls are liable to fouling, they are smellier than vented systems and the risk of ground water contamination is greater because of their depth.

—The bore-hole is 35-45 cm in diameter and any depth up to 7 m.

—If being bored by hand to a considerable depth, pipe grips may be needed to turn the auger, and a tripod and block and tackle to act as a guide and withdraw the auger: see Figure 21/d.

—A fly-proof seat structure should be provided (this also reduces fouling and smells).

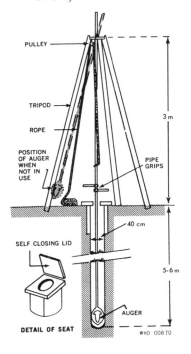

PULLEY

TRIPOD

ROPE

POSITION OF AUGER WHEN NOT IN USE

PIPE GRIPS

3 m

40 cm

SELF CLOSING LID

5-6 m

AUGER

DETAIL OF SEAT

WHO 00870

Figure 21/d
Sinking a deep bored-hole latrine

(Reproduced from ref. d)

Adapted from: O'Hara, A. S. (1967) *Environmental health in disaster,* Ottawa, Department of National Health and Welfare, Canada, p. 86.

355

Bucket latrines

Latrines in which excrement is collected directly in buckets to be taken away for composting or fish ponds tend to be very insanitary. *Very* careful attention is needed to minimize smells and flies: the bucket must be well enclosed—the squatting hole be kept covered—urine and wash wastes be drained to a soakage pit—regular emptying and maximum cleanliness be assured. See refs. a and c on p. 350.

Composting latrines

Such latrines render excreta harmless with time and produce fertilizer. Figure 21/e shows one of proven effectiveness, the Vietnamese double septic bin, suitable for a family of 5-10. Urine does not enter the bin, being diverted into a separate container.

—After each defecation ashes are sprinkled over the faeces.

—Once filled, the bin is sealed (e.g. with lime cement or clay) and the adjoining bin used.

—A full bin is left to compost for at least two months and the contents then removed through the rear access door, which has also been hermetically sealed during composting.

Figure 21/e **Double-bin composting latrine**
(ENCLOSURE NOT SHOWN)

TWO SEPARATE BINS WITH
SEALED REAR ACCESS DOORS

COVER FOR BIN IN USE

BIN IN USE

BIN NOT IN USE
I.E. COMPOSTING,
SEALED & DATED

URINE DRAIN

URINE CONTAINER

(Reproduced from UNHCR *Handbook for emergencies*)

Water seal latrines

Water seal ("pour-flush") latrines are cheap, simple in technical design but require a permeable soil for their soakaway and a ready supply of water. (Pit latrines can be modified to become water seal latrines where soil conditions allow.)

The water seal is made by a U-pipe filled with water below the squatting pan or seat. It is flushed by hand with some 1-3 litres of water into a pit or soak-away.

—A large water container with a 3 litre dipper should be close by the latrine.

—This system is suitable where water is used for anal cleaning and where the people are used to flushing.

—It is *not* suitable where paper, stones, corncobs or other solid materials are used for anal cleaning.

If flushing is inadequate or solid anal cleaning materials used, the U-pipe quickly becomes blocked.

In areas with impermeable soil such as clay, it is not possible to use a soakage pit. The liquid run off can be carried in pipes to an area suitable for disposal: see Table 21/1.

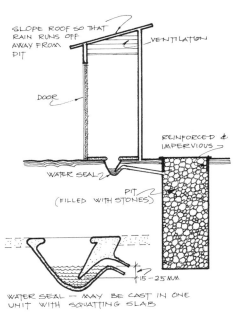

Figure 21/f
Water seal (pour-flush) latrine

(Reproduced from UNHCR
Handbook for emergencies)

357

Table 21/1

Disposal of liquid effluent when soil is impermeable

Effluent can be disposed of fairly simply and cheaply using waste stabil-
ization (oxidization) ponds—in which the wastes are broken down and
rendered harmless by natural processes:

—Ponds are particularly effective in hot climates as the rate of treatment increases with temperature.

—Required pond area depends on population and mean temperature:
possibly 1 sq.m per person.

—They must be properly constructed, controlled and securely fenced
off.

See referenced publications and get technical advice.

Aquaprivies

Aquaprivies consist of a squatting plate or seat above a small septic tank from
which effluent drains to an adjacent soakage pit.

—A minimum water tank volume of one cubic metre (1,000 litres) is
required.

Figure 21/g **Aquaprivy (example with a seat)**

—About five litres per user *must* be added daily to maintain the water seal and avoid serious odour and insect problems.

Aquaprivies are less easily blocked than the cheaper water seal latrines but are not recommended where solid materials are used for anal cleaning. They must be kept topped up: sufficient water must be readily to hand and regular supervision be assured.

Emergency sanitation units

The Oxfam sanitation unit is an example of a complete, packaged system able to be delivered to an emergency site. It comprises a communal treatment system with 20 squatting plates, two flexible tanks made of nylon-reinforced butyl rubber for sewage treatment, and all necessary pipes and fittings.

—It is a proven system which can be assembled quickly and is not affected by soil conditions.

—One unit can serve up to 1,000 persons per day.

—It requires about 3,000 litres of water a day at full design capacity: the water must not be saline.

—A good soakaway or alternate effluent disposal is required.

—It is not suitable for communities using solids (stones, corn-cobs etc.) for anal cleaning and has therefore been used widely in Asia but little in Africa.

The main disadvantages are cost (about $7,000 in 1985), problems of unfamiliarity, and the quantity of water required. A reliable operator is essential. The effluent contains as many bacteria as raw sewage and must therefore be carefully disposed of.

ANNEX 22

PERSONAL AND ENVIRONMENTAL HYGIENE

Objective

- **To minimize the risks of disease by assuring the best possible personal and domestic hygiene, and an environment free from major health hazards.**

Priorities

Together with access to reasonably safe water and sanitary means for the disposal of excreta (see Annexes 16-21), personal, domestic and general environmental hygiene are essential to protect the health of people in general, and of children in particular. This includes ensuring that:

—Appropriate facilities, soap and utensils are available for personal hygiene;

—Food is handled in as sanitary manner as possible, and food stocks inspected where necessary;

—Stagnant and waste water is quickly drained away;

—Garbage is collected and disposed of in an appropriate manner;

—Dust is controlled to be extent possible; *and*

—Health education campaigns emphasize the importance of hygiene in all these domains.

A rapid survey should be made—jointly by health and sanitation personnel and community leaders if at all possible—to:

—Assess the general state of hygiene in the community, and

—Identify immediate, practical measures which might improve the situation.

Personal hygiene

Ensure that, to the extent possible, households have or have access to facilities to wash themselves and their clothes:

—At the simplest level this requires a sufficient supply of buckets and soap (hard bar types).

—In some crowded situations, in camps or urban areas, it might be necessary to repair or establish communal washing facilities: some degree of supervision of their use and maintenance may then be required.

—In many cultures, separate facilities are needed for men and women.

In conjunction with the provision of any necessary supplies, it will normally be essential to organize, as quickly as feasible, a campaign to emphasize the importance of personal hygiene—particularly in the prevailing, emergency situation.

Food hygiene

Health and sanitation services should, to the extent practicable, try to ensure the best possible levels of food sanitation at the **communal** level, in stores, etc.:

—Medically screen all personnel handling food (other than in sealed containers): anyone with an infectious disease should be excluded, and treated;

—Inspect any food of which the containers have been damaged: control sales/distribution if necessary;

—Destroy any food which has been in contact with flood water and not in hermetically sealed tins: clean and disinfect tins which have been in flood water; *and*

—Check hygiene measures in any slaughterhouses.

Through supervision of any communal kitchens and feeding centres, and health/nutrition education to improve **domestic** practices, try to ensure that:

—Food is protected from flies;

—Fresh foods are not kept too long, unless refrigeration is available;

—Cooks and others handling food wash their hands well;

—Water used for washing vegetables is safe;

—All foods (except thick-skinned fruits) are cooked: raw meat, fish, vegetables or soft-skinned fruits are avoided: milk is boiled;

—Prepared food is consumed quickly: long delays between cooking and eating are avoided; *and*

—All utensils are cleaned as thoroughly as possible.

Waste/stagnant water

Drain waste and stagnant water away as quickly as possible to soakage pits or habitual water courses: dig channels, pump or otherwise carry the water away. It not only smells unpleasant but also provides breeding places for insects, especially mosquitoes, and spreads infections.

If removal of stagnant water cannot be achieved quickly, it may be necessary to reduce risks by chlorinating it to kill pathogens—see Table 18/6—and/or spraying to prevent mosquitoes breeding.

Waste water generated from washing, bathing and food preparation should be localized at its sources and drained directly into local soakage pits, as far as possible.

Solid refuse/garbage

The accumulation of refuse/garbage—and animal manure—is both unpleasant and unhealthy. Rodent and insect-borne diseases increase with improper disposal. Appropriate arrangements must therefore be made and routines be (re-)established for its storage, collection and disposal. Note that free range chickens, goats and pigs, when available, help control garbage. Dogs spread it.

The suggestions that follow particularly concern areas of high population density—urban areas or camps—where the problem and dangers are greatest.

Storage and collection

For the initial cleaning up of accumulated garbage:

Mobilize labour and some means of transporting the garbage to selected disposal sites/dumps.

To contain/collect each new day's garbage:

Place metal or plastic containers—e.g. 200-litre oil drums cut in half—in appropriate locations: provide lids, if possible, and punch drainage holes in the bottom.

For market areas and large institutions:

Construct large rectangular bins with floors sloping down to a door at one end (from which the garbage can be shovelled out). Keep them covered, if possible, whenever garbage is not actually being deposited or removed. Spray the sites with insecticide daily.

Arrange for the garbage to be collected regularly, perhaps daily, from all containers. Give special attention to provisions for hospitals, health and feeding centres, and similar community service institutions.

Assar, ref. a, suggests that one truck of capacity 10 cubic metres making 3 trips each day can clear the garbage produced by 5-8,000 people.

UNHCR recommends a ratio of one container per 10 families in camp situations, with such containers being placed throughout the site in such a manner that no household is more than about 15 metres away from one.

Disposal

Means of disposal will depend on the space and equipment available, and previous practices. Normally garbage should be buried at designated locations or burned—using incinerators if possible. In either case the location should be well away from any dwellings and, preferably, fenced to restrict access. (It is, in an emergency phase, rarely feasible to segregate different types of garbage and organize the composting of degradeable/organic material.)

If space and bulldozers are available, **sanitary landfill** disposal may be possible:

—The waste is dumped, under supervision, in large, specially dug/bulldozed trenches in flat areas, on small slopes, in hollows, or the edge of marshy land.

363

—Sites should be 1 km or more downwind of major habitations, and not close to water courses.

—Deposited refuse should be compacted and finally covered with 50 cm of soil.

—The operation should, where appropriate, be integrated into any local land reclamation programme.

On a smaller scale, in rural areas, waste may be **buried** in hand-dug pits or trenches:

—A typical trench might be 1.5 m wide and 2 m deep.

—At the end of each day, refuse should be covered with a little earth.

—When full to within 40 cm of ground level, fill in completely with earth, compact it and mark the site.

The contents can usually be dug out after 6 months and used on fields. Assar, loc cit, suggests that 1 m length of such a trench might be filled in one week for every 200 people.

In many situations, it will be best/necessary to **burn/incinerate** all solid wastes. An example of an incinerator improvised with corrugated iron sheets and iron bars is shown in Figure 22/a

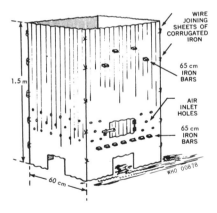

Figure 22/a
Open corrugated iron incinerator

(Reproduced from ref. b)

Adapted from: United Kingdom, Ministry of Defence (1965) *Manual of Army Health,* London, H.M. Stationery Office, p. 240.

Where there is, initially, no alternative to **dumping** garbage in open areas:

—Fence off the area;

—Crush tins to inhibit mosquito breeding in them when they fill with rain-water;

—Burn the waste as quickly as possible; *and*

—Cover the burned refuse with a little earth.

Medical waste should be treated separately, burning as much of it as possible without delay. Needles and scalpels are especially dangerous.

Dust

Large amounts of dust carried in the air can cause eye irritations, respiratory and skin problems, and contaminate food. Dust can also harm some types of equipment.

The best preventive measure is action to stop the destruction of vegetation in the vicinity. Dust control can be achieved by spraying roads with water or oil, and controlling traffic. This will rarely be possible on a large scale but might be considered around health facilities and feeding centres.

Possible UNICEF inputs

Depending on the assessment of actual needs and possibilities, some of the following inputs might be considered:

— Expertise to help plan and implement appropriate arrangements.
— Materials for the (re-)establishment of washing facilities and garbage collection systems.
— Local costs, shovels, etc. for the removal of accumulated garbage.

Further references

a. *Guide to sanitation in natural disasters*, M. Assar—WHO (1971) E/F/S

b. *Guide to simple sanitary measures for the control of enteric diseases*, S. Rajagopalan & M. Shiffman—(WHO) 1974 E/F/A

VECTOR CONTROL
(CONTROL OF DISEASE-CARRYING INSECTS AND RODENTS)

Objectives

- **To reduce the transmission of specific communicable diseases by directly or indirectly destroying — or at least containing — the carriers ("vectors") concerned.**

- **To reduce losses and contamination of food stocks by rodents.**

Priemities

Likely problems

Emergencies often create environments typically favourable to the proliferation of disease-carrying insects and rodents, which can also spoil or destroy large quantities of food.

Table 23/1 lists common vectors, related diseases and the environments/conditions under which the vectors are likely to proliferate. Note also that:

— Crowding—of displaced persons and others—greatly increases the risks of exposure to vectors and of disease transmission.

— Previous long-term control operations, if any, may also have been interrupted by the emergency.

Organizing a response

Essential initial actions are:

— Assessment by a locally experienced professional of the influence of events on the status and breeding potential of various prevalent vectors.

— A population survey for lice, fleas and ticks if many people appear to be suffering from such infestations.

— A survey to determine the extent and location of rodent (rat) infestations— their major harbourages and runs.

— A review of the problems with members and leaders of the community including explanation/education on the significance and possible means of vector control and improved personal hygiene.

Don't underestimate the difficulty of reducing the numbers of flies, mosquitoes and rodents quickly in the aftermath of an emergency!

Actions

● **Give top priority to improving general environmental sanitation (disposal of excreta, garbage and waste water), personal hygiene (requiring adequate soap and water) and the careful storage of food and water.**

● **Intensify/initiate appropriate chemical control measures against mosquitoes and rodents where necessary.**

Physical screens may be used against flies, especially in health and feeding centres.

Professional expertise with local knowledge and experience is necessary to plan and supervise control measures, especially the choice and use of chemicals taking account of any insecticide resistance in local vectors and pests.

Control measures should be undertaken as part of, or at least in close co-ordination with, the relevant national programmes and practices. The measures used in   **367**

Table 23/1

Vectors which may pose significant health risks

Vector	Health risks	Favourable environments
Flies	Eye infections (particularly among infants and children); diarrhoeal diseases	Exposed food; excreta; dead animals.
Mosquitoes	Malaria; Filariasis, encephalitis;	Stagnant water, especially in the periphery of inundated areas; pools and slow-moving water.
	Yellow fever, dengue;	Stored water in or around dwellings; accumulations of rain water in old tins and other containers.
Mites	Scabies, scrub typhus	
Lice	Epidemic typhus, relapsing fever	Overcrowding and poor personal hygiene
Fleas	Plague (from infected rats), endemic typhus	
Ticks	Relapsing fever, spotted fever	
Rats	Rat bite fever, leptospirosis, salmonellosis	Inadequately protected food; exposed garbage; covered spaces.

The insects also cause bites and/or annoyance!

(Adapted from *UNHCR Handbook for emergencies*)

previous long-term programmes should normally be maintained, but operations may need to be refocused and rescheduled/accelerated in relation to the new circumstances.

Priority should be given to areas of high population density and those subject to particular seasonal factors (such as inaccessibility during rains). Follow-up surveys are essential to evaluate the effectiveness of measures taken.

Specific control measures

Mosquitoes

Essential actions:

- Spraying important resting places of adult mosquitoes with specific insecticides.
- Spraying standing water with larvicides or growth inhibitors.
- Space spraying by air or ground (e.g. vehicle-mounted) equipment, particularly for yellow fever and dengue vectors.
- Elimination, to the extent practicable, of habitats—especially stagnant water, empty tins, etc.

Flies

Essential actions:

- Good general sanitation, especially the disposal of all organic waste including dead animals.
- Making latrines as fly-proof as possible.
- Physical screening of windows in hospitals, health and feeding centre kitchens.
- Spraying garbage containers occasionally with insecticide. (It is often advisable to rotate between different chemicals in spraying operations.)

Rodents (rats)

Essential actions:

- Dusting specifically identified rat "runs" with an appropriate rodenticide.
- Baited traps in warehouses.

Attention should be given first to any crowded temporary camp settlements, food warehouses in ports and elsewhere, markets and hospitals. Rodenticides, if used, should normally be "chronic" (slow acting) rather than "acute".

In areas where *plague* or other arthropod-borne diseases are endemic, action must be taken to control the fleas, ticks or other vectors caried by the rats *before* any large-scale control of rodents is attempted—especially through the use of large **369** numbers of snap traps. Otherwise an epidemic of plague may be precipitated by fleas transferring from the dead rats to humans!

Care must be taken in disposing of dead rats which may be carrying plague-bearing fleas. Wear gloves. Incinerate the bodies if possible, otherwise bury them in a deep hole well away from any water including ground water.

Lice

Essential actions:

—Improved personal hygiene!

—Mass delousing of people, clothes and bedding by dusting with insecticide (e.g. 1 per cent lindane) if problems severe.

Lice are found mainly on collars, waistbands and seams. Washing clothes is only effective if the water temperature is maintained at at least 54 °C, which is rarely possible. Dusting is best done using compressed air equipment.

Fleas

Essential actions:

—Dusting of rodent runs and fumigation of their burrows with appropriate insecticides.

—Insecticide treatment of bedding may be necessary; but infants' bedding should not be treated, only washed.

—Where flea-borne diseases are prevalent, applications to persons bodies and clothes may be required.

Where no flea-borne diseases are prevalent, fleas may be removed by hand from bodies of persons infested, and by combing from bodies of infested domestic animals; they should be immediately crushed.

Ticks

Tick problems may be able to be reduced by acaricide applications in outdoor areas where ticks are prevalent or by clearing vegetation for 50-100 metres around camps/villages. Indoor applications of acaricides may be necessary where large numbers of ticks are found inside dwellings.

Bed-bugs

Simple methods such as beating bedding and furniture outdoors, well away from dwellings, or pouring hot water over bed frames, can reduce infestations. With heavy infestations it may be necessary to apply insecticide to beds, mattresses, crevices in walls and furniture—but infant bedding, including the crib, should not be treated with insecticide. Treated bedding must be dried completely before reuse.

Possible UNICEF inputs

Depending on the assessment of actual needs and possibilities, some of the following inputs might be considered:

—Appropriate chemicals and sprayers.

—Personal equipment for survey teams (collection jars, protective clothing, lamps, etc.)

—Transport, local operating costs.

—Soap for domestic and institutional use; detergent and disinfectant for institutional use.

—Appropriate essential drugs for treatment, especially Benzyl Benzoate against scabies and lice.

—Materials and local costs for health education campaigns

Further references

a. *Emergency vector control after natural disaster*, Scientific publication No. 419—PAHO (1982) E/S

b. *Guide to sanitation in natural disasters*, M. Assar—WHO (1971) E/F/S

c. *Chemical methods for the control of arthropod vectors and pests of public health importance*—WHO (1984) E/S (F expected 1986)

ANNEX 24

SHELTER

Objective

- **To assure necessary shelter for families in order to safeguard the lives of young children.**

Emergency shelter

Priorities

Only the necessary minimum of time, effort and resources should be committed to temporary, emergency shelter. Permanent reconstruction should be promoted as soon as possible.

When provision does have to be made for emergency shelter:

— Provide materials which can be reused later in permanent reconstruction;
— Make maximum use of materials which can be salvaged from damaged buildings;
— Give highest priority to roofing;
— Avoid "temporary" and prefabricated/relief housing.

Materials

Tough *plastic sheeting* and/or *tarpaulins* and *rope* are often useful for constructing/improving emergency shelter arranged by the survivors themselves. They are also materials which can usually be reused later.

Tents may be available in stockpiles and — if robust — can provide temporary shelter where such is a necessity (due to the weather) and the improvisation of other shelter is not feasible. Tents do, however, deteriorate in use and in some conditions have a short useful lifespan.

Table 24/1 provides some suggested specifications for sheeting and tents.

Notes for tent suppliers: Tent specifications are to be understood as minimum in material weight and floor space. Only quality, heavy-duty tents should be offered; white or lightly dyed (olive, green, brown).

Canvas must be equally strong in warp and weft. Treatment of the canvas: salamander flame retardant, rot and water-proofing process or equivalent; chemicals used for treatment must not smell offensive. Stitching: by machine with extra strong, weatherproof thread. Ridges: reinforced with canvas or cotton tape. Hems: wide enough to accept eyelets. Eyelets: non-ferrous. Cabs and taps: strongly stitched at outer and inner ridge for upright poles.

Ventilation and window openings: protected with mosquito netting. Flaps: with good overlap unless zippered. Zippered door flaps to have ties sewn on (in case zipper breaks). All entrance fastners, zippers, clips and ties to be heavy duty and, where appropriate, non-ferrous.

Anchorages for tent and fly sheet every 50 cm. Guy ropes: equivalent in strength to 12 mm sisal rope and ultra-violet stabilized. Pegs for guys: 40cm long, iron or steel. Pins for walls and groundsheet: 15 cm long, iron or steel. Poles: tubular steel (not wood or bamboo), standard sections not more than 1.5 m long.

Packing: tent, poles, accessories and hardware bundled in a single packsack.

"*Temporary housing*" (usually prefabricated) is to be avoided. It is rarely in fact replaced. The units are often very expensive, especially when of imported components — absorbing resources which might better be directed towards permanent reconstuction — and may require special expertise for erection. Services, including water and sanitation arrangements, markets, etc. also have to be provided at the site.

373

Where such units and/or the siting of them have been unsuitable for local patterns of family life, or necessary services have not been provided, the housing has either been little used or rapidly become slums. Experience with special, prefabricated "emergency shelters"—e.g. polyeurethane igloos—has so far not been encouraging.

Table 24/1

Specifications for plastic sheeting and tents

Reinforced polythene tarpaulin/groundsheet material

UNIPAC 50-860-10: 4 m wide, 50 m long (200 sq. m total area) in centre-folded rolls 2 m wide, 25 cm diameter, approx 55 kg—reinforced ultraviolet ray resistant—0.25 mm thick (275 g/m²)—plastic eyelets both sides every metre, double row of eyelets across every 5 m—colour green.

Plastic sheeting

Where it is immediately and cheaply available, seamless polythene sheeting (preferably black) can also be useful although less strong than the above and without eyelets: 0.25 mm thick—4-8 m wide supplied in double-folded rolls of 100 m or more in length—approximately 1 kg/m².

Rope

Essential for use with tarpaulins: minimum l m rope for every square metre of tarpaulin—e.g. UNIPAC 50-700-00 (7.6 m coils).

Family tents

12 sq.m tents are usually supplied. See UNIPAC catalogue.

Round, bell-type tents (e.g. 50-880-02 made of 300 g/m² cotton or cotton/polyester canvas, total approximately 22 kg) are suitable if air-freighting is necessary and/or there are high winds, and if camp beds are *not* being used. 8 persons/tent.

Otherwise rectangular, ridge-type tents are usually preferable (e.g. 50-880-04 made of 400 g/m² cotton or cotton/polyester canvas, total including flysheet approximately 50 kg). 6 camp beds/tent or 8 persons without camp beds.

Hospital ward tents

80 sq.m ridge (e.g. 50-880-05) or frame tents with centre height 3.6-4.0 m and high side walls can accommodate 10 hospital beds or 40 patients without beds. Windows with mosquito nets and flaps are essential.

N.B. All tents must be supplied complete with poles (sectional steel tube), all necessary ropes/guy-lines, sufficient iron or steel pegs and pins (including spares), and mallets.

Reconstruction of dwellings

Priorities

Initial pre-programming surveys and investigations must thoroughly consider: land ownership—structural designs—type and availability of materials—methods of financing. Knowledge of pre-existing housing conditions, life styles, existing co-operative mechanisms and normal house building processes is vital to planning any assistance.

Families may be assisted to (re)construct small "core" dwellings initially—one or two rooms—which can be enlarged/extended later, if and when the family can afford it.

Assistance should be spread over an extended period to allow for proper planning and gradual/phased implementation with full community participation.

Land ownership and tenure

These legal aspects are crucial and must be investigated and settled before any programme is initiated. People are usually reluctant to invest their own resources (including effort) in reconstructing property they do not own or in installing non-movable structures on land they do not own.

If assistance is to benefit the needy population rather than landlords, inputs may need to be of materials which can, if necessary, be removed later to be used on another site—e.g. corrugated sheets.

Structural designs and construction techniques

Be cautious about proposing fundamental changes but encourage adaptations of normal practices which would help to reduce future vulnerability of the buildings to floods, winds and/or earthquakes, and which:

—Are based on proper technical advice and proven experience;

—Are "affordable"—do not greatly increase the cost compared with a traditional building;

—Do not depend on materials which are not normally available in the country; *and*

—Can be incorporated in traditional construction processes by local craftsmen.

375

Where changes are sought, ensure that:
— The community is thoroughly involved and agrees in advance;
— Appropriate demonstration constructions are arranged; *and*
— Local craftsmen are trained on the job.

Any "model" building should be for community purposes—e.g. a clinic or community hall. "Model villages" are to be avoided.

Materials

Use/supply only materials which will be available, at a reasonable price, in the country in the long term. Otherwise ongoing maintenance and repair will not be possible.

In some situations, government price controls might be necessary to forestall profiteering in such materials in the aftermath of a disaster.

Financing/distribution

If *free distribution* of materials is considered appropriate, carefully establish and enforce distribution criteria to ensure that the maximum benefit is derived—in terms of numbers of particularly needy families enabled to establish at least a minimum of suitable housing.

In many situations it has been found to be better, and possible, for materials to be *sold* at subsidized prices and/or against *credit* with repayments being made into a revolving fund from which further development projects in the community are then financed.

Good knowledge of local social structures, co-operative experiences, banking, etc. is essential. The specific objectives of any assistance programme must be carefully defined in agreement with the community itself and the local authorities.

Construction processes

In some situations it may be useful to constitute "*work teams*" to undertake all or part (e.g. the roof) of the actual construction work. Means and rates of payment for such teams must be agreed with the community and the local authorities at the outset.

Necessary *tools* may be provided to such teams, or co-operative groups, or be sold (perhaps at subsidised prices or on credit) to individual artisans. Tools must be appropriate—ones to which local craftsmen are accustomed.

Possible UNICEF inputs

Depending on the assessment of actual needs and possibilities, some of the following inputs might be considered for emergency shelter:
—Plastic sheeting and/or tarpaulins and rope.
—Tools, nails, etc.
—Tents.

However, other organizations are often ready and able to provide emergency shelter. UNICEF resources should be committed for such purposes only if the need is urgent and others are not able to act quickly enough. The reimbursable procurement facilities of UNICEF may be made available to the government and other agencies.

UNICEF would not normally be involved in the long term reconstruction of private dwellings. Strictly limited inputs of a catalytic or "bottle-neck-breaking" nature—e.g. tools, nails—might, however, be made where such are needed and not being provided quickly enough by others.

Further references

Shelter after disaster—UNDRO (1982)   E/S

PERSONAL AND HOUSEHOLD SUPPLIES

Objective

● **To assure the availability of adequate personal protection (clothing and blankets) for young children, and basic household items to enable the households to which they belong to function.**

Clothing and blankets

Where people are exposed—especially at night—to cold/wet conditions and do not have adequate personal protection, the rapid provision of blankets and/or appropriate clothing will be a real and urgent need. Alternatively, provision might need to be planned in anticipation of a forthcoming seasonal change in climate.

In other circumstances, the early commitment of scarce resources to the procurement, transportation, handling and distribution of such items is generally neither necessary nor appropriate. (Such items are not always lost in emergencies and, even when they are, the replacement of them may not be high among the survivors' own immediate priorities.)

Blankets

Blankets are versatile and may also be used as shawls (i.e. clothing). They should be durable and able to withstand getting wet. Cotton or synthetic ones are generally more appropriate than wool in tropical climates.

If blankets are produced/available locally, or in the region, they are probably more likely to be kept and used by the intended beneficiaries than ones of a quite different quality from elsewhere.

Clothing

Clothing, where needed, must be culturally appropriate. If the need is not immediate, consider supplying cloth and ensuring the means for clothes to be made up locally—sewing machines for tailoring co-operatives, spare parts for local textile mills, etc.

Funds spent on shipping even donated/second-hand western-style clothing to countries where such is not customary would generally be better used buying clothing locally, if available in necessary quantities, or providing cloth.

Where the immediate provision of clothing is not an absolute necessity, the importation and distribution of made-up clothes also makes the process of rehabilitation much slower and more difficult for local tailors and artisans.

Household supplies

Priorities

Cooking utensils, water carriers/containers and stoves may be needed for family units and/or any communal kitchen facilities—especially for displaced people and those who cannot salvage their own after a sudden, cataclysmic disaster.

Utensils and stoves in particular should normally be of a type already used in the area: this may indicate local procurement. If improved, fuel-efficient stoves are to be promoted, ensure their acceptability to women—through local trials and demonstrations—*before* relying on their widespread adoption and use.

Buckets are often needed and useful: they are more suitable for storing water if provided with a lid. Plastic jerry cans are very useful for carrying and storing water: traditional wood or earthenware pots may also be used. **379**

In some situations, pre-packed "family kits" have been found useful. Such might include: 2 cooking pots, a kitchen knife, and bowls, spoons, mugs sufficient for the average household; a suitable stove, lantern, soap and other essential hygiene supplies. Such supplies are needed quickly, if at all, but the need for them should not be exaggerated nor the practical difficulties of distribution be underestimated.

The light-weight emergency family cooking set UNIPAC 20-365-10, with the addition of cutlery if necessary, may be appropriate if deliveries by air from outside the country are necessary.

Communal facilities

Where communal facilities are intended to be a very short-term measure, supplies for them must be delivered quickly, or not at all.

Improvisation may be called for: e.g. the use of cleaned, empty oil drums for boiling water and cooking cereals rather than investing in the procurement of special large (and expensive) pots which may not arrive on site before the kitchens are due to be disbanded and family utensils are required instead.

Possible UNICEF inputs

Depending on the assessment of actual needs and possibilities, some of the following inputs might be considered:

—Blankets—by rapid local/regional procurement or ex-UNIPAC.

—Clothing—appropriate children's sizes—and/or cloth and thread.

—Sewing machines (if there are suitable co-operative/community organizations to ensure good use of them).

—Cooking utensils, possibly in sets.

—Stoves; possibly also fuel for them.

—Buckets, water containers.

However, other agencies are often ready and able to provide such "relief" items when needed. If so, UNICEF resources should be conserved for "rehabilitation" and interventions which contribute to development in the long term.

DISPLACED POPULATIONS
(SPECIAL CONSIDERATIONS FOR)*

Objectives

- To avoid the congregation of people in temporary camps, if possible.

- To minimize health hazards, assure basic needs are met, and make life tolerable for displaced children and families until they can return home or be permanently resettled.

- To help displaced families and communities to return to their homes or resettle elsewhere, if necessary.

Temporary camps of displaced persons

Refugee/relief camps are almost invariably demoralizing and, initially at least, insanitary with high levels of disease and apathy. Once people have left their

---

* The guidelines provided in this annex are largely derived from the *UNHCR Handbook for emergencies,* UNHCR (1982), and, in *Disasters,* vol. 5, No. 3 (1981): "Camps as communities", J. Holt, and "Camp lay-out and the siting of facilities".

homes and congregated in camps, possibilities for re-establishing self-support, self-respect and healthy community life and environments are considerably reduced/retarded.

Camps must therefore be avoided if at all possible:

—Promote and support evacuations only where absolutely necessary to pre-serve life in the face of a specific and immediate threat;

—Deliver necessary assistance and services to people where they live, to the extent possible.

Where camps are temporarily unavoidable, give attention to:

—Social organization within the population;

—Site selection, layout, shelter and sanitation arrangements;

—Provision of basic services (including food, water, health care, social services and stimulation for children); *and*

—Promoting whatever level of self-support and useful employment is poss-ible.

The UNHCR *Handbook for Emergencies* (ref. a) provides guidelines for the organization and management of a refugee camp. The requirements for camps of internally displaced persons are similar, apart from issues of international pro-tection.

Social organization

- **Promote and support social mechanisms which encourage the formation of effective communities and provide a basis for collective decision-making and action.**

- **Try to identify leaders who have genuine popular support and a commitment to the well-being of the community as a whole.**

Don't assume that displaced populations are integrated communities. They often comprise abnormally high proportions of women, children and old people. Tra-ditional hierarchical relationships are sometimes, but not always preserved. There is, however, often a degree of solidarity and cohesion arising from the shared experience of insecurity and dependence.

Individuals generally emerge who seek to lead/organize the population—or sub-groups within it—and present themselves as representatives of the population vis-à-vis local authorities and the providers of aid. They often include traditional leaders, political leaders and young educated persons. They may or may not have the confidence and support of the majority of the population. Educated youth in particular are in fact often alienated from their own society.

Women leaders must always be mobilized and supported in the organization of activities specifically for women and young children. Their full participation in all aspects of camp organization should also be promoted but, in some societies, it may not be realistic to expect to bring about an immediate and radical change in their status and role in matters traditionally the preserve of men.

Site selection, layout, shelter and sanitation

Table 26/1 lists the characteristics of the ideal site. In practice, compromises usually have to be made. Conditions should be as similar as possible to what the population is accustomed to, and rights to the use of the land be assured.

Site layout will always be a compromise between the needs of public control and service provision on the one hand, and the social needs of the people on the other. Military precision and the appearance of order are not necessarily appropriate, but the location and accessibility of facilities—latrines, water points, clinics, feeding centres—is crucial to their use and very high population densities are to be avoided, if possible, for health and social reasons.

Involve community leaders in developing a site plan which:

—Is appropriate to the needs, preferences and traditions of the population, particularly its make-up in terms of individual and extended families, clans, villages, distinct ethnic and/or religious groups, etc.

Table 26/1

Site for a displaced persons camp

To the extent possible, any camp should be located where:

☐ Adequate water is available all year round;

☐ Space is sufficient for the number of persons expected (30 square metres per person if possible);

☐ There is adequate drainage (avoiding flat and marshy ground);

☐ There are no major environmental health hazards, high winds, extremes of weather or risks of flooding;

☐ There is fairly easy access to road and other communications, and to supplies of food, cooking fuel and shelter materials;

☐ Vegetation provides shade and soil conditions permit water infiltration and possibilities for vegetable gardening; and

☐ There is good security and little possibility of the population being affected by hostilities, or coming into conflict with local residents.

—Encourages the organization/formation of small community units/sectors (of perhaps 5,000 people) with decentralized community services: health clinic—primary school—supplementary feeding centre (if required)—social service centre—recreation space;

—Ensures access within each such community unit/sector to latrines (within 50 m of each family), water supplies and washing facilities (within 100 m if possible);

—Includes central facilities necessary for the camp as a whole: administrative and service co-ordination offices—warehouses—tracing service—hospital; *and*

—Minimizes fire risks by avoiding overcrowding and incorporating fire breaks (gaps without buildings).

It is generally best to establish distinct residential clusters with central services either at the centre or near the main entrance to the site. Plans must, however, be adapted to: the terrain—existing rivers, roads and land use—the number of people and space available.

Allow space to receive additional people (e.g. extended family members) if necessary within the area assigned to each distinct community group. Ensure that space allocated for community services is indeed reserved for such use.

Delivery of basic services

In all cases, committees or other mechanisms of community participation must be established from the earliest possible moment and take as much responsibility as possible for planning and organizing all services—including introducing any new arrivals to the arrangements in the camp, services available and opportunities for participation.

Issues of basic food supplies, special feeding, health care, water supplies and social services are dealt with in other annexes. In each case arrangements need to be adapted to the camp context—in particular the abnormal social situation, environmental health risks and lack of existing infrastructure—and the standards of provision available to the local population.

The establishment of schools for children—teaching literacy and numeracy in the language of the population itself—should have high priority. The lack of stimulation in a camp can otherwise be very detrimental to the development of children.

Careful attention is necessary to ensure that standards of provision for different groups are reasonably uniform, and that all involved organizations observe common practices with regard to the remuneration of workers recruited from the population for various service operations.

Promoting self-respect and self-support

Support activities which:
- —Help families to establish some control over their own lives;
- —Enable families to produce at least a little food and earn income in other ways; *and*
- —Provide opportunities for constructive use of people's time and abilities, and relieve boredom;

Petty trading should not necessarily be discouraged, unless it is suspected that large volumes of food rations or other relief assistance are being diverted.

Helping people to return home/resettle

After a period of evacuation or forced displacement, special help may be needed for some time to enable people to settle back into their previous homes and lives, or to resettle elsewhere when return is impossible.

UNHCR frequently supports programmes of assistance to refugees being repatriated/resettled in developing countries. Similar assistance may be needed by families who return home or resettle in another location after a period of displacement within their own country, e.g.:
- —Food assistance and/or employment programmes until the next harvest;
- —Agricultural tools and inputs;
- —Raw materials/tools/equipment for cottage industries;
- —Tools/materials for reconstruction of dwellings.

At the community level, assistance may be needed to:
- —Re-establish water supplies and sanitation systems;
- —Restore basic health services, schools, etc. including community service premises.

Special assistance may be needed for families who are destitute, especially when able-bodied adults and means of livelihood have been lost. The rapid (re-)establishment of social services can be important to identify and help such families, see Annex 27.

Reception centres may, in some circumstances, be needed to provide shelter, food, water, and basic health care for returnees during the first days/weeks. Special **385** arrangements may be needed for unaccompanied children within the returning population, see Annex 28.

Possible UNICEF inputs

Depending on the assessement of actual needs and possibilities, some of the following inputs might be considered:

To prevent displacements:

—Inputs to help meet the basic needs of people in their own localities, to the extent possible: see Annexes 2-25.

For people in temporary displaced persons camps:

—Materials/tools for erection of family shelters: see Annex 24.

—Utensils/cooking fuel, clothing, blankets (where necessary): see Annex 25.

—Supplies and/or funds to support programmes to assure access to food supplies, special feeding programmes (where necessary), health services, water supplies and sanitation: see Annexes 2-23.

—Support for initiatives aimed at achieving a degree of self-support, and education programmes.

For returnees/resettlement:

—Assistance for families (especially the destitute and single-parent families) to re-establish productive activities.

—Assistance to the re-establishment of local production, water supplies, community services, etc.

—Basic materials and equipment (utensils, etc.) for any necessary reception centres.

Further references

a. *UNHCR Handbook for Emergencies*—UNHCR (1982)   E/F/S

b. *Medical care in refugee camps, Disasters,* vol. 5, No. 3—International Disaster Institute, London (1981)   E

ANNEX 27

COMMUNITY-BASED SOCIAL SERVICES*

Objectives

- **To help people to meet their own needs, resolve personal problems and inter-personal conflicts, where necessary.**

- **To prevent family separations, where possible.**

---

* The guidelines provided in this annex are derived largely from the *UNHCR Handbook for social services,* provisional edition, UNHCR, 1984.

Priorities

Help may be needed by individuals, families and/or community groups. Help is most needed by:
- —Unaccompanied children (see Annex 28);
- —Single-parent families;
- —Destitute families;
- —Families of which the mother and/or bread-winner is sick/injured/in hospital/in prison;
- —Disabled persons;
- —Psychologically disturbed individuals;
- —Unaccompanied young women;
- —Unaccompanied elderly persons;
- —Ethnic minorities.

Table 27/1 lists some of the areas in which help may be needed. In addition to practical services, policies are necessary—must be advocated—which protect and promote the integrity of the family.

Where sufficient help is not able to be provided by traditional community mechanisms, culturally appropriate social services may be reinforced/established.

Mechanisms and services to help meet these needs should not be forgotten and starved of resources as attention is focused on more obvious material needs, some of which may in fact be less important!

Helping the community to help itself

Wherever possible, actions should be community-based. They should:
- —Draw personnel and other resources from within the community as much as possible;
- —Be designed, carried out and evaluated, as far as possible, by members of the community;
- —Be based on the culture and traditional coping mechanisms of the community; *and*
- —Be decentralized with as much authority as possible for decision making and using resources given to the participants.

This also helps to assure that there is a focus on what the people consider to be their priority needs.

Table 27/1

Priorities for social services

Possible needs to be met:

—Providing information to community members about the situation and the resources/services available;

—Helping individuals/families to solve problems, and those with special needs to receive and use assistance available to them;

—Helping the destitute, single-parent families, disabled persons and others to find suitable places to live and to support themselves to the extent possible;

—Helping individuals and families under stress to adjust to a new environment and any loss experienced;

—Helping resolve conflicts that may arise within families and the community; *and*

—Promoting measures and activities, where possible, to prevent or mitigate the effects of foreseeable problems within the community.

Activities may thus include:

—Establishing and operating information centres;

—Making the services of trained social workers available to help individuals in dealing with authorities and outside organizations, and to provide counselling services for individuals and families;

—Helping to organize community self-help activities of all kinds, including income generating activities for women and the destitute, cooperative child care, etc.;

—Organizing activities—educational, recreational, perhaps daycare—for children;

—Arranging group support and special services for disabled persons, especially children, and those suffering emotional and psychological problems;

—Providing rehabilitation therapy and training for those recently disabled.

Close co-ordination with health workers is essential as problems are often brought to their notice in the first instance.

The government and outside assistance should, as necessary, offer encouragement and support—including appropriate professional guidance, resources and training—to efforts within the community.

Reaching the needy

The most needy individuals are often hesitant to come forward themselves:

—Arrangements must be made to systematically look for and identify those who have particular needs and ensure that they receive food and other available assistance; *and*

—Community social workers should make themselves "available" regularly at known locations to talk informally with people and listen their problems and requests.

Where formal social services did not previously exist, or have been completely disrupted, the function of screening the community may initially fall on general relief personnel working with community leaders. Where and when feasible, this function should be integrated with other social support services within the community and community-based social workers work closely with those directly organizing food and other emergency assistance.

Table 27/2

Criteria for selecting social workers

Basic factors:

—Age; sex; previous work experience;

—Ability to read and write the local language;

—Ability to read and write, or at least speak, a common language with other national and international personnel;

—Educational background; social position.

A high level of education and/or social position may help or hinder a community worker depending on the requirements of the job and the way these characteristics will affect relations with members of the community. The ability to read and write is useful, but not necessarily essential for *all* workers.)

Personal factors; each individual should:

—Be respected as honest and trustworthy by other members of the community;

—Be concerned about the needs of others;

—Show initiative and good judgement;

—Be able to communicate easily with those requiring help;

—Be a good listener; *and*

—Have an agreeable personality.

He/she should be willing to continue in the job for the foreseeable future.

Initiating social service programmes

Activities may initially focus on only one or two immediate problems/issues: others may be included later to evolve a comprehensive programme. Ensure, however, that:

— All social service activities are properly integrated;

— Participation includes as broad a range as possible of community sub-groups (but without unduly delaying action); *and*

— Special efforts are made, where necessary, to ensure the full participation of women in planning and organizing activities.

Identify and mobilize existing community structures, services or NGOs to promote, plan and organize appropriate programmes within the community. Establish a special community board/committee if necessary.

Staffing

Selection: Arrange for community social workers to be carefully selected by professionals, already serving social workers and/or the community itself. Table 27/2 suggests some criteria.

Training: Define needs for and arrange appropriate initial (pre-service) training, also ongoing in-service training. Choose formal training methods carefully and consider apprenticeships — placing a new worker with an experienced worker for an initial period.

Assigning: Individuals should be assigned either functionally (for specific functions in a large community) or geographically (all functions in a small community); possibly in small teams (usually a man and a woman together). Avoid assigning individuals to the particular localities in which they live. Rotate them between functions/areas occasionally.

Identifying specific needs

The responsible community committee/body should establish priorities for action. Assigned community social workers may start by undertaking an initial needs survey as the beginning of a continuous process of identifying needs and helping to find solutions. Check-lists for screening and assessment at the household level are suggested below.

391

Check-list for social service screening

House-to-house investigations should determine whether there is anyone within the household facing the problems listed or knowledge of anyone elsewhere who faces such problems.

General household screening

☐ Anyone who has an illness or injury that needs treatment?

☐ Anyone having trouble: taking care or him/herself—getting enough food, water, cooking fuel?

☐ Anyone who does not have the things needed for daily living, e.g. cooking utensils, sufficient clothes or blankets?

☐ Anyone who does not have an adequate place to live?

☐ Any children separated from their parents, unaccompanied?

☐ Anyone who has difficulty: walking—using arms or legs—seeing—hearing—speaking—learning?

☐ Anyone who has behavioural or mental problems, or problems because of sometimes acting in a strange way?

☐ Anyone who needs help with contacting family members in another place, or finding family members who have become separated?

Single-parent (and destitute) families

☐ What has happened to the husband/wife who is not present?

☐ Can the family provide any information that could help with family re-union?

☐ Do the children and parent seem to be: healthy—adequately fed—adequately dressed?

☐ If anyone has been sick: when—were they treated by a doctor—what was the illness—is anyone still taking or in need of medecines?

392 ☐ Have the children been fully immunized (in line with local EPI)?

☐ If the parent is the mother, is she breast-feeding or pregnant? If so, does she attend a clinic? Does she receive/need any special help which is available?

☐ What skills and possibilities does the parent or any older child have to work and support the family? Are they aware of and able to use appropriate services and/or training opportunities?

☐ What special problems is the family facing?

☐ Are there any friends, neighbours or relatives who can help solve some of the problems?

Single-parent families

Problems likely to be faced by single-parent families include:

— Difficulty of achieving self-support due to domestic responsibilities, lack of time and/or skills to cultivate land or earn an income;

— Restricted mobility and problems of access to assistance and services due to due to child-minding responsibilities;

— Difficulties in arranging a reasonable place to live and physical security, especially where the single parent is a woman.

Problems, if unresolved, often lead to family disintegration, especially where the single parent is a man.

Actions which can help to resolve some of these problems include:

— Promoting arrangements for the care of young children, co-operatively among families or through centres at places of work or where services are provided. (A meal may need to be provided for the children during the day.)

— Ensuring that community services—health clinics, feeding/food distribution centres, etc.—are delivered close to all communities (through small static units or mobile operations).

— Assisting cottage industries providing work which can be done at home.

— Providing relevant training, credit or other assistance to enable groups to establish co-operative income generating projects.

— Arranging practical help and encouragement to single parents from neighbours, religious and community leaders as well as social workers, and counselling to help them (especially men) accept their role as single parents.

393

Unaccompanied young women

Young women who are separated from their families—including women who are heads of families—may face problems of unwanted advances, rape, temporary relationships and unwanted pregnancies as well as difficulties in finding places to live and protect their belongings.

Mutual support groups and residential centres can help and also provide opportunities for co-operative child care, training and income generating activities.

Disabled children (and adults)

To the extent possible, ensure prompt and appropriate medical care for the sick and injured (and a safe physical environment) to *prevent* physical impairments and consequent disabilities.

Where children (and adults) already suffer handicaps as a result of specific disabilities, promote services to help them integrate into society: see Table 27/3.

Table 27/3

Impairments, disabilities and handicaps

Impairments include: amputated limb—paralysis—burn scars—hypertension—blindness—deafness—mental retardation—disturbed thought processes.

These may result in *disabilities* such as a decreased ability to: walk—speak—hear—see—lift—learn—maintain contact with reality.

These in turn may result in *handicaps* such as:
—Inability to perform usual work/hold a job;
—Decreased capacity for household tasks;
—Inability to have normal social relationships;
—Inability to attend school.

Appropriate therapy, aids and rehabilitation training may reduce actual disabilities. Such actions plus social/psychological help and occupational/vocational training can then reduce/eliminate the handicap by enabling the person—child or adult—to fulfill a more normal role in society.

Action to help disabled children (and adults)

Arrange for physical aids—artificial legs, crutches, wheel chairs, etc.—to be pro-duced locally to meet the specific needs of individuals, see ref. e. Apart from advantages in cost, speed of delivery and individual tailoring as compared with imported aids, locally produced items can also be repaired by local craftsmen (or the users themselves).

Arrange rehabilitation therapy/training. Ref. 'b' provides detailed guidelines for rehabilitation training which can be provided by family members, neighbours, etc. ("trainers") with a minimum of guidance and supervision. Essential actions are:

—Assessing needs and developing a plan;
—Translating the materials in ref. b into the local language, where necessary;
—Mobilizing/appointing and training local supervisors;
—Mobilizing community leadership, teachers and others to support the pro-gramme;
—Finding, for each disabled child/person, a trainer who is willing and can understand the training materials;
—Arranging initial orientation of each trainer, and providing ongoing guidance and supervision;
—Assuring referral services, especially for those with behavioural problems and/or requiring medical treatment.

Where special rehabilitation expertise and services are available in institutions, use them to help plan the programme, train local supervisors and provide special services for the minority of individuals who do not respond to community-level training.

Try to ensure/arrange for disabled children to be integrated into the local school wherever possible, and provide appropriate training and employment opportu-nities for the older ones.

Psychological problems

Children suffering severe trauma—and many who have become unaccompanied as a result of the emergency—need psychological assessments and assistance. This can include help in re-associating with adults for children who have been abused, severely deprived, witnessed killings, etc.

Help should be offered in the context of the individual's existing system of beliefs and rituals. It might include one-to-one counselling by trained professionals in **395** association also with traditional/religious leaders, and mutual support groups of individuals with similar problems.

Possible UNICEF inputs

Depending on the assessement of actual needs and possibilities, some of the following inputs might be considered:

—Expertise to help plan and implement programmes, including training.

—Local operating costs for surveys of need, training and operations of community-based social workers, rehabilitation supervisors, etc.

—Materials/funds for local production of aids for disabled children.

—Recreational and educational materials for cooperative child care arrangements/centres.

Further references

a. *UNHCR Handbook for social services,* provisional edition—UNHCR (1984) E (some parts also F/S)

Specifically on rehabilitation of disabled persons:

b. *Training disabled people in the community*—WHO (RHB/83.1) (1983) E/F/A (parts also available in many other languages, consult WHO and/or HQ)

Also draft companion guides: *Guide for intermediate level supervisors* and *Guide for translation and adaptation*—WHO (RHB drafts 1983) E

c. *Rehabilitation for all—a text book on the management of community-based rehabilitation*—WHO (expected 1988) E

d. *Childhood disability: rehabilitation and prevention at the community level*—Rehabilitation International/UNICEF (1982) E

e. *Aids for disabled children*—Appropriate Health Resources and Technologies Action Group (London) E

f. *Disabled village children: a guide for community health workers, rehabilitation workers and families,* D. Werner—Hesperian Foundation (1987) E

ANNEX 28

UNACCOMPANIED CHILDREN*

Objectives

- **To reunite each unaccompanied child with his/her family wherever possible and not harmful to his/her emotional, social and psychological needs.**

- **To assure appropriate care for children while they are unaccompanied — care which meets their particular needs, especially emotional and developmental needs — and any protection necessary for them.**

Care includes both temporary arrangements (interim care) while family tracing efforts are made, and long term care until adulthood for those for whom family reunion is not achieved within a reasonable period of time.

---

* The guidelines provided in this annex are largely derived/adapted from the findings and recommendations of the *Study of unaccompanied children in emergencies* undertaken 1982-85 by E. Ressler, N. Boothby and D. Steinbock, funded in part by UNICEF. See ref. a.   **397**

What is an unaccompanied child?

An "unaccompanied child/minor" has been defined as a child/individual who is under the legal age of majority and not accompanied by a parent, guardian or other adult who by law *or custom* is responsible for him/her.

Children of all ages are often found to be "unaccompanied" in emergencies, but their particular needs for care and protection have not always been recognized.

Table 28/1

Reasons for children becoming "unaccompanied"

Before, during and after an emergency a child may become separated from his/her family or adult next-of-kin in various ways:

Against parents' will, a child may be:

Lost　　Accidentally separated from other family members, e.g. during population movements (spontaneous or organized);*

Abducted　　Deliberately taken away from parents by other adults/organizations;

Runaway　　Choosing to leave and live apart from their parents without parental consent;

Orphaned　　Both parents (or legal guardian) and close adult relatives in "extended" families having died.

With parents' consent, a child may be:

Abandoned　　Deserted by parents who have no intention of subsequent reunion (this can include "unwanted" babies);

Entrusted　　Placed voluntarily in the care of another adult, or institution, by parents who intend to reclaim him/her eventually; **

Independent　　Living apart from parents (alone or with others) with parental consent.

In conflict situations, children may also be:

Conscripted　　Enlisted in fighting units with or without their parents' consent, or their own.

---

* Children are sometimes also "lost" in emergencies (a) due to inadequate or inaccurate hospital records and tagging, and the movement of patients between institutions; and (b) when taken away from apparently dangerous situations by service personnel or volunteers seeking to protect or arrange medical treatment without first finding and informing the parents.

** A child may be "entrusted" or even "abandoned" when parents believe that his/her chances of survival will be improved by being with the other people, or when facilities and services are established for unaccompanied children which are significantly better than those otherwise available.

(Adapted from ref. a)

The circumstances in which children may become separated from parents and other adult relatives are listed in Table 28/1.

Priority actions

Figure 28/a summarizes the essential components of any programme, and the actions required—sequentially—in respect of each child identified as unaccompanied.

Prompt *programme* action is needed to:
- —Establish arrangements (e.g. in social service information offices/centres) to receive reports of and systematically register and document children who are unaccompanied, and parents searching for children;
- —Search for unaccompanied children within the community;
- —Arrange to provide help, where necessary, to families currently caring for unaccompanied children to enable them to continue to do so in an appropriate manner;
- —Arrange to provide shelter, food and medical care for other unaccompanied children for a few days, if necessary initially, in simple community-level "emergency care" centres;
- —Find and screen families in the community willing to foster unaccompanied children; *and*
- —Establish mechanisms to place each child in interim care appropriate to his/her particular needs, and to record the placement and any subsequent movements.

Arrangements must ensure that unaccompanied children are quickly identified and that *for each child*:
- —Immediate care and supervision is provided;
- —As much information as possible is gathered on his/her background and the circumstances of the separation from his/her family;
- —Medical and psychological screening is arranged; *and*
- —Tracing efforts are initiated to find and reunite the child with his/her family wherever possible.

Simultaneous action is also needed to:
- —Prevent further, avoidable family separations: see Annex 27;
- —Confirm and publicize policies and provisions for unaccompanied children including responsibilities for protecting their interests and supervising arrangements for their care;
- —Mobilize available child welfare expertise and train other workers/volunteers; *and*

399

Figure 28/a

Programme actions required for the care and protection of unaccompanied children in emergencies

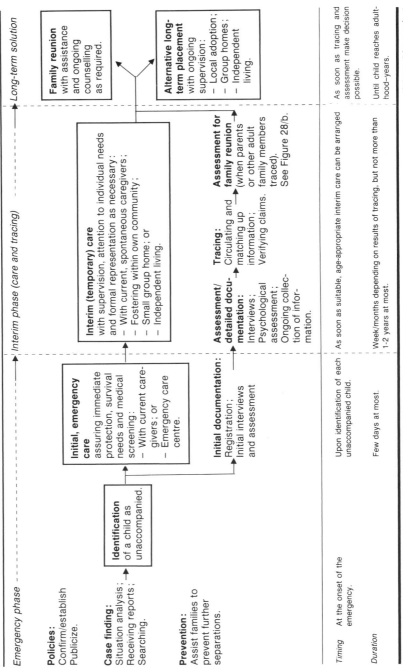

(Adapted from ref. a)

—Remove administrative, political or military barriers to family reunion, where necessary and possible.

Principles

Children's needs

Unaccompanied children should be (a) cared for in ways which best meet their individual emotional and developmental needs, see Table 28/2, and (b) protected from possibilities of abuse. This applies to both temporary, interim care and long-term care where needed:

—Stable, *long-term* arrangements should be made for each child as quickly as possible—by reunion with his/her family or alternative long-term placement if reunion is not achieved within a reasonable period;

—In the mean time, suitable *interim* care and protection must be assured for each unaccompanied child regardless of the cause or duration of the separation from his/her family;

—Time spent by children in emergency care centres should be only the minimum necessary to arrange appropriate, interim placements for them;

—Sibling groups should be kept together;

—Children should, wherever possible, be kept in their own cultural environment and care be arranged within the communities where they are found;

—Children should not be moved around any more than absolutely necessary between different care arrangements, nor be isolated from the rest of the community in institutions; *and*

—Older children should participate in decisions regarding arrangements for themselves and their younger siblings.

Resources and effort must be concentrated on interim care arrangements, tracing and assisting family reunions. Emergency centres should be provided with only the minimum facilities necessary.

Care within "extended" families and/or according to local traditions should generally be encouraged—except where the child would be treated as a servant (see below, p. 409). Narrow and limiting definitions of "family" must be avoided.

Provisions and basic services for unaccompanied children should be similar to— and not separate from—those for other children in the community. Special psychological and legal assistance should, however, be provided where needed on the basis of thorough individual assessments.

Table 28/2

Emotional and psychological needs of children

Children need:
— Emotional security and stability;
— Individual and sustained care of at least one adult, preferably some-one of a similar linguistic and cultural background;
— Continuity in existing relationships with other adults and children;
— Continuity in societal relationships, education, cultural and religious practices; *and*
— Specific help to overcome particular, individual problems.

Unaccompanied children in particular need environments which provide as many stablizing factors as possible and minimize possibilities for additional stress. Continuity of community and cultural ties is all the more important in the absence of the family.

The stable, nurturing care of an adult is especially important for infants and young children.

While efforts to trace members of a child's family being made, avoid actions—however well-intentioned—which may hinder eventual family reunion including: adoption—change of name—movements to places far from the likely locations of family reunion. But also ensure that children are not be held "in limbo" and denied new, permanent ties too long: see below, p. 410 and Figure 28/b.

UNICEF and other concerned groups should resist any proposals for an early transfer of unaccompanied children to other countries.

The evacuation of unaccompanied children—especially to another country—should be considered only in the most exceptional circumstances when their lives are in immediate danger. All movements of each child should be formally recorded.

N.B. The assertion by a child that his/her parents are dead must be treated with caution. Experience has shown such assertions to be unreliable—particularly in certain conflict situations (guerilla fighting and civil wars).

Organization

Local child welfare expertise must be mobilized to define needs, recommend and establish appropriate programmes, train other personnel and assure ongoing professional supervision.

Protection of the children's interests may in some circumstances, especially in the case of displaced populations, be facilitated by the designation of representatives or guardians for them recognized by the appropriate national authority.

NGOs are often best suited to organize programmes for unaccompanied children but should be carefully selected/vetted:
— Any from outside the community itself must have demonstrated competence in child care and agree to abide by the principles stated.
— Agencies oriented towards international adoption should *not* be involved in arranging care for unaccompanied children during emergencies.

In some cases a special unit may be needed within the **national child welfare service** to manage or oversee the necessary programme(s).

International consultants with previous experience in similar operations can provide valuable advice, but the involvement of outside personnel should be limited to supporting roles.

Identification, documentation and tracing

Finding and registering

Centres/offices should be designated/established where:
— Parents who have lost children can register;
— Members of all communities can report unaccompanied children for whom they are caring;
— Young unaccompanied children can be brought by people who find them but are unable to care for them; *and*
— Older unaccompanied children can present themselves.

Searches/enquiries should also be made within the community—by community social workers, volunteers, community and religious leaders—to identify other unaccompanied children and parents searching for children.

Make it clear, however, that no status or facilities beyond those available to other children are to be provided for unaccompanied children. Otherwise parents may be encouraged to abandon, temporarily or permanently, their children into such special care.

Arrangements must ensure that, as soon as each unaccompanied child is found/reported, action is taken to:
— Register the child and establish an individual file/dossier;   **403**

—Record all information available concerning the child's circumstances (including exactly where and when the child was found) from those who brought the child forward or with whom the child was when found (this is especially important for infants and very young children); *and*

—Photograph the child holding a small board on which his/her name, location and assigned reference number are clearly marked. Use a camera and film from which subsequent copies can be made for tracing purposes. If feasible, also take an "instant" picture to put immediately in the file.

Unaccompanied children may be found: in homes other than that of their parents—at hospitals and clinics—at food distribution centres—in temporary camps/relief centres—as street children and beggars—in orphanages—alone.

If a census of the entire population is being made—especially in the case of displaced populations—this can be a good opportunity, without making any special separate enquiries, to identify unaccompanied children and others for whom tracing assistance or other special services may be necessary.

Documentation

Table 28/3 provides a list of the aspects on which information should be sought and recorded in respect of each child. Translate/adapt it to the particular needs of the situation, prepare and distribute appropriate forms so that information is recorded systematically and in a manner to be useful for tracing and other purposes.

Similar details should also be recorded for parents who have lost children: personal details of the child(ren)—family structure—circumstances of the family/child separation—history of the child before separation—medical history of the child—the family's intentions, wishes and plans—other information relevant for tracing.

For each child identified, interview and record as much information as possible, as quickly as possible, from:

—The child him/herself (interviewed by trained personnel from his/her own community, if possible someone the child already knows and trusts);

—Adults currently caring for the child;

—Brothers, sisters, friends with the child;

—Teachers, health workers, community and religious leaders; *and*

—Other adults in the community who know the child, including neighbours and relatives.

Also accumulate and record information on an ongoing basis, especially from those caring for the child, e.g. foster parents, staff in emergency centres and group **404** homes.

N.B. Adults coming forward at any site to identify/claim particular children may also be able to provide information concerning other children found at the same location.

Tracing

Investigative procedures are needed to:
- —Determine, as quickly as possible, the identity of each child, the identity and location of his/her parents and/or other close family members;
- —Match parents seeking children with known unaccompanied children; *or*
- —Establish that tracing and family reunion is unlikely or impossible.

Speed is vital as young children do not sustain emotional ties to absent family members to the same extent as older children and adults. Special documentation and decentralized action-oriented searches are needed for children within—or separate from—any larger family tracing programme (e.g. that of ICRC in conflict situations).

Actions which have been found to be very useful in determining children's identities and tracing their families include:
- —Posting photographs and brief details on bulletin boards and circulating the same within communities;
- —Interviewing parents who have lost children, and recording details which can be compared and matched up with those of children found elsewere;
- —Taking the children (individually or in groups) to locations they have described/remembered—possibly after arranging in advance to meet there with parents who have reported having lost children.

Inform the child of progress in tracing efforts.

However, in some conflict and refugee situations the asking of questions and the circulation of information might endanger the child or the family. The potential benefits of tracing must then be weighed against the risks that the process would impose on the child and family.

HQs can advise concerning NGOs which have experience in implementing tracing activities for unaccompanied children.

Verification

Whenever adults claim children, or family members appear to have been traced, their identities and claims must be verified. Before bringing the adults and children together: exchange photographs—compare descriptions—check knowledge/accounts of events and family composition.

Table 28/3

Basic information required for the documentation of unaccompanied children

Basic personal data:

Family name—forename/given names—sex—age/date of birth—place of birth—tribe/caste/ethnic origin—nationality—languages spoken—religion—education—particular identifying features (disabilities, scars, etc.)—personal belongings.

Accompanying siblings (brother/sisters/other child relatives):

Names—sexes—ages—relationships.

Circumstances when identified:

Location/address where found—date and time;

If found/reported by other adults: the adults' names—address—relationship to child;

If in care of these adults: how the association came about—the length of time the child has been with them;

If with other unaccompanied children: the names and assigned reference/registration numbers of the other children—how long they have been together.

Family structure:

Name—age/date of birth—relationship to child—occupation—last known location/address of: father, mother, brothers, sisters, grandparents, aunts, uncles, other relatives, other persons normally living in the family household.

Circumstances of the family/child separation:

Reasons for separation (see Table 28/1)—date and place of separation—when and in what circumstances child last saw parents/other family members—if death of parents is presumed, why child believes this to be so.

History of the child before separation:

Important events in the child's life—description of people and places remembered.

History of the child since separation:

Places of residence—legal status of any formal placements—length of time spent in each place—important events, people and places remembered—how shelter food and water have been obtained.

Health status and past medical history.

Psycho-social assessment:

Appraisal of the child's current emotional state—the importance of current relationships—extent to which the child's (age-specific) developmental needs are being met.

Other information of importance concerning the daily care of the child.

The child's intentions, wishes, plans:

With whom the child wishes to be reunited if they could be located— their relationship—where and how they might be traced.

Other information relevant for tracing:

Names and locations/addresses of other persons who may provide additional information about the child—other information that might be helpful in locating family members or understanding more fully the circumstances of the family/child separation.

Information relevant to the determination of *refugee status* and wishes for repatriation or resettlement, where appropriate.

(Adapted from ref. a)

Emergency and interim care

Initial emergency care

If a child is already being cared for by a family other than his/her own, the child should stay with that family, at least temporarily, but the arrangement be registered and monitored. The family should be assisted if necessary.

Try to arrange immediate fostering for any child not already being cared for spontaneously by other adults—especially for infants and young children.

Arrange shelter, food and water in temporary emergency care centres under the supervision of social workers for any children for whom fostering is not immediately possible. Arrange appropriate interim care within a few days.

Arrange medical screening and establish initial documentation within the first few days. Arrange psychological screening as soon as practicable: simple techniques can be used by social workers and others when professional services are lacking, see ref. d.

When there is no alternative to moving children to another location—because their lives are in immediate danger or to provide medical treatment—full records must be kept. Formal agreements should be established with those taking custody of the children to assure that appropriate care and protection will be provided and that the children will be returned if and when families are traced or other suitable arrangements made for their care within their own community.

Table 28/4

Possibilities and preferences for the interim care of unaccompanied children

For all infants and young children (0-5 years):
—Fostering with adult relatives;
—Fostering with the families of friends; *or*
—Fostering with other families in their own community;

For older children (6-14 years):
—Fostering as above for as many as possible, especially those who express a wish for a family environment; *or*
—Group care in small, community-level homes, especially for any for whom rapid family reunion is assured.

For adolescents (over 14 years):
—Fostering for those who wish it;
—Group care; *or*
—Supervised independent living (in small groups).

For older children and adolescents, their individual needs and preferences should be the determining factors.

For sibling groups, make arrangements—in consultation with the oldest child—to keep them together (with the same foster family or in a group home), or at least for the older children (possibly living independently) to remain in close contact with the younger ones (in a foster family).

Arrangements for *independent living* must take account of cultural attitudes. It may be appropriate for boys at an earlier age than for girls.

Group care or supervised independent living may be necessary, initially, for children who:
—Have special problems;
—Are not used to family living—having been without any family care for more than a year; *or*
—Have been severely deprived or abused and need to be helped, gradually, to accept and trust adults.

Care in large *institutions* (e.g. orphanages and other arrangements which isolate the children from the normal life of the rest of the community) should be considered only as a last—and temporary—resort, and for children who have major individual problems.

Interim care

Table 28/4 lists the possible and preferred arrangements for interim care. Any children who are already in other kinds of placement—especially in institutions—should be transferred into more appropriate care as soon as possible.

The children's need is for security and stability in relationships rather than physical comforts. The establishment of close, emotional bonds with the persons caring for them—whether foster parents or house parents—is vital. Large centres with special facilities often fail to meet this need and, on the other hand, actually attract the placement there of children who are not in fact unaccompanied, thus splitting families!

Supervised fostering

Placing a child in the care of a stable family from the same cultural heritage and social background is the best way to meet the need for emotional security, especially but not only for young children.

Foster families should:
— Be carefully screened in advance and carefully matched with the individual personalities and needs of the child(ren);
— Agree to release the child(ren) if and when family reunion becomes possible, but be willing (if possible) to care for the child(ren) until adulthood in case family reunion is not able to be achieved within 1-2 years; *and*
— Be provided with additional rations and/or other material assistance where necessary.

Placements should be on a formal basis, properly documented. Trained social workers should supervise all placements on a regular basis to help and advise both the child and the foster family, and to ensure that the child's best interests are safeguarded.

The child must not be considered as a servant. In societies where families find it hard to conceive of taking in a child except as a servant, special care is needed. Unless satisfactory supervision is available, group care may be preferable.

Group care

Group care centres/homes, where needed, should:
— Be limited, ideally, to 5-8 children of mixed ages (and sexes);
— Have facilities similar to the typical household in the community;
— Have "house parents" appointed/chosen from respected adults in the local community who have reared their own children and are willing to continue in the job for the foreseeable future; *and*

409

—Be integrated into the local community as much as possible.

Continuity of relationships should be assured and an environment as close as possible to a "normal" home and family be created. Assistants might be chosen from among unaccompanied young women in the community who may need a secure place to live, see Annex 27.

Necessary training and instructions must be given to the house parents and other staff, and the operation of the units and the relationships within them be supervised by trained community social workers.

Material provisions for the children should be similar to those for other children in the community:
—The children should attend the community school and participate in the normal recreational and other activities of children in the community;
—They should *not* be provided with special, distinguishing clothing;
—Separate services and elaborate facilities should *not* be established.

Independent living

Arrangements must prepare the adolescents for independent adult life while assuring professional adult help and supervision, and continuity of their own relationships.

Family reunion and alternative long-term placements

Possible arrangements for long-term care of children (i.e. until adulthood) are listed in Table 28/5 in usual order of preference.

Experience has shown that a high proportion of unaccompanied children are usually able to be reunited with family members. Alternative long-term arrangements will, however, be necessary for those for whom family reunion proves not to be possible within a reasonable period, and any for whom it is judged that reunion would be harmful to the child's interests.

Each case must be considered and decided individually in the light of child welfare policy, legislation and practice in the country concerned. Children—especially infants and young children—should not, however, be kept "in limbo" for periods of years in the vague hope that family reunion may eventually prove possible.

Figure 28/b suggests the kind of decision criteria which might be considered—those proposed by the authors of the study of unaccompanied children in emergencies, ref. a. They suggest, as a general rule of thumb, that alternative long-term care should be arranged for children whose parents/families cannot be traced within 2 years (1 year for children under 5).

Table 28/5

Arrangements for long-term care of unaccompanied children

Possible arrangements in usual order of preference are:

—Reunion with parents if possible within a reasonable period (not more than 1-2 years?) and if not harmful to the child's emotional and developmental needs: see p. 402 and Figure 28/b;

—Reunion with other adult relations;

—Adoption/integration into the family which has fostered the child on an interim basis;

—Adoption/integration into a family of friends;

—Adoption/integration into another family within the child's own community;

—Group care in small, community-level group homes (for older children and some of those with special problems); or

—Supervised independent living in small groups (for adolescents).

Decisions for each child must be based on his/her age, any special individual problems/needs, the expressed wishes of the child (if over 5 years), and the success or otherwise of interim care arrangements.

Assessment for family reunion

Once identities and relationships have been confirmed:

—Inform the parents about the state of the child and find out whether they wish and are able (with help if necessary) to care for the child until he/she reaches adulthood;

—Inform children about the circumstances and wishes of their parents; *and*

—Check any accounts of previous abuse or neglect.

Decisions on whether to proceed with family reunion should be taken by professional child welfare officers and sanctioned by customary law. They must be based on: the wishes of the parents—the age and wishes of the child—the length of separation—the strength of the child's new psychological attachments—the previous family-child relationship.

411

Figure 28/b

Possible criteria for decisions concerning family reunion or alternative long-term placement

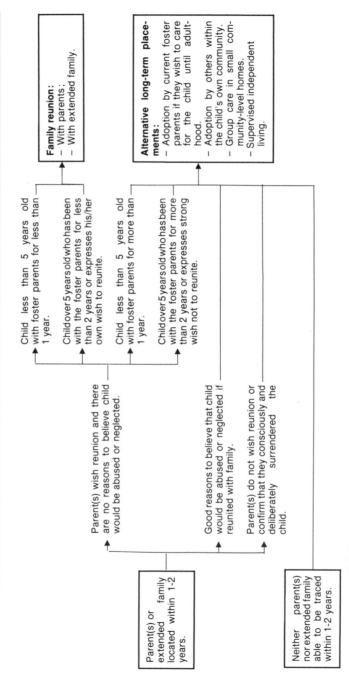

Family reunion:
- With parents;
- With extended family.

Alternative long-term placements:
- Adoption by current foster parents if they wish to care for the child until adulthood.
- Adoption by others within the child's own community.
- Group care in small community-level homes.
- Supervised independent living.

Child less than 5 years old with foster parents for less than 1 year.

Child over 5 years old who has been with the foster parents for less than 2 years or expresses his/her own wish to reunite.

Child less than 5 years old with foster parents for more than 1 year.

Child over 5 years old who has been with the foster parents for more than 2 years or expresses strong wish not to reunite.

Parent(s) wish reunion and there are no reasons to believe child would be abused or neglected.

Good reasons to believe that child would be abused or neglected if reunited with family.

Parent(s) do not wish reunion or confirm that they consciously and deliberately surrendered the child.

Parent(s) or extended family located within 1-2 years.

Neither parent(s) nor extended family able to be traced within 1-2 years.

N.B. Each case must be decided on the basis of an individual, professional assessment. The above assumes that where a child has been fostered, the foster family is able and willing to continue to care for the child until adulthood. If this is not the case, a child who has been fostered for more than 1-2 years may still be considered for family reunion, or an alternative long-term placement.

(Schematic representation of criteria suggested in ref. a)

Preparation for family reunion

If the child is to be reunited with his/her family after a long separation, the process of re-establishing relationships must be carefully planned and nurtured:
— Provide counselling to allay any fears on the part of the child;
— Carefully plan arrangements for transport and actual meeting; *and*
— Provide assistance to the family, where necessary, and ongoing counselling.

Assistance and counselling will be particularly important if the child is handicapped, the family weakened, or the community as a whole improverished.

Alternative long-term placements

Where family reunion is not possible, or judged to be contrary to the child's best interests, adoption/integration into families within their own communities is generally to be preferred, especially for young children. This may be with the families who have fostered them on an interim basis. Support and assistance as well as follow-up supervision may need to be provided to adopting families for an extended period.

In some situations it may be necessary, especially for older children, to maintain small group homes or supervised living arrangements, and to make special efforts to provide them some form of training for employment and income generation as well as integration in formal and non-formal education and recreational activities within the community.

Large, institutionalized orphanages should be avoided. They are often very expensive as well as being dehumanizing. Cross-cultural/international adoption should be considered only if no suitable form of adoption, group care or independent living can be arranged locally.

Possible UNICEF inputs

Depending on the assessment of actual needs and possibilities, some of the following inputs might be considered:
— Child welfare expertise to help plan and organize appropriate programmes.

413

To prevent family separations:

—Assistance to vulnerable families, see Annex 27.

For children who are already unaccompanied:

—Material assistance for foster families.

—Stationery, office supplies and transport for tracing activities on behalf of unaccompanied children.

—Materials for the repair of premises to be used for small, community-level emergency care centres or group homes, and basic equipment (sleeping mats, blankets, utensils, etc.) for such units.

—Local operating costs for: the appointment and training of community-based social workers and personnel for any necessary emergency care centres, group homes and tracing service—purchase of necessary food items not available from general feeding programmes or fuel for cooking—fuel and maintenance for supervisory vehicles.

Further references

a.　*Unaccompanied children—care and placement in wars, natural disasters and refugee movements,* E. Ressler, N. Boothby & D. Steinbock—draft Redd Barna (1985); (expected Oxford University Press 1986)　E

b.　*UNHCR Handbook for social services,* provisional edition—UNHCR (1984)　E (some parts also F/S)

c.　*Post-disaster programmes, International Child Welfare Review* No. 17/18—International Union of Child Welfare, Geneva (1973)　E/F

d.　*Guidelines for interviewing unaccompanied minors and preparing social histories,* preliminary version—UNHCR social services section (1985)　E

EDUCATION

Objective

- **To restore and promote the further development of education in the community, especially for young children and women.**

Priorities

Immediate, preliminary repairs to school premises may be necessary if they are required to serve as temporary shelter and/or centres for other priority relief activities. This may be the case where there has been considerable destruction of dwellings and other premises.

Once survival needs have been assured, encourage and support community initiatives to rehabilitate and reopen schools—particularly primary schools—wherever:

—The community itself accords high priority to the re-establishment of regular school activities as an important aspect (and symbol) of normality and stability;

—Schools previously served as centres for community and extension services, and are a natural focus for relief and rehabilitation programmes; *and/or*

—Schools might now assume such a role in the absence of other existing structures at community level.

Subject to overall priorities, determine the *rehabilitation* needs of primary schools, teacher training institutes, etc. Develop plans and budgets for necessary reconstruction, re-equipment and re-staffing to enable normal educational activities to be resumed.

Clearly identify and give priority to the most basic needs—those without which the schools cannot function effectively at all.

Displaced populations

Teachers may be present but no premises, books or any other necessary materials.

Unless the population is expected to move again in the very near future, support by the provision of essential equipment, books and other basic supplies any efforts made within the community itself to restart schools.

In instances of long stay or permanent resettlement:
- The establishment and staffing of schools should be planned carefully and jointly between the community and the local education authorities;
- Established local practices and standards (including curricula and books) should, in general, be followed; *and*
- Primary schools should be small and decentralized within the community(ies): premises should be of construction similar to that of the dwellings and be erected by community effort to the extent possible.

Women's education

Ensure that, during the rehabilitation phase, specific education components for women are integrated wherever appropriate in all programme interventions: in food production—health and nutrition—sanitation, etc.

Possible UNICEF inputs

Depending on the assessement of actual needs and possibilities, some of the following inputs might be considered:
- Materials and/or tools to enable preliminary repairs to be made quickly to school premises where they are needed for shelter and relief purposes.

During the rehabilitation (or resettlement) phase:

—Essential materials and tools for reconstruction and the replacement of furniture in primary schools and teacher training institutions.

—Basic equipment, books and initial quantities of expendable supplies (probably set-packed in standard kits) for primary schools and for institutes training primary school teachers and trainers for women's programmes.

—Assistance to re-establish the local production and distribution of text books, teachers guides and teaching aids for primary schools, and materials for women's education.

—Transport necessary for the implementation of any rehabilitation/reconstruction programme and to replace any for normal supervisory purposes which may have been lost: spare parts for damaged vehicles.

—Local operating costs for reconstruction work and the restarting of teacher and instructor training courses, especially the initial training of any newly recruited teachers and instructors for women's programmes.

ANNEX 30
PLANNING AND MANAGEMENT OF LOGISTICS

Objective

- **To assure the delivery of material assistance to and within the affected area as quickly and efficiently as feasible.**

Defining needs and priorities

As soon as any requirement for the movement of a substantial quantity of supplies has been established:

1. **Mobilize logistic expertise and local knowledge.**

2. **Tabulate data on the quantities of different supplies which need to be delivered month-by-month to different locations, and from where they must be transported.**

3. **Map-out the logistic requirements and possibilities on a large-scale map or diagram of the country.** Show:
   — Planned distribution locations and the number of target beneficiaries at each.
   — Points of origin of supplies (ports/airports/local suppliers).
   — Available transport routes noting (a) any points where transshipments are needed, (b) specific constraints (ferries, damaged bridges, etc.) and the maximum daily capacity, and (c) the number of days for a round trip on each route.
   — Storage capacities needed and available at different locations.
   — Fuel depots and distribution points.
   — Vehicle maintenance facilities.

4. **Evaluate all available possibilities for transporting and storing the planned quantities of supplies.**

5. **Draw up a short-term plan for the deployment and scheduling of immediately available means of transport on specific routes, and the use of available storage capacity.**

6. **Identify actions which could be taken to increase capacity and/or reduce costs or delays, and specify for each: the materials and expertise needed — likely cost — time to implement — expected capacity increase or savings.**

7. **Evaluate possibilities and initiate actions to assure the maintenance of capacity and to increase it (if necessary) as quickly and efficiently as possible.**

Then

Monitor the situation and revise operational plans as the requirements and possibilities change.

Ensure continuity in management. Avoid a proliferation of short-term personnel.

Short-term consultants/missions on logistics can make valuable contributions in some situations — including bringing a "fresh look" at problems and focusing attention on specific issues — but continuity of executive and operational personnel and an ongoing process of assessment and response are vital.

Mathematical techniques exist to calculate the optimum deployment of capacity. In a major operation it may be worth getting operations research workers from a university, government agency or private company to help plan deployment.

Scheduling and stockpiling

Requirements for use/distribution of supplies will often be uneven with peaks in one or several months. If supplies can be obtained sufficiently in advance, plan to **419**

Figure 30/a **Components of a typical logistic system**

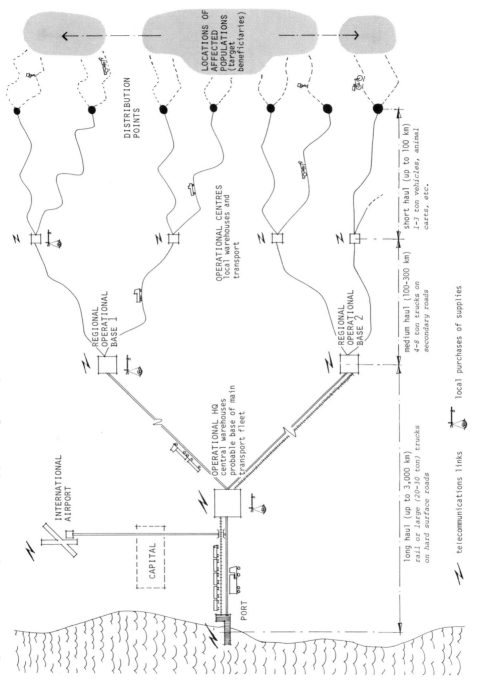

build up stocks in the area/region in advance of the peak requirements so that the long-haul deliveries can be made at a more steady rate throughout the period.

If seasonal/weather conditions are expected to make transportation along certain routes—including those for final distribution—difficult during particular periods, build up stocks sufficiently close to the point of end-use before further deliveries become impossible. (Stocks should be sufficient to cover expected requirements for the entire period during which further deliveries may not be possible.)

Assessing transport and handling possibilities

Knowledge of previous local arrangements and facilities is essential. Get the advice and assistance of individuals and organizations (including commercial companies) operating in the area. Complement this with specific technical expertise (from outside the country if necessary).

Give particular attention to:
- Off-take from ports—which often represents a greater constraint than discharge in the port itself.
- Local access roads and means of transport—including animals—to actually get supplies into the affected area and to the (often scattered) communities in need.

Don't underestimate the time it takes to load, unload and manoeuvre supplies, especially by hand. While the provision of employment may be an important, subsidiary objective, the use of mechanical equipment—fork lifts and (especially for bagged food) conveyor belts—can very significantly increase handling rates *and* reduce damage and consequent losses.

See Annexes 31, 32, 33, 34 and 35 for particular considerations concerning ports, airports, in-country transport, warehousing and mechanical handling. Figures 30/b, 30/c and 30/d suggest formats which might be useful for:
- Recording data on individual routes between key locations (comparing alternative modes available);
- Summarizing the alternatives over all routes;
- Recording data on storage and handling facilities at various locations.

In assessing the capacity available note that, in many situations, it may not be realistic to expect that trucks will in fact be dedicated to one function or purpose alone. They are likely to be used for other purposes from time to time. **421**

Figure 30/b **Format for recording data on individual routes between key locations**

ROUTE from: to: distance:					
	Road	Rail	Water	Air	Remarks
General characteristics					
Present constraints					
Seasonal considerations					
No. units available	*(trucks)*	*(wagons)*	*(barges etc.)*	*(planes)*	
Unit capacity (tons)					
Total capacity (tons)					
Travelling time (days)					
Days to load & unload					
Total days/round-trip					
No. round-trips possible per month					
Total carrying capacity per month per unit (tons)					
Possible actions to increase capacity					
- likely cost					
- likely time to effect					
- expected outcome					
Compiled by: Sources of data: date:					

Actions to increase capacity/efficiency

The most immediate, productive and economical actions to increase capacity might be:

— Redeployment of available transport units (trucks etc.) between sectors and/or between alternative routes.

—Minor/temporary repairs to vital bridges, roads and ferries.

—Limited repairs to warehouses—especially roofs and doors.

—Repairs to handling equipment and/or the provision of additional equipment including generators to provide lighting for night working.

Purchasing/importing more trucks, and more substantial repairs to infrastructure might follow.

In extreme cases there may be no alternative to mounting a major airlift, at least in the short-term, but this should be avoided if at all possible on account of the enormous cost and the limited quantities which can in fact be moved by air.

As a last resort, it may have to be acknowledged that the required quantities of supplies will not be able to be delivered to the area in the time required. Consideration may then have to be given to moving some of the communities temporarily to other, more accessible locations, and rescheduling the supply pipeline.

Buffer zones

In some circumstances, especially following severe, localized disasters, local authorities have established a "buffer zone" around the affected area to which access by non-essential personnel and transport is restricted.

Warehouses are set up *outside* that zone to receive supplies coming from further afield, and supplies forwarded into the affected area only as and when required for immediate distribution/use. The majority of emergency assistance personnel are also housed outside that zone.

Figure 30/c **Format for summarizing transport possibilities and capacities of various routes**

SUMMARY OF THE CARRYING CAPACITIES OF TRANSPORT ROUTES

from	to	No. round-trips/month				Unit capacity (tons)				Total tons/month/unit			
		Road	Rail	Water	Air	Road	Rail	Water	Air	Road	Rail	Water	Air
(A)	(1)	6	2	—	30	10	20	—	4	60	40	—	120
(A)	(2)												
(B)	(2)												
(B)	(3)												

423

Figure 30/d **Format for recording data on storage and handling facilities at transshipment/storage locations**

FACILITIES AT TRANSSHIPMENT/STORAGE LOCATIONS

location: _____   transport routes (by road/rail/water/air) available to: _____

Site / premises	(1)	(2)	(3)
site name ownership			
Access (road/rail/water) Distance from rail yard etc.			
No. buildings Type of construction Type of floor No. loading doors			
Floor area (sq.m.) Useful height (m)			
Open stacking area (sq.m.)			
Security			
Power supplies			
Handling equipment available			

Compiled by: _____   Sources of data: _____   date: _____

In this way rescue operations, self-help and assistance programmes among the affected communities are not unduly hampered by the need to arrange facilities for more supplies and outside personnel than are absolutely necessary in the immediate area at any time.

Communications

Unless telephone/telex connections are both extensive and reliable, it will probably be necessary (in any major operation) to establish a radio network between all key points: central control unit—ports—airports—major warehouses:

—Such a network must be authorized by the appropriate government agency;
—It might be operated under direct government control or by an approved organization;
—Discipline must be established for the use of the system: set times for contacts between particular locations and record all messages.

If the situation is such that trucks (and possibly river craft) must move in convoys on certain routes, mobile radios may be provided for convoy leaders.

Further references

General descriptions of and guidelines for logistic operations:
a. *Emergency supply logistics handbook*—licross/volags steering committee for disasters, Geneva (1982) E/F/S
b. *Red Cross cargo*—ICRC, Geneva (1985) E/F
c. *Aspects of logistics in the Somalia refugee relief operation*—International Disaster Institute, London (1983) E [Analysis of a case study.]

PORT OPERATIONS

Objectives

- **To determine for each sea and river port: the types/sizes of vessels able to be received — the current discharge, handling and storage capacities.**

- **To increase cargo handling/through-put capacity, if necessary.**

Possible actions

Priority

If sea and/or river ports are congested, try to secure priority for vessels carrying emergency supplies. It has been useful in some situations to reserve specific berths for such vessels, and this also makes it easier to control the supplies.

Handling equipment

The availability and proper use of mechanical handling equipment (cranes, fork lifts and conveyors) can not only considerably increase the rate of discharge of vessels but also reduce the damage and loss caused by rough handling.

If fork lifts are available advise shippers that, where appropriate, cargoes can be shipped "palletized". If not, consider repairing/providing such equipment: see Annex 35.

If wharf cranes are *not* available or not functioning in sufficient numbers in any port it may be necessary to:
— Instruct that cargoes are sent there only on vessels with self-unloading capability;
— Arrange for the repair of existing but out-of-service equipment and/or provide additional mobile cranes, etc.

At a more basic level, ensure the availability of sufficient rope slings and nets.

If warehouses are more than 30 m from the ship side—and if most handling is manual—ensure sufficient trolleys and tractors (or light trucks) to move cargo to them.

Self-unloading capability may be particularly important for heavy items—trucks, etc. Most vessels can unload bagged food and small cases a ton at a time, but not all have "heavy lift" derricks. Get technical advice and full specifications for any parts or new units required.

Storage

Make immediate/temporary repairs to warehouses (especially roofs and doors), and/or supply tarpaulins where necessary to protect supplies. In the case of major operations arrange for specific sheds/warehouses to be reserved for emergency supplies, if possible.

Night working

The through-put of cargo is a function of the hours worked. Where necessary, promote and facilitate the operation of night shifts. Generators and lighting may be needed: see Annex 35.

Demurrage

Make every effort to see that vessels (and their cargoes) are not held up at the ports **427** but, in many situations, general congestion and poor organization often makes some demurrage inevitable:

— Approach the appropriate authorities to waive port/demurrage charges.
— If a general waiver cannot be obtained, ensure that some budget provision is made for such charges.

Assessment check-list: ports

The best *sources of information* are likely to be the port/harbour authorities themselves and local shipping agencies. Check the current state of on-shore facilities by direct inspection.

Identification

☐ Name and exact location (especially if the port was previously little used by international agencies and shipping lines).

Access

☐ Current depth restrictions in approach channels, turning basin, etc. and those expected in the coming weeks/months? (Water levels may change significantly with seasons.)

☐ Are any new obstacles (e.g. wrecks) restricting access?

☐ Are pilots and/or tugs needed and available? Pilot vessels?

☐ Depth alongside wharves/piers?

☐ Depth in any anchorages used for discharge into lighters?

Berths/mooring facilities

☐ Number, length and general condition of berths alongside wharves and piers?

☐ Number of anchorages: number and capacity of available lighters?

Handling equipment

☐ Number, capacity and condition of fixed cranes, mobile cranes, forklifts?

☐ Number and capacity of trolleys (both hand- and tractor-drawn), tractors and in-port trucks?

☐ Are fuel and operators available for the equipment?

☐ Can containers be handled? If so: What sizes? At how many berths?

☐ What limits therefore on the size/weight of packages able to be handled?

Storage

☐ Number, size/capacity and condition of sheds/warehouses? Security?

☐ Area of open, hard-stand space? Are sufficient tarpaulins available?

☐ Quantity of cargoes presently stored: balance of space available? (What prospects for removing currently stored cargoes?)

Operations

☐ What was the normal monthly through-put previously? What maximum discharge rates were achieved?

☐ Number of shifts and hours of working of (a) port, (b) customs: Previously? Presently?

☐ Present average waiting time for vessels?

☐ What other major cargoes are to be handled in the immediate future: imports—exports?

☐ Is lighting available: in warehouses—on quays? What source of power (mains or generators)? For what hours is power presently available?

☐ Number of staff: customs—berth/warehouse supervisors—tally clerks—foremen—stevedores?

☐ What actions are being taken/planned to restore/increase capacity? What further actions could quickly increase capacity? What cost? How much time? Who would have to approve them?

Off-take

☐ Rail: Where are wagons loaded? (Are sidings on the quays?) Are shunting locomotives available?

☐ Road: Are road connections open? What trucks and transporters are normally used? Are they still available?

☐ River: Number and capacity of self-propelled craft, barges and tugs? **429**

Possible UNICEF inputs

Specific, limited inputs necessary to ensure that supplies being provided by UNICEF, WFP and others for the benefit of children (and their families) can in fact be delivered. Depending on the assessment of actual needs and possibilities, some of the following inputs might be considered:

— Technical assistance: practical expertise to help organize port operations.

— Repairs to roofs, doors, etc. of warehouses needed for emergency supplies.

— Repairs to or replacement of cranes, fork lifts, generators, lighting installations, etc.

UNICEF would not be involved in rehabilitation of facilities *per se,* but only to the extent necessary to ensure the timely delivery of emergency assistance to children.

ANNEX 32

AIRPORT OPERATIONS

Objectives

- To determine, for both international airports and small airstrips in the affected area, the type of aircraft able to land and take off, and the operational facilities available.

- To increase capacity, if necessary.

Possible actions

Runways

Runways may be repaired to enable the full length to be used. Small, rural airstrips may be extended to take larger aircraft through works projects using local labour and a minimum of heavy equipment (graders/bulldozers).

Handling equipment

If appropriate fork lifts are lacking it may be impossible to (safely) unload large/heavy items from the majority of cargo aircraft (with doors 3-6 m above the ground). A few aircraft carry self-unloading devices but, apart from these, it may be necessary to insist on only military-style cargo aircraft with ramps (e.g. Hercules C.130) being used, at least for heavy items including any vehicles which it is necessary to airlift.

If large quantities of cargo are to be airlifted, high-lift forklifts may be repaired or provided.

Storage

Specific parking bays and sheds may be reserved for emergency carriers and supplies. Sheds may be repaired if necessary, local constructions be erected, or prefabricated warehouses be provided (in the case of major airlift operations): see Annex 34.

Assessment check-list: airports

The best *sources of information* are likely to be the civil aviation authorities and the airlines/air transport companies (especially the pilots themselves) operating in the area.

Identification

☐ Name and exact location: official designator: elevation/altitude?

Landing and take-off facilities

☐ Usable length of runway: type of surface—nature and position of any damage/obstructions?

☐ Are runway and approach lights available and working?

☐ What navigational aids are available and operating?

☐ What air traffic control and communications arrangements?

Aircraft servicing facilities

☐ What types of aviation fuel are available? What cost?

☐ Availability and condition of start-up generators/other ground equipment?

432 ☐ Aircrew rest facilities?

☐ What types of aircraft are therefore able to operate?

Cargo handling

☐ Availability and condition of taxiways and parking areas?

☐ Number, capacity and condition of forklifts?

☐ Number and capacity of trolleys and tractors?

☐ Are fuel and operators available for the equipment?

☐ What limits therefore on size/weight of packages able to be received?

Storage

☐ Number, size, capacity and condition of sheds/warehouses? Security?

☐ Area of open, hard-stand space? What tarpaulins are available?

☐ Quantity of cargoes presently stored—balance of space available?

☐ Is lighting available: in warehouses—in loading/unloading areas? What source of power? For what hours is power presently available?

Operations

☐ What was the normal monthly through-put previously?

☐ Number of shifts and hours of working of airport and customs personnel: previously—presently?

☐ Number of staff available including tally clerks and labourers?

☐ How are landing rights granted? What airport charges are normally levied?

☐ What royalties are charged on non-scheduled carriers? Can these be waived for emergency charter flights?

☐ What actions are being taken/planned to restore/increase capacity? What further actions could quickly increase capacity? What cost? How much time? Who would have to approve them?

Possible UNICEF inputs

As for ports (see p. 430) with the possible addition of support to the repair/extension of rural airstrips.

ANNEX 33

IN-COUNTRY TRANSPORT

Objective

- **To deliver supplies to locations within the affected area as and when needed.**

Deliveries must be organized having regard to considerations of speed (where this is crucial), reliability and cost.

Choices

Rail and *river* transport are usually cheapest. Use them wherever possible for moving bulk commodities on major routes. Arrange special supervision if necessary. (They may not be the fastest means but this may not matter if the objective is a steady flow.)

Trucks are more flexible (provided roads are open) and will almost certainly be needed for local distribution at least.

Air transport—other than of personnel and urgent medical supplies and spare parts—should be considered only as a measure of last resort. It is usually possible to move only very limited quantities of supplies and is always very expensive. In a few situations there may be no short-term alternative but, in most, available funds would be better spent providing the means to move much larger quantities by surface.

Road transport

The possibilities are, in order of preference: use government trucks—borrow others—repair out-of-service government trucks—use contractors—rent trucks—buy new units for a special emergency fleet.

Government trucks

- **Use existing government trucks wherever available and feasible. Assure necessary fuel, tarpaulins, tyres, spare parts, maintenance and repair facilities, and administrative controls.**

If some trucks are out of service for lack of spare parts:
- —Get a technical assessment specifying the parts and any technical assistance required to rehabilitate them.
- —Don't waste time on "derelict" vehicles.
- —Ensure that trucks repaired will in fact then be used for intended programme purposes!

Repairing existing trucks can be the quickest and cheapest way of increasing capacity if: there are not too many different types—they have not been out-of-service for too long—and the necessary workshop and supervisory capacity exists. If very large expenditures would be required, short-term programme objectives may be better served by using the funds to pay local contractors to move the necessary supplies.

Contract transport

- **Where there is a reasonably well-developed private transport sector with reliable contractors, use those services rather than buying trucks.**

Problems of maintenance, insurance, driver selection and discipline etc. are then borne by the contractors, not added to the problems which hard-pressed field personnel and central administrations have to cope with. Greater flexibility is **435** provided to meet the inevitable peaks and troughs in actual requirements for transport.

For the movement of bulk supplies on well-established routes:

— Issue contracts on the basis of defined rates per ton delivered to specified locations (perhaps different rates for different commodities);

— Make provision separately for the carriage of light but bulky supplies, e.g. sets of clinic equipment (payment may have to be made on the basis of volume or simply the nominal capacity of the trucks used); *and*

— Consider including provision to enable the receiving officer at a regional warehouse to send trucks on to unload directly at specified distribution sites if desired: define the additional amount to be paid for extra distances involved.

For local distribution within the affected area:

— As above, *or*:

— Establish contracts under which the contractor will provide a specified number of trucks each day, and additional ones if and when required.

For the latter it may be necessary to pay a daily/weekly rental plus an additional amount for each "ton-km" for goods actually carried. (The number of ton-kms performed = weight of load in tons × distance from warehouse to destination in kilometres.)

In all cases:

— Select contractors to ensure that delivery is reasonably assured even if the conditions are difficult; *and*

— Ensure that responsibility for insurance and losses are defined.

Buying new trucks

Trucks may have to be purchased *if* sufficient capacity is not otherwise available *or* if the need is expected to continue for a long period, the organizational capacity to manage the fleet can be assured, and it will be preferable to contracting. If so:

— Consider what types of truck are most appropriate for different routes/sectors and the supplies involved;

— Get advice on specifications and standardize to the extent possible.

— Get the best possible assurance that any trucks provided will in fact be used for the intended programme purposes.

Annex 48 provides guidelines concerning the choice and specification of trucks.

Organizing a truck operation

- Use/expand any suitable existing government organization to manage the fleet itself and dispatching operations.

- If there is none, consider co-operating with an existing transport organization — grafting the emergency fleet onto an already functioning operation, such as a bus company.

- If necessary, establish an independent operation: get an experienced transport manager to set it up and run it.

Select and train drivers carefully. As far as possible assign them to and make them responsible for individual trucks. Ensure that reasonable working hours are not exceeded. This, as much as anything, can maximize performance in the long run by minimizing accidents and breakdowns due to carelessness, misuse or inadequate maintenance.

Don't underestimate the time, technical and management skills needed to establish a trucking operation from scratch: recruiting drivers, supervisory and other staff — organizing parking, fuel supplies, maintenance, etc. Begin as quickly as ever possible in a small way and expand progressively.

Convoys

- Avoid using convoys unless absolutely necessary. More supplies will be moved in less time if trucks move individually — or only in very small groups.

- If, however, there are long distances to be covered through remote areas or particular problems of security on certain routes, appoint convoy leaders able to enforce discipline and resolve problems, breakdowns, etc.

If a convoy is delivering to a number of different locations along a route, establish a discipline whereby any truck which has discharged all its load either waits at that point for the rest of the convoy to return (if returning by the same route), or continues with the convoy (if making a circuit).

Ensuring fuel supplies

- Check actual availabilities in field locations and discuss possible arrangements with oil companies and distributors themselves.

If fuel is not available in sufficient quantities in the areas of operations:
- Try to make arrangements directly with oil companies whereby specific **437**

quantities will be guaranteed—at specified locations—for emergency vehicles.

—Otherwise arrange to buy fuel directly from oil depots and to transport and store it where needed.

At any major operational base, try to get the use of large (preferably underground) storage tanks and pumps, and organize deliveries using bulk tankers. In many situations, however, supplies will have to be transported and stored in drums (200 litres or 44 gallons each). See p. 449 concerning the handling and storage of fuel.

Maintenance and repairs

- **Establish and enforce regular preventive maintenance schedules for all vehicles.**

- **Use local workshops where they exist and are adequate: establish own workshop if necessary.**

- **Ensure that adequate supplies of lubricating oils, brake/clutch fluids and spare parts are available.**

- **Ensure that breakdown/crane trucks are available to recover any trucks which break down or get stuck in the field.**

Facilities for regular maintenance and minor repairs should be available as close as possible to the operational base(s) of the trucks. It will usually be easier to plan to bring each truck in for maintenance on a certain day each month rather than at fixed intervals of kms/miles.

Get an experienced workshop manager to plan and organize any workshop operation. Order tools, equipment, oils and necessary spare parts as quickly as ever possible. Give special attention to needs for tyres and batteries. Tyres can wear out in 10,000 kms on the roads sometimes experienced. Ensure strict control of stocks and issues.

Road and bridges

Bridges

Army engineers are well-equipped to undertake initial, temporary repairs (or reinforcement) of bridges. In some situations, Bailey Bridge parts may need to be imported.

If the local military is unable to undertake the task quickly, small groups of army engineers from donor countries approved by the government may be brought in to do the job. (Such personnel have in some operations worked in civilian clothes under the direction of the UN or the appropriate government ministry.)

Access roads

In some instances—especially where populations have been displaced and significant numbers are now located in areas which were previously sparsely inhabited—it may be necessary to improve local access roads. Much can often be done using local labour—perhaps on a food-for-work basis—but some heavy equipment (graders, bulldozers) are likely to be needed if the job is to be accomplished quickly.

Air transport

The characteristics of some aircraft often used in emergency operations are summarized in Table 33/1.

Types of contract

Normal airfreight: Fixed rate/kg on established routes with national or other established airlines.

Trip charters: Normally a basic rental charge plus the cost of fuel actually used for a round trip to a specified destination. Cargo can be loaded up to the allowed capacity of the aircraft for the airports concerned and the conditions prevailing.

Time charter: For a specified number of days, weeks or months. Normally on the basis of a defined rate per hour of actual flying time, subject to a guaranteed minimum number of hours per week or month. (Costs vary considerably with types of aircraft and the actual situation but may be of the order of $ 100-200 per hour for small, propellor-engined aircraft.)

Trip or time charters may be possible with the national airline, other local companies or international companies. An NGO, "Aviation Sans Frontière" (ASF) frequently assists other NGOs and international organizations in setting up and running light aircraft operations in emergencies. ICRC also has considerable experience. Ask EOU for advice if necessary.

439

Table 33/1

Capacities and characteristics of some aircraft

	Maximum load capacity (kg)	Usable volume (cu. m)	Minimum length of runway (m)	Special aspects
Pilatus Porter	950	3	120	Small door
Twin Otter	1,800	12.4	220	Small door
Skyvan	2,100	22	500	Ramp: can take a Land Rover
DC-3	3,000	21	1,200	
Fokker F.27	5,000	65	1,200	
DC-6	11,000	80	1,500	
Transall	17,000	140	1,000	Ramp for trucks
Hercules L.100-30	21,000	170	1,400	Ramp for trucks: can use earth/ grass air-strips
B.707/320C	36,000	255	2,100	
DC.8/63F	44,000	302	2,300	"Stretched" version
DC.10/30F	66,000	412	2,500	
B.747	100,000	460	3,000	

N.B. The minimum length of runway required and the maximum load capacity depend on the altitude of the airports concerned and the temperature. Capacity is reduced for long distances as more fuel has to be carried.

(Adapted from *Red Cross Cargo* ICRC, 1985)

Possible UNICEF inputs

Depending on the assessment of actual needs and possibilities, some of the following inputs might be considered:

—Technical assistance: experienced logistic, workshop or warehouse managers—practical mechanics.

—Funds for: additional (national) personnel—operating costs of co-ordinating units—stationery.

— Funds for contracting in-country transport for the movement of programme supplies.

— Spares and/or funds for the repair of out-of-service vehicles and ongoing maintenance of programme vehicles.

— Provision/rental of additional trucks/boats.

— Materials/funds for repair or improvisation of warehouses for programme supplies. (Exceptionally, prefabricated warehouses.)

— Materials/funds for minor repairs to access roads and bridges.

— Tools and equipment (possibly some construction materials) for field workshops.

UNICEF-assisted programmes might make use of air transport arranged by the government or other agencies for the emergency operation as a whole. UNICEF might participate in cost-sharing arrangements with other organizations and/or finance occasional air deliveries. Only in exceptional circumstances would UNICEF consider itself organizing an operation involving multiple flights over an extended period.

Further references

a. *Vehicle workshop operations,* R. S. Stephenson—International Disaster Institute, London (1984)   E

WAREHOUSING

Objective

- To ensure that materials provided by UNICEF, and those provided by others for programmes of concern to UNICEF, are appropriately stored and handled at all locations where temporary storage and/or stockpiling is necessary.

Warehouse premises

- The possibilities, in order of preference, are: use existing government/ UNICEF stores—borrow—repair—requisition—rent—improvise—construct locally—import (prefabricated).

If it is necessary to establish any warehousing operation from scratch, or to assist the government in improving an existing operation, mobilize personnel with experience in warehouse management as soon as possible. Table 34/1 lists the factors to be considered in choosing a warehouse.

Wherever possible:
- Obtain the use of existing warehouses: arrange repairs (roofs, doors, locks, lighting) if necessary.
- Improvise using abandoned factories, schools, etc.

If no suitable buildings are available:

- Build stores using local materials—wood, bamboo and thatch—and/or tarpaulins, or use tents for short-term purposes and small, local stores. (Ensure that stacks within such stores are raised off the ground and covered with plastic sheeting.)
- Use empty shipping containers (if containers are being received in the ports and can be transported to and unloaded at the sites where stores are needed) or old railway wagons.
- Consider providing (importing) prefabricated structures for long-term operations and large capacity stores.

Establish a proper basis for use of premises. Define responsibility—in writing—for making any necessary repairs or alterations, and for making good any alterations at the end of the operation, if necessary.

Arrangements should be made with local authorities if the premises are publicly owned or if the private owner cannot be located. Interior partition walls might be removed or machinery be moved if the premises are expected to be used for several months at least.

Table 34/1

Choosing a warehouse

Each warehouses should, ideally:

- Be of sound, non-combustible construction;
- Have floors which are level, strong and watertight;
- Be dry and well ventilated: free from rodents;
- Be secure (in doors, windows and the perimeter fence/gates);
- Have easy, but controlled access;
- Have platforms or ramps for ease of loading/unloading;
- Have adequate electric power supply and lighting (available 24 hours-a-day);
- Have an office room/enclosure and secure rooms or cages for small, high-value items; and
- Be as close as possible to the major transport facilities being used in that location—roads, ports, airports, railway sidings.

A single, large building—with sufficient doors for the loading/unloading of several trucks simultaneously—is usually best. Separate buildings can be useful if a variety of commodities are being handled which should be kept well clear of each other.

A secure parking area may also be needed for trucks. Ideally this should be attached to the warehouse (or workshop), but it could be separate.

Size/capacity required

Estimate the volume (cubic metres) and floor area (square metres) required:

a. For temporary/transit storage; *and*
b. For contingency/reserve stocks.

Depending on the situation it may be desirable to maintain a stock equivalent to 60 days expected distribution/consumption for foodstuffs, drugs and other "consumables", plus a reserve of other items (utensils etc.) if any deterioration of the situation—e.g. increases in numbers of displaced persons—may be anticipated.

Table 34/2 provides an example of calculating storage space required. It uses food grains as the example. Indications of the volume equivalents of other commonly handled supplies are given in Table 34/3.

Table 34/2

Calculating storage capacity requirements

E.g. to calculate the space required for 60 days' supply of food grains for 1,000 people based on a ration of 400 g/person/day:

1. Rations of 400 g per day for 1,000 people amount to 400 kg/day = 0.4 MT/day. Thus 60 days' stock = 24 MT.

2. 1 MT(metric ton = 1,000 Kg) of food grains occupies approximately 2 cu m. If bags are stacked 2 m high, 1 m² of floor area is needed for each ton.

3. Space actually occupied by 24 MT = 48 cu m, or 24 m² of floor area, assuming stacks 2 m high.

4. For the total warehouse floor area required, add 20% (multiply by 1.2) to allow for necessary access aisles and ventilation within the warehouse:

$$24 \times 1.2 = 28.8 \text{ m}^2$$

Prefabricated warehouses

These may either consist of fabric stretched over a frame, or be "inflatable"—reinforced, shaped fabric kept raised by air pressure created by a small fan driven by either electric power or a small diesel engine. In either case, a concrete base is desirable: as a minimum, small concrete foundations must be made.

Such units can often be delivered and erected within a matter of 3-4 weeks and, if carefully maintained, can last for several years. Specify: the volume capacity required—any limits on length, width and the position of doors—the means available to deliver the components to the site—whether technicians should be provided to supervise erection.

Figure 34/a **A large frame-and-fabric warehouse in use**

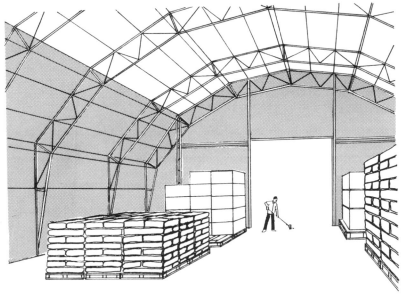

A *frame-and-fabric* unit typically costs (in 1985) about $25 per square metre of floor area, excluding freight, and weighs about 10 kg/sq.m. Delivery time 2-3 weeks (for a unit 15 m × 20 m).

An *inflatable* unit (in 1985): $40 per square metre of floor space, excluding both the electric fan (and necessary generator if power supplies not regular) and freight. Weight is about 8 kg/sq.m. plus the accessories. Delivery time 6-8 weeks (for a unit 15 m × 25 m).

Organizing a warehouse

Staffing and responsibilities

- Select and appoint the best available personnel and give them clearly defined job descriptions, responsibilities and instructions.

- Ensure day and night-guards and, if necessary, labour and supervisory personnel for 24-hour coverage.

The storekeeper/manager must understand that he/she is accountable for all supplies received and for the control and safety of all personnel.

Tools, equipment and warehouse supplies

All stores should have:

—Adequate stationery, pocket calculators, etc. for keeping proper records.
—Steel cutters (UNIPAC 40-850-07), hammers (40-575-05) for opening cases.
—Spare bags and cartons/cases to recouperate and repack supplies from packages damaged during transport and handling.

For large stores, hand-operated banding tools (self-crimping) and a stock of the necessary steel strapping will be useful, say 10 coils (200 Kg). Buy locally or ask UNIPAC. Mechanical handling equipment (fork lifts, conveyors, etc.) can greatly speed up and reduce damage during handling. See Annex 35.

Pallets/dunnage

Wherever possible, raise all supplies off the ground/floor by first laying down pallets or dunnage (sawn timber or beams of any kind). If these are not available with the warehouse:

—Ask UNIPAC and other shippers to state on Bills of Lading that pallets and dunnage used on vessels should be delivered to the consignee;
—Borrow, rent or, if necessary, buy; *and/or*
—Use traditional, woven mats.

This is to avoid the bottom layer being damaged by any water or other fluids which might enter or be spilt, or dampness which might rise through the floor. It is especially important in stores lacking proper floors, and for bagged food even on apparently dry floors in order to permit circulation of air.

Stacking of supplies

- **Build stacks neatly and carefully to ensure stability. With rectangular bags/boxes, orient alternate layers in different directions (at right angles to each other).**

- **Limit stack heights so that dismantling is not difficult and to limit the risk of pressure damage either to the commodities themselves (e.g. bagged food and cement) or to cartons (which might cause a stack to collapse).**

Aisles between stacks should be:

- —Straight and at least a metre wide—more if large packages are to be moved within them;
- —Not more than 6 metres apart; *and*
- —Positioned to gain the maximum benefit from available lighting (both windows and electric fittings) and to avoid stacks obstructing any ventilators.

In tents and improvised shelters, stacks must never touch the fabric of the tent, or the thatch. In open areas, keep stacks away from perimeter walls.

Maximum stacking heights depend on the commodities, the packing and the means of stacking (and dismantling). In general, heights should be limited as indicated in Table 34/3.

Positioning of commodities

Items which are difficult to move and those which are required frequently should be placed near the door(s). Ones which are generally issued together might usefully be placed close together.

Foodstuffs should normally be stored separately from other items. Fuel and oil must be kept separate from everything else.

Label each stack as to its contents. If the space is large and the items many, keep an up-to-date plan showing what supplies are stacked where in both the warehouse and stacking area.

Rotate stocks

- **For all supplies, issue the oldest stocks first—"first-in-first-out".**

- **Don't stack new consignments on top or in front of similar items received previously.**

Even if the items themselves may not deteriorate, the packaging might do so making further handling difficult. Cartons rot quickly in hot and humid climates. Direct sun as well as moisture adversely affects many materials.

Small and valuable items

Shelving—perhaps with bins—may be needed for small items. Ensure that shelves are stable, preferably fixed to the wall or floor. Locked cupboards, rooms or cages within the warehouse may be required for high-value items. **447**

Control of rodents

- Ensure general cleanliness: clean up any spillages, especially of food, promptly.

- Get professionals to deal with any serious problems.

Table 34/3

Volume and stacking heights of common items

Commodity/item	Normal unit package	Approx. volume per ton (cu. m)	Typical maximum stacking height[a]
Food grains, beans	50 kg bags	2	20-40 bags
Flour and blended foods	25 kg bags	2	20-30 bags
DSM in bags	25 kg bags	2.4	20-30 bags
DSM in tins inside cartons	20 kg/ctn (4 tins each)	4	8 ctns if stacked individually
Edible oil in tins inside cartons	25 kg/ctn. (6 tins each)	2	20 if palletized
Oil in drums	200 litres	1.4	2 drums upright: place wood between rims 3 drums on their sides
ORS	35 kg ctns	2.4	3-4 m [b]
Other mixed drugs	45 kg ctns	3.5	3-4 m [b]
Clinic equipment and teaching aids	35-50 kg ctns	4.5	3-4 m [b]
Kitchen utensils	35-40 kg ctns	5	3-4 m
Family tents	35-60 kg each	4.5	Depends on means of lifting/stacking
Blankets (compressed)	bale of 70 85 kg	4.5	

[a] Maximum stacking height depends on the packaging materials (including outer packages/cartons) as well as the climatic conditions, the equipment used for stacking and the skill of the workers. The figures shown above are only rough guidelines: check any specific recommendations given by the suppliers (possibly printed on cartons).

[b] The approximate, average packed weights and volumes of drug and clinic shipments (based on 1985 UNIPAC prices) are:

	Weight	Volume
$1,000 worth of mixed drugs	400 kg	1.4 cu.m
$1,000 worth of ORS	660 kg	1.6 cu.m
$1,000 worth of clinic equipment	125 kg	0.65 cu.m

Rodents and insects are an obvious danger to foodstuffs but also damage fabrics (tents, blankets, etc.) and the packaging of other items. Baiting with poison must, however, be done only with great care, especially when foodstuffs, children and animals are around. If bagged food becomes insect-infested (by weevils, etc.) it should be fumigated.

Handling of fuel/oil

Drums of fuel and lubricating oils must always be stored separately from other items, especially food:

— They should be kept well away from other buildings and frequently used paths;

— If not in a building, they should at least be shaded from sun and rain;

— No smoking must be allowed within a clearly marked perimeter of at least 10 metres; *and*

— Foam fire extinguishers and sand buckets must be placed nearby.

Drums should be opened using non-ferrous tools, and the fuel preferably be drawn from upright drums using semi-rotary hand pumps. Otherwise brass taps which screw into the drums should be used, and wooden frames be constructed to prevent drums rolling when tilted.

Funnels will always be useful, also measuring jugs for dispensing oil.

General safety measures

Inspect all stacks regularly. Dismantle and rebuild any which show signs of collapsing. Clean up spillages of all kinds promptly, especially oils.

Ensure that all mechanical equipment is properly maintained and operated only by authorized users. Personnel should never ride on fork lifts.

Ensure that first aid supplies are available—and someone who knows how to use them. Keep an accident book.

Fire precautions

● **Define responsibilities and actions to be taken by individual personnel in case of an outbreak.**

● **Ensure that fire-fighting equipment is readily accessible both inside and outside buildings.**

449

Establish liaison with the local fire department (if any). Practise fire drills regularly.

Provide water and sand buckets, plus foam extinguishers if fuel and oils are present. Instruct personnel in the use of extinguishers.

Strictly control smoking by all personnel—including visitors and contractors' drivers.

Never store any flammable material in the main store—not even temporarily. Place all combustible waste in metal bins and clear them out regularly.

Security

- **Regularly check the security of all gates, doors and windows, especially if the building was not designed as a secure store.**

Weld bars across window frames if necessary. Put padlocks on the *inside* of as many doors as possible. Establish strict control of all keys.

Do not allow non-employees to linger, especially in areas where supplies are being received and dispatched. Check vehicles leaving the store/compound.

Stocktaking

- **Regularly check the stocks on hand—make physical counts and check quantities against the paper records.**

Thoroughly investigate any discrepancies and take appropriate action to improve security, the supervision of documentation, or the physical arrangement of the store as necessary. If theft is suspected, report it to the local police authorities.

Writing-off and disposal

If any supplies are lost or damaged beyond use/recuperation, the storekeeper should prepare a written report and obtain the approval of the relevant supervisory authority before formally writing off the items in the records. Damaged items/commodities should then be disposed of.

In the case of foodstuffs, consult the local health authorities to determine whether the commodities can and should be made available for animal feed, or must be burned/buried.

In the case of any UNICEF supplies not formally and finally handed over to the government but still in the custody of UNICEF or another agency, the report must be made to the local UNICEF Property Survey Board.

Possible UNICEF inputs

Depending on the assessment of actual needs and possibilities, some of the following inputs might be considered:

— Materials/funds for repairs and/or local construction of warehouses for programme supplies.

— Tools and other supplies for warehouse operations (see Annex 36 for forms required).

— Repair/rental/provision of mechanical handling equipment for major programme operations (see Annex 35).

— Funds for staff and other operating costs.

— Technical assistance—warehouse management.

Assistance should be limited to stores under UNICEF control and/or necessary for programmes assisted by UNICEF.

Where it is necessary for UNICEF offices in the capital, port and/or regional centres to establish and operate warehouses under UNICEF's direct control—to facilitate consolidation and repacking of consignments as well as controlled distribution:

1. Establish necessary agreements with the government.
2. Obtain HQs approval for the budget necessary for the setting-up and operation of a suitable store.
3. Find and obtain the use of suitable premises and establish appropriate records and control systems.
4. Telex details and the store(s) and the stocks held to Chief of Operations/UNIPAC for insurance to be arranged if necessary.

Provide regular reports to appropriate government departments on the movements of supplies and stock balances. If the warehouse will need to be operated over an extended period, plan to train government personnel and hand over the operation to an appropriate government body in due course.

Further references

a. *Food storage manual*, 2nd ed.—WFP (1983)
b. *Guidelines to materials management*, P. Bannister, Field Logistics Advisor— UNICEF/NYHQ (1982)

451

ANNEX 35

GENERATORS AND MECHANICAL HANDLING EQUIPMENT

Objective

- **To increase the rate of handling supplies in ports and warehouses and/or to (re-)establish capacity to lift and move heavy items.**

Priorities

Where electricity supplies are not available, or not reliable, the provision of generators (and lighting sets if necessary) to operate electrical conveyors and permit night working can greatly increase cargo handling rates in ports, airports and any other warehouses.

Where large quantities of supplies and/or heavy items have to be received, the availability of suitable forklifts and conveyors (for bagged food) can greatly speed up handling and reduce damage, especially when goods are delivered pal-letized.

Where existing, functioning equipment is not sufficient, the possibilities, in order of preference, are: borrow—repair—rent—buy. Get the best possible technical advice if any assistance is being envisaged to repair or provide such equipment. The following notes are provided only to indicate what must be specified.

Defining specifications for equipment

Generators

Specify:

- —Required output: watts, volts, number of cycles *and* number of phases.
- —Diesel or petrol engine—should normally be diesel for any unit greater than 2 kw or one intended for long and continuous use.
- —Whether with hand or battery starter.
- —Whether to be used as a completely independent source or as a stand-by to be plugged into an existing installation.
- —What connecting wires and related equipment (e.g. lighting sets) may be needed.

If for stand-by use, full specifications of the existing installation will be required to ensure compatability. In all cases, voltage, cycles and phases should be compatible with those generally in use on the country to avoid the need for transformers.

Provide 30-40% spare capacity (watts) for any units which will be run for long periods.

Fork lifts

Specify:

- —Load capacity (e.g. 2 tons): add 30% over and above what is expected to be the heaviest actual load.
- —Height of lift (3 m sufficient for most operations but 5-8m may be required in airports and some stores.)
- —Length of forks.
- —Diesel or electric: normally diesel in ventilated areas or outside—electric in enclosed areas and if recharging facilities are available (specify voltage and phases of the power supply).

Conveyors

Specify:

—Whether "flat" (to move supplies over a distance on flat or low inclines, e.g. between vessels and warehouses) or "inclined" (to raise or lower packages to/from trucks, stacks, etc.).

—Length—width of belt—maximum weight of individual packages to be carried—capacity (tons/hour).

—Volts, cycles and phases of available electric supply.

If necessary, a generator may need to be supplied to run several conveyors.

WAREHOUSE AND DELIVERY RECORDS

Records required

Record systems need not be sophisticated but must be established at the outset and be understood by those required to operate them. Storekeepers may need to be trained.

Someone must always be responsible for supplies: the storekeeper while goods are in storage, the driver/transporter while they are in transit. At each handover, consignments should be checked for any losses or damage which should then be recorded.

If adequate systems and forms exist within government operations, use them rather than developing new ones. The following records are needed:
—Goods inward record.
—Consignment note (waybill/dispatch note).
—Goods outward record.
—Stock cards.

Goods inward record

A complete, sequential record of all supplies received into the store. Use a hard-back ledger or, for small stores, a simple exercise book. A typical format is shown in Figure 36/a.

File the supply notes/waybills received with each consignment either by source (e.g. one file for each supplier and other point of origin) or in a single series corresponding to the goods inward ledger.

Figure 36/a Goods inward record

Date	From	Ref.	Items / commodity	No. and type of packages	Units/weight per package	Total units/ net weight	Remarks (incl. special marks)

Consignment notes

For each individual dispatch to a particular consignee, issue a "Consignment Note" (or "waybill") which:

— Describes the goods (nature and quantity) and, if necessary, the purpose for which they are issued;

— Identifies the specific consignee and address to whom the supplies are being released, or to be delivered;

— Provides for the driver/transporter taking responsibility for delivering the supplies to sign for them;

— Provides for the consignee to acknowledge receipt, noting the condition of the goods received and any specific shortages/damages.

Consignment Notes (CNs) should be numbered sequentially and normally be produced in triplicate.

— One copy, bearing the original signature of the immediate recipient (transporter) is retained for the store records.

— The original and one copy accompany the consignment.

— The original will be retained by the consignee while the duplicate is returned, via the transporter, to the dispatching store as a final receipt and proof of delivery.

In some cases—e.g. deliveries of UNIPAC sets—the characteristic markings on the packages, including individual box numbers, should be noted. The dispatcher and receiver then have a record of exactly what is being transferred and can relate it to the relevant packing list.

The example of a simple CN provided in Figure 36/b may be used/adapted for most emergency warehousing operations. A more detailed format may be necessary in the case of pharmacies, etc.

Figure 36/b Consignment note (simple)

C O N S I G N M E N T N O T E	Serial no.

Originating Store: _____   Date: _____

CONSIGNEE

(blank box)

GOODS

No. & type of packages	Units/weight per package	Description of items	Remarks/discrepancies

AUTHORIZATION

Reference/signature: _____   Date: _____

WAREHOUSE DISPATCH

Goods described above dispatched in good order except as noted, in custody of:

transporter: *(contractor/individual)* _____   carrier: *(no. of truck/boat etc.)* _____

signature: *(storekeeper)* _____   time: _____   date: _____

RECEIPT FOR TRANSPORT

Above mentioned goods received for transportation and delivery to the designated consignee.

signature: *(driver/contractor)* _____   time: _____   date: _____

CERTIFICATION OF RECEIPT BY CONSIGNEE

Certified that the above mentioned goods have been received in good order except as otherwise noted.

signature: *(consignee)* _____   stamp   date: _____

(original to consignee: copy no.1 to be returned to the originating warehouse duly receipted by the consignee: copy no.2 to be retained in warehouse records.)

Goods outward record

A complete, sequential record of all dispatches made. Use a hardback ledger, or a simple exercise book, similar to that for the goods inward record. Sample format in Figure 36/c.

Figure 36/c Goods outward record

Date	C.N.	Items / commodity	No. and type of packages	Units/weight per package	Total units/ net weight	Consignee	Remarks (incl. special marks)

Stock cards (for different items)

Stock cards provide a record of all transactions (receipts and dispatches) and the balance on hand at all times for each distinct type of item: e.g. 50 kg bags of rice; tyres of a particular size; 20-ft lengths of 2" pipe; etc. A typical format is shown in Figure 36/d.

In some cases it may be desirable to keep separate records not only for different commodities but, within a particular commodity type, for consignments of different origin. (E.g. to establish one stock card for UNIPAC dispensary kits ex "Carrier/SR X" and a different one for similar kits off a subsequent carrier.)

A more detailed format may be required for the operation on a long term basis of, for instance, a spare parts store when part numbers, monthly usage rates, reorder details, etc.

Figure 36/d Stock card

Store: _____   Commodity: _____

Special marks: _____ Type of packages: _____ Units/weight per package: _____

Date	Received from ... / dispatched to ...	Receipts (incoming)		Dispatches (outgoing)		Balance
		Ref.	Quantity	C.N.	Quantity	

may also need to be included. An example may be found in the *Guidelines to materials management* prepared by the Field Logistics Advisor, Supply Division.

Control systems

Authorization of dispatches

If the storekeeper or some other person at the same location is empowered to authorize the release of supplies, he/she may prepare and sign the appropriate Consignment Notes as the authority for the dispatch.

If authority rests elsewhere, the person responsible must issue necessary instructions—usually in writing, by telex or a formal, recorded radio message—to the storekeeper who references that instruction on the Consignment Note.

Verification of correct delivery

Only a limited number of individuals should be authorized to receive supplies at each destination. Their specimen signatures and copies of any rubber stamp they use should, if possible, be provided to the relevant dispatching storekeepers. Storekeepers should check the signatures and stamps on returned CNs.

If necessary, and especially if payment is being made to transporters on the basis of evidence of delivery, get confirmation of delivery directly from the consignee, independently of the duplicate CN presented by the transporter. Do this by:

a. Storekeepers sending lists (perhaps once a week) to each consignee quoting, for each dispatch made to them: the CN No.—the number of the truck or boat—the nature of the goods—the number of packages. The consignee should reply promptly confirming the correct receipt or otherwise of each consignment. *Or*

b. Sending an extra copy of the CN with each consignment (making 3 in all). The consignee should sign and return one copy to the transporter and send the extra copy, signed directly back to the dispatching storekeeper by other, independent means.

Monthly stock and movement reports

For most situations, each location handling supplies (ports, airports, transshipment and storage sites) should prepare, at the end of each month, summary reports **459** showing the quantities/consignments of different goods received, the quantities dispatched (possibly also listing these by destination), and the balances on hand. Copies should be sent to the central logistics control point. A format such as that in Figure 36/e may be appropriate.

Figure 36/e **Monthly stock and movement report**

MONTHLY STOCK MOVEMENT REPORT

Warehouse / location: _____ Reporting period: from _____ to _____

Item/commodity	Units / type of packages	Stock at start of period 'a'	Receipts during period			Dispatches during period			Losses 'd'	Stock at end of period =a+b−c−d	Remarks
			From	Ref.	Quantity 'b'	To	C.N.	Quantity 'c'			

Practical aspects

Printing/copying of Consignment Notes

An original and two (or three) copies will be required of each Consignment Note. If large numbers of CNs will be required, have them printed in pads, possibly pre-numbered and with different colours for the different copies. In many situations, however, it will be necessary—and sufficient—to use stencilled sheets. If the paper is not too thick, two legible copies (carbons) should be possible.

Photocopying completed CNs would be expensive and it would be unwise to have a system which depended on the operation of a photocopier! If forms are printed in pads, control the use of them by establishing a simple register and recording all pads issued.

Loading for different destinations

If supplies for different destinations are being loaded on the same truck or boat, separate CNs must be issued for each consignee.

If the packages are not all identical (especially in the case of UNIPAC sets which comprise several different packages per set), it can be useful to paint special marks on the different lots—e.g. "A" on all items for one consignee; "B" on those for another.

Part 6 REFERENCE
ANNEXES

This part provides a number of sample formats and notes/suggestions concerning aspects of internal UNICEF operations. Most are reproduced directly from the relevant chapters of the *UNICEF Field Manual,* Book E, *Emergencies.*

FORMAT FOR SITREP 01

Prepare the telex in the following format. Include the headings shown (PRIMO—NATURE AND . . .) and present the points under each heading as paragraphs AAA), BBB), etc. Leave a blank line after each heading and between each paragraph. Send it simultaneously to NYHQ, GEHQ and the Regional Office.

FOR (. . . Chief/EOU . . .)/(. . . Chief programme desk . . .)
INFO (. . . Emergency officer/GEHQ . . .)/(. . . Regional Director . . .)

PRIMO—NATURE AND IMPACT OF EVENTS

—The nature of the situation, its primary cause and any immediate secondary effects. The date, time and location.

—The geographic area affected and the estimated total population thereof.

—The general social and economic impact, and particular effects on children. Quote the sources of any official or other reports.

—The reported numbers of dead, injured, hospitalized, and the proportion of the population believed to be affected in specific ways.

—The projected evolution of the situation, including any possible secondary effects (e.g. further flooding or population movements).

SECUNDO—SECTORAL ASSESSMENTS

Brief summary of the main findings of initial investigations/assessment to date in terms appropriate to the situation, possibly as follows:

AAA) Food supplies and nutrition

BBB) Health

CCC) Water and sanitation

DDD) Shelter and household needs

EEE) Special child problems

TERTIO—ACTIONS TAKEN AND PLANNED BY GOVERNMENT AND OTHERS

—The financial and organizational capacity of the government to cope. Whether an official request made for international assistance.

—Actions already taken and/or planned by the government and others. Any needs remaining unmet.

—The mechanisms that exist for co-ordination between concerned agencies and with the government.

QUARTO—UNICEF ACTION AND RECOMMENDATIONS

—Whether any UNICEF staff member has visited the area and/or been temporarily assigned there.

—What immediate relief, if any, has been arranged within the representative's own discretion: how distributed/used.

—What, if any, further UNICEF action/assistance is proposed. Outline the:
Specific nature of the proposed action/assistance;
Estimated cost;
Operational means of implementation;
Time frame/schedule envisaged for implementation;
Suggested method of financing;
Relationship to regular UNICEF programme.

—Whether any further assistance from UNICEF might be proposed later.

QUINTO—ORGANIZATIONAL AND OTHER ASPECTS

—Any security problems for UN/UNICEF personnel. Whether any additional staff support is needed: if so, what and when. Any other matters of internal UNICEF management and organization.

—What documents and other materials are being sent (by pouch, mail, courrier).

—When the next Sitrep (02) will be issued.

REGARDS (Signature)

FORMAT FOR SITREPS 02, 03, etc.

Address as for Sitrep 01, Annex 37. Include the following aspects, as appropriate, in the order presented here:

PRIMO—NEW DATA

—Particular events, developments or new information since the last report.

SECUNDO—PROGRESS OF OPERATIONS

—Progress and problems in implementation of each programme activity of concern to UNICEF since the last report; mention specifically any programme components supported by particular donor contributions.

—Any changes in previously announced plans/intentions, with reasons.

TERTIO—FINANCIAL POSITION

—CFs and POs issued, and expenditures incurred since last sitrep. Balance of funds uncommitted.

QUARTO—NEW PROPOSALS

—Any proposals for new/additional UNICEF assistance:
    Specific nature of the proposed action/assistance;
    Estimated cost;
    Operational means of implementation;
    Time frame/schedule envisaged for implementation;
    Suggested method of financing;
    Relationship to current efforts of UNICEF and others. **465**

QUINTO—INTERNAL UNICEF MATTERS

—Changes in the security situation for UN/UNICEF personnel.

—Personnel movements since last report: present disposition of involved staff.

—Specific problems/questions/needs in matters of supply, finance, personnel, administration.

SEXTO—MISCELLANEOUS

—Particular human interest stories useful for public information and fund raising purposes.

—Any notable visits/contacts with journalists and other visitors.

—What documents, etc. are being sent.

—When next sitrep will be issued.

REGARDS (Signature)

ANNEX 39

REQUEST FOR ADDITIONAL PERSONNEL

Telex simultaneously to NYHQ, GEHQ and the regional office as follows:

FOR (Chief/EOU) / (Chief budget section) / (Chief RSDS-DOP)
INFO (Emergency Officer GEHQ) / (Regional Director)

FOR (Ruritania flood) EMERGENCY, FOLLOWING ADDITIONAL PERSONNEL REQUIRED:

PRIMO—INTERNATIONAL PROFESSIONALS

AAA)... title of post
LEVEL:... proposed L- (or NPO-) level.
DUTY STATION:... location where individual to be based.
MAIN RESPONSIBILITIES:... brief indication of job description and extent of responsibilities to be exercised.
QUALIFICATIONS REQUIRED:... the practical/techncial qualifications and experience necessary.
DURATION:... the length of time for which the person should *initially* be appointed: state if extension is likely or possible.
TARGET EOD:... the date by which the individual's services are required: if particular urgent tasks cannot be initiated before their appointment/arrival, say so; also say if work is dependent on any other actions.

467

OTHER INFO: . . . any other relevant information, e.g. whether local candidates available or HQ should identify candidates; language requirements; ability to use/operate certain equipment; difficult living/working conditions; etc.

FUNDING: . . . BAL/CCF reference or proposed source of funding—whether against special funds or general resources.

BBB) CCC) DDD) etc. . . . . as above for any other international professional-level posts.

SECUNDO—NATIONAL PROFESSIONAL LEVEL POSTS

As above except that it is understood that candidates will be sought and proposed locally.

TERTIO—GS-LEVEL POSTS

Summary of posts by functional title, location, proposed level and duration: e.g.

AAA) ONE WAREHOUSE SUPERVISOR, DISTRICT X, GS6, 6MTHS FROM 01 JAN

BBB) FOUR MECHANICS, DISTRICT X, GS4, 4MTHS FROM 01 FEB

CCC) TEN WATCHMEN, DISTRICT Y, GS1, 6MTHS FROM 01 JAN

GRATEFUL YR PROMPT ACTION AND APPROVAL.
REGARDS (signature)

ANNEX 40

PROPOSING CANDIDATE FOR PROFESSIONAL-LEVEL POST

Telex simultaneously to NYHQ, GEHQ and the regional office as follows:

If for an international post:

FOR   (Chief/EOU) / (Chief RSDS-DOP)
INFO   (Regional Director)

If for a national professional officer post:

FOR   (Regional Director)
INFO   (Chief/EOU)

FOR (Rurutania) EMERGENCY, RECOMMEND IMMEDIATE RECRUIT-MENT FOLLOWING CANDIDATE FOR POST OF ... (title and PAT number if already available) IN ... (duty station) DURATION ... MONTHS START-ING ... (proposed starting date) AT LEVEL ...

FAMILY NAME: ... individual's family name.

OTHER NAMES: ... individual's first, second names.

NATIONALITY: ... current nationality and any previous nationalities.

DOB: ... individual's date of birth

PERMANENT ADDRESS: ... permanent residence, possibly in another coun-try.

469

DEPENDENTS: SPOUSE:... name and date of birth, CHILDREN:... names and dates of birth.

EDUCATION:... list degrees/technical diplomas obtained including main subject, year, name and place of school—e.g. BA SOCIOLOGY 1964 CORNELL UNIV NY USA.

LANGUAGES:... abilities/fluency in different languages.

EMPLOYMENT:... state years of employment, title of post, name and location of employer: for each post indicate "R" if that experience was professional and relevant to the post for which the candidate is now proposed, "NR" if not relevant: e.g.

1985-86 NUTRITION PROGRAMME SUPERVISOR, ITALIAN SAVE CHILDREN AGENCY, DISTRICT X, RURITANIA—R.

1984-85 PUBLIC HEALTH NURSE TRAINER, ITALIAN SAVE CHILDREN AGENCY, BANGLADESH—R.

1981-84 COMMUNITY NURSE, ROME, ITALY—R etc.

[List sufficient to justify the level proposed for the appointment; for recruitments to L-3/4 posts the last 15 years might be appropriate.]

MEDICAL CLEARANCE:... state whether certificate presented and/or examination by UN physician arranged.

OTHER INFORMATION:... any additional information relevant in support of the appointment at the level and step proposed.

GRATEFUL YR PROMPT ACTION. RGDS (signature)

REQUESTING SUPPLIES/LOCAL PROCUREMENT AUTHORIZATION

Requesting supplies from offshore sources

Telex simultaneously to Copenhagen and NYHQ as follows:

FOR   (Chief Procurement/UNIPAC)   INFO (Chief/EOU)

FOLLOWING SUPPLIES URGENTLY REQUIRED FOR (Ruritania flood) EMERGENCY:

AAA)   Description of item(s) and the quantity of each required. For standard warehouse items: the stock number and short description. If supplies are to be set packed, state number of sets at the beginning then list items stating number to be in each set, e.g. 50 DISPENSARY KITS EACH CONTAINING: 01-455-50 SCALE INFANT HANGING 1 KIT, etc. For non-standard items provide necessary minimum specifications (see Chapter 18, pp. 147-148).

BBB)   Background information on intended use. This is particularly important for non-standard items for which complete specifications may not be available.

CCC)   Estimated total cost. (State basis of estimate if appropriate).

DDD)   Mode of transport requested. If airfreight, give justification. Indicate your assumption regarding transport costs or ask UNIPAC for an immediate rough estimate if required.

EEE)   Target arrival date (TAD). State any special considerations such as "NOT USEFUL UNLESS RECEIVED BEFORE ..."

FFF)   Port of entry: seaport or international airport.

GGG) Consignee. State the appropriate number on the established consignee/distribution list held by Supply Division or, if different, the complete name and address.

HHH) Type of packing required: e.g. "WOODEN CRATES, NO PACKAGE TO EXCEED 50 KG"

III) Any special markings required.

JJJ) The BAL/SCF/project code references if available, otherwise ask EOU/NYHQ to provide/advise.

PLS ADVISE ASAP WHETHER SPECS AND TAD CAN BE MET.
RGDS (signature)

Requesting authorization for local procurement

Telex simultaneously to Copenhagen and NYHQ as follows:

FOR (Chief Procurement/UNIPAC)
INFO (Chief/EOU) / (Director/Supply Division)

AUTHORIZATION FOR LOCAL PROCUREMENT OF FOLLOWING SUPPLIES URGENTLY REQUESTED FOR (Ruritania flood) EMERGENCY

AAA) Description of item(s) and quantity of each required: provide reasonable technical specifications for items of equipment.

BBB) Brief explanation of intended use.

CCC) Estimated cost based on local market survey: quote costs for any major items individually, otherwise total cost for the list.

DDD) Target delivery date: if supplies are produced locally, confirm that suppliers can meet this target date: if supplies are imported, confirm that the required quantities are available duty free from stocks already in the country.

EEE) Reasons and justification for local procurement, including date/period when items are expected to be put into use.

FFF) BAL/SCF/project code.

472 GRATEFUL YR PROMPT AUTHORIZATION. RGDS (signature)

ANNEX 42
ORGANIZING AND REPORTING ON FIELD VISITS

Check-list for field visits

Other participants

Try to arrange a joint mission with representatives of relevant government departments and/or other organizations.

Information and instructions

Obtain, *before* leaving for the field:

- [ ] Baseline data available on the area.

- [ ] Information available on the current situation as a result of investigations and enquiries already made.

- [ ] Listing of government officials and other organizations to be contacted. (Have any already been informed of your mission?)

- [ ] Information on vehicles or other means of transport arranged and/or expected to be available in the field.

- [ ] Knowledge/lists of others (organizations/individuals) to whom requests not appropriate for UNICEF should be referred.

- ☐ Guidelines on personal security.

- ☐ Guidelines for contacts with journalists.

- ☐ Definition of the extent and limits of any personal authority to commit UNICEF, to allocate supplies or disburse funds.

Leave behind details of your proposed itinerary and possible contact points.

Things to take

Consider the following:

- ☐ Any permits or letters of introduction necessary—or at least desirable—to travel to and within the area. (In some high risk situations it may be necessary to have an official escort.)

- ☐ Maps.

- ☐ Cash.

- ☐ First aid kit; flashlight and spare batteries; candles; water bottle.

- ☐ Other personal needs: be as independent as possible in food and all other respects.

- ☐ If travelling by road—sufficient water (for drinking and the radiator), fuel, oil and basic spare parts.

Things to do

On arrival and/or as quickly as possible thereafter:

- ☐ Establish means of communication back to the country office (unless returning the same day).

- ☐ Contact local officials, community leaders, representatives of local and other outside organizations already present, etc.

- ☐ Visit, to the extent possible: family dwellings—any temporary camps/settlements—health and social service institutions—water and sanitation facilities—food stores—logistics facilities.

- ☐ Report back regularly to the country office.

- ☐ Take reasonable precautions to safeguard your own health and security.

Sample format for a field trip report

1. Date and itinerary:

2. Participants:

3. Purpose/terms of reference:

4. Persons contacted:

5. Summary findings/observations:
   a. Health and nutrition status;
   b. Food and income: food availability—local production—access of different groups to available supplies;
   c. Shelter and household functioning;
   d. Water and sanitation;
   e. Health service operations;
   f. Community social services;
   g. Special problems of children: unaccompanied—traumatized, etc.

   (Within each sector, note any significant differences between different communities/localities.)

6. Special information concerning particular areas/institutions:

7. Summary conclusions:

8. Follow-up actions required:

475

ELEMENTS OF A PLAN OF ACTION

1. Background and context

Briefly summarise the origin, nature and extent of the situation; the findings and conclusions of the assessment. (The kind of information specified for Sitrep 01, see Annex 37.)

State any assumptions being made. Assumptions typically concern the evolution of the situation itself; the resources to be mobilized from other sources; the behaviour and responses of the affected population, etc.

2. Objectives

Define short-term objectives very precisely and in "operational" terms. Specify:
- —The target areas/populations (defined in terms which enables them to be identified and selected in practice).
- —The outcomes which are hoped for (in measureable terms).
- —The period during which the objectives should be achieved.

Normally, specific training and capacity development objectives should also be included.

Also specify the long-term objectives towards which the emergency intervention is expected to contribute. Envisage the kind of long-term programme which should continue when the emergency assistance is phased out.

3. Intervention strategy

Describe the means by which it is hoped to achieve these objectives—what will in fact be done—what inputs and services be provided.

Specify how the intended target groups will be identified and beneficiaries be selected.

4. Phasing of operations and deliveries

Establish a specific time schedule for implementation of activities, including the termination of "emergency" assistance, phasing out into long-term regular programmes.

Clearly distinguish any separate phases within the overall operation and define the sequence of activities involved within each phase.

Prepare flow charts showing the sequence of decisions and actions, and/or a bar chart showing the phasing of activities over time and the inter-relationship between them.

A "critical path" analysis may help to determine the best, feasible schedule and to identify exactly when particular decisions and actions should be taken/completed in order that others can start/continue as planned.

5. Mechanisms and responsibilities for implementation

Specify how the various activities will be organized, who will be responsible for particular actions and decisions. Ensure that all aspects of operations are covered.

Define the criteria to be used for allocations, and the practical arrangements for actual distributions, accounting and supervision.

Specify what, if any, special units will be established, what their authority will be and how they will be staffed—what arrangements will be made to strengthen existing structures—what the role of community institutions and NGOs will be—etc.

The government, or indigenous organizations designated by it, should normally be responsible for implementation. Where local capacity and resources are limited:

— Include (within the UNICEF budget) assistance to strengthen/augment capacity as necessary at all levels; *or*

— Consider collaboration with an NGO in a joint project—if the government agrees. **477**

Assistance to strengthen capacity might include funds for the establishment and operation of special project units, for the appointment of additional, locally available personnel and/or technical specialists from outside.

Where there is no reasonable alternative, UNICEF may itself undertake certain operational responsibilities. This *might* include the establishment and operation of warehouses; the operation (including maintenance) of small truck fleets; contracting for other in-country transportation (including aircraft); the organization and supervision of distributions; disbursing funds for field operations; etc.

In such cases, clearly define the role and responsibilities for UNICEF as a whole, and of personnel to be appointed/seconded by UNICEF, and make necessary provisions in the budget for all operating costs.

6. Logistic requirements

Based on a thorough analysis of requirements and possibilities (see Annex 29), specify:

—The transport (truck, rail, boat and/or aircraft) capacity which will be needed at different periods, how and from where it will be obtained (by borrowing, contracting and/or purchasing);

—The storage capacity which will be needed at different locations at different periods and how it will be provided;

—The requirements and arrangements for: the purchase and delivery of fuel; maintenance of vehicles; stock control, etc.

Note, however, that while capacity can often be increased by one means or another, the logistics system may—initially at least—impose limits on the quantities of supplies which can be delivered. Take account of the demands of other priority programmes.

7. Personnel requirements

Specify the type and numbers of personnel, including technical experts, who will be required at different periods—and from where they will be obtained (and paid):

—Don't underestimate the manpower required for implementation both from within the community and from outside.

—Remember that the start-up phase requires a greater concentration of experience and expertise that the continuing management of an ongoing programme.

Specify job descriptions and the types of appointments to be given to any personnel to be recruited.

Plan to use the existing resources (expertise) of national bodies, UN and other agencies to the extent possible and available. Envisage bringing in additional foreign personnel only if in-country resources are inadequate.

If short-term consultants are envisaged, specify the number of months required at different periods. Plan for continuity—repeat visits by the same consultant and adequate staff to follow-up after and between their missions.

8. Arrangements for monitoring and evaluation

Specify arrangements for monitoring implementation on a continuous basis. See Chapter 6.

Outline the kind of final evaluation which should be made when the emergency programme is being phased out; how and by whom it should be done. See Chapter 7.

9. Budget

Prepare the total, estimated budget for the programme. Show the requirements during specific time periods and the breakdowns between different contributors. Double-check to ensure that nothing has been overlooked!

Where operations are to be undertaken in different areas, prepare separate budgets for each area plus one for central functions. Then prepare an overall, consolidated budget with the individual components attached. Consider the following budget headings:

Programme Supplies	Specify quantities *and* estimated costs. [Include detailed list, with specifications, in an annex.]
	List items to be obtained locally separately from those to be imported.
Transport of supplies	Purchase and/or rental of trucks or other means of transport. [Attach a list of the vehicles required.]
	Fuel, spares and maintenance for trucks/boats.
	Contracting commercial transport (including aircraft).
Storage and handling	Repair/construction/renting of warehouses.
	Equipment and materials for use in warehouses.
Port charges	Clearance and handling charges in ports and airports.
	Include contingency for demurrage charges!

479

Personnel	Salaries, allowances and travel expenses for all personnel (recruited or seconded) for whom any such payments will have to be made. [Attach a list of personnel including levels and specific time periods of appointments.]
Short-term consultants	Fees, travel expenses—international and in-country. [Attach a list of anticipated requirements stating the particular type of expertise and number of man-months required at specific periods.]
Office establishments	Repair/rental of office and other premises.
	Essential office equipment and supplies.
	Office running costs—expendables, telephone charges, equipment maintenance, etc.
Personnel vehicles	Purchase and/or rental if necessary. [Attach a list of the vehicles required.]
	Fuel, spares and maintenance.
Contingency reserve	Probably 5-10% of total estimated costs.

Include in the budget for UNICEF, "operating costs" to cover all the direct costs of UNICEF's own related operations, staff appointments and travel, vehicle operating costs, and incidental expenses.

ANNEX 44

SAMPLE PROJECT AGREEMENT BETWEEN UNICEF AND AN NGO

PROJECT AGREEMENT

This agreement is made between the ... RURITANIAN CHILDREN'S AGENCY ... (hereinafter referred to as "the AGENCY") and the UNITED NATIONS CHILDREN'S FUND (hereinafter referred to as "UNICEF").

Whereas certain resources have been made available to UNICEF for programmes of co-operation in ... Ruritania ..., and whereas the AGENCY disposes of the capacity to implement programmes in ... Ruritania ... with the approval of and in co-operation with the Government of ... Ruritania ..., it is hereby agreed that UNICEF and the AGENCY will co-operate in the project entitled:

PROVISION OF WATER TO THE DISPLACED
POPULATIONS IN DISTRICT 'X'
....

as described in the Project Description attached as Annex A to this Agreement, and as follows:

Article 1:   Responsibilities of the AGENCY

1.1   The AGENCY shall:

(*a*)   Implement the project and utilize the funds, equipment and supplies provided by UNICEF in accordance with the project description attached as Annex A and with the budget attached as Annex B;

(*b*)   Make available the personnel, supplies and services which represent its own contribution in accordance with Annexes A and B;

481

(c) Be authorized to make variations not exceeding 10 per cent between the items of the budget funded by UNICEF as shown in Annex B providing that the UNICEF allocation is not overspent; any variations exceeding 10 per cent that may prove necessary for the successful implementation of the project shall be subject to prior consultation with UNICEF and signature by both parties of an appropriate amendment to Annex B;

(d) At all times act in consultation with UNICEF and its staff in ... Ruritania ... and avail itself of the advisory services of UNICEF and other United Nations organizations in the country;

(e) Return to UNICEF all vehicles and non-expendable equipment made available to the AGENCY by UNICEF or purchased by the AGENCY using funds provided by UNICEF, and any UNICEF funds unspent when this Agreement expires or at the end of the project; separate loan agreements will be concluded between UNICEF and the AGENCY for vehicles and equipment made available by UNICEF;

(f) Deliver the supplies and equipment listed in Annexes A and B as being part of the AGENCY's contribution and undertake the procurement of other supplies, equipment and services using funds made available by UNICEF as also detailed in Annexes A and B. The sources of such supplies, equipment and services shall be mutually agreed between the AGENCY and UNICEF.

(g) Ensure that its procedures for placing orders or awarding contracts for the purchase or hire of all supplies, goods, equipment and services under the present Agreement, safeguard the principles of economy and efficiency, and that the placing of orders is based on an assessment of competitive quotations or bids.

(h) Maintain separate accounts recording all receipts and expenditures under this project relating to UNICEF's contribution and ensure that any obligations entered into and all disbursements made are satisfactorily documented; for each payment a voucher will be established bearing the project designation, the name of the payee, the amount, purpose and date of the disbursement; original bills, invoices, receipts and any other documentation pertinent to the transaction will be attached to the voucher in support thereof; these vouchers and the attached documentation will be systematically filed in dossiers specifically established to hold the financial documentation of the project;

(i) Facilitate inspection and audit of the project by the UNICEF Internal Auditors or any other person duly authorized by UNICEF on behalf of the United Nations; should they at any time wish to do so, the United Nations Board of Auditors may also carry out an audit of the project;

(j) Facilitate visits to the project site(s) by UNICEF staff or any other person duly authorized by UNICEF to review the operations and achievements of the project during its period of implementation and thereafter;

(k) Submit to UNICEF monthly narrative reports on the progress of operations, and financial and stock reports on the use made of all funds and supplies provided by UNICEF, submit an internal evaluation report on the project every 6 months; each report should reach UNICEF within 20 days of the ending of the period concerned.

Article 2: Responsibilities of UNICEF

2.1 UNICEF shall:

(a) Assist in the implementation of this project by making available the co-ordination services of its staff;

(b) Contribute as total amount of . . . R$123,000/= . . . towards the implementation of the project in accordance with the budget attached as Annex B. The first installment of . . . R$41,000 . . . will be remitted to the bank account designated by the AGENCY within five working days following the signing of this Agreement by the parties hereto. Second and subsequent instalments will be remitted when satisfactory reports and accounts have been submitted covering disbursement of at least 70 per cent of the preceeding instalments.)

(c) Make available supplies and equipment as detailed in Annexes A and B.

2.2 UNICEF:

(a) Shall not be liable for any expenditure incurred in excess of the contribution specified in this agreement;

(b) Shall not be liable to indemnify any third party in respect of any claim, debt, damage or demand arising out of the implementation of this Agreement and which may be made against the AGENCY;

(c) Will not accept liability for compensation for the death, disability or other hazards which may be suffered by employees of the AGENCY as a result of their employment on work which is the subject matter of this Agreement.

Article 3: General provisions

3.1 The schedule of payments referred to above is subject to revision to take into account any contributions in kind as may be made available through UNICEF towards the requirements of the project.

3.2 Should the number of persons for whom assistance is foreseen under this Agreement decrease significantly below that originally envisaged or if, for any reason, circumstances change to reduce the the need for assistance compared with that originally foreseen, the AGENCY shall immediately inform UNICEF; the **483** agreement may then be amended after mutual consultation and the UNICEF contribution be adapted to the new situation or be discontinued as the circumstances may warrant.

3.3 The project governed by this Agreement shall be deemed to have commenced on the ... First of April 1985 ... and shall terminate on the ... Thirty First of March 1986 ...

3.4 Should it become evident during the period of project implementation that an extension of this Agreement beyond the termination date will be desireable, the AGENCY shall immediately initiate consultations with UNICEF so as to ensure that, should it be so agreed, an appropriate amendment to this Agreement may be made before its expiration.

3.5 Any income derived by the AGENCY from funds provided by UNICEF, such as interest on bank accounts or profit from the sale of goods purchased with the UNICEF funds, will be entered into the AGENCY'S accounts as income credited to the Project and may only be utilized for purposes specified in this Agreement.

3.6 If during the period covered by this Agreement, it is considered appropriate to revise or vary any terms of this Agreement including the Project Description, consultations will be arranged among the parties; revisions or variations shall require signature by all parties to the Agreement.

3.7 If during the period covered by this Agreement, the AGENCY is prevented from carrying out its obligations under this Agreement, the AGENCY will report this immediately to UNICEF who shall decide what arrangements, if any, shall be made to further implement or curtail the project.

IN WITNESS WHEREOF the undersigned, being duly authorized thereto, have on behalf of the parties hereto signed this Agreement at the place and on the day below written.

For: RURITANIAN CHILDREN'S   For: UNITED NATIONS
.... AGENCY ....   CHILDREN'S FUND

Signature: ....   Signature: ....

Name: ....   Name: ....

Title: ....   Title: ....

....

Place: ....   Place: ....

484 Date: ....   Date: ....

ATTACHMENTS

Annex A—Project description
This should provide full details of the project along the lines of a Plan of Action—including specification of arrangements and responsibilities for organizing implementation: see Annex 43.

Annex B—Project budget
This should provide a breakdown of the whole budget for the project—along the lines suggested in Annex 43, section 8—and clearly showing which amounts will be covered by the UNICEF contribution and which be the responsibility of the NGO concerned and/or any other parties.

ANNEX 45

SKILLS REQUIRED OF PERSONNEL

A wide variety of skills may be required in emergency operations depending on the role being assumed by UNICEF. This will normally include programming and management skills and, possibly, functional specialists and field assistants.

Programming

Assessment, programme formulation and implementation in emergency situations requires a blend of:

—Previous experience in such operations;

—Good understanding both of the local social, economic and cultural milieu, including the capacities of governmental and other organizations;

—Skills in situation analysis, planning, programming and personal relations; *and*

—Operational abilities (to get things done).

Functional Specialists

Depending on the nature of the assistance to be provided and whether UNICEF itself has to assume any operational responsibilities, specialists may, for instance, be required in: feeding programmes—nutrition surveillance—health care—water supply/treatment—logistics—transport management and maintenance—supply operations—administration and accounting—personnel administration—overall programme management.

Field assistants

In major operations it can also be useful to have, in addition to functional specialists, one or more mature, young staff—with energy, ideas and at least some relevant previous experience—to serve as field assistants working in close contact and communication with the Representative/team leader.

Qualities required

All staff must be very *practical*. Other important personal qualities required are:

—Maturity and a well-structured approach to work and problems;

—A capacity to work under pressure;

—An ability to work as a member of a team (both within UNICEF and with staff of the government and other agencies), being always sensitive to the needs and reactions of other as well as the operational imperatives of the situation;

—Political sensitivity, avoiding hasty judgements and rash statements;

—An ability and willingness to take initiatives and decisions when necessary within the general framework of assigned responsibilities;

—An interest and ability to empathize with the affected community while also preserving a general attitude of detatched objectivity;

—A robust constitution and good health.

ROLES OF OTHER ORGANIZATIONS IN EMERGENCIES

This annnex provides only *very* brief notes. See *UNICEF Field Manual,* Book E, *Emergencies,* reference note R2 for more details.

UNDRO

... HQ, Geneva, unless otherwise decided (see p. 9) co-ordinates UN system response and acts as a focal point—at the international level—for information concerning current disaster situations. Details of outstanding assistance needs of the government and the funding requirements of other agencies—to the extent that these are communicated to UNDRO—are telexed to many potential donors and other organizations.

... can release up to $50,000 for an emergency. In some cases, donors contribute additional, special funds to the organization. UNDRO may use such funds directly, or reallocate them to other agencies.

... may second staff members or consultants to assist the UN Resident Co-ordinator in his responsibilities to co-ordinate UN action at the country level.

... also seeks to promote disaster prevention, mitigation and preparedness, especially in disaster-prone developing countries.

The UNDP Resident Representative is the representative of UNDRO at country level.

UNDP

. . . can release up to $30,000 for immediate relief following a natural disaster.

In the cases of major disasters up to $1 million may, in certain circumstances, be made available for technical assistance in support of rehabilitation and reconstruction projects.

The UN Resident Co-ordinator (usually the UNDP Resident Representative) is responsible to convene meetings of the UN "Team" and co-ordinate UN response at the country level.

WHO

. . . may provide/reassign staff, consultants and/or transport on a temporary basis, and is often also able to offer inputs of medical supplies and equipment. Such inputs may be considerable if special contributions are obtained.

. . . also promotes disaster preparedness and training for health service personnel.

WFP

... may provide emergency food aid where necessary and, in certain cases, make a contribution towards the in-country transport costs of that food and/or the mobilization of transport and storage capacity (and expertise) for its handling within the country.

. . . normally aims to provide an appropriate staple/cereal, a source of protein (e.g. dried skim milk or beans), and a concentrated source of energy (a fat or oil). WFP may, on an ad hoc basis, be able to make special provision for additional items.

Initial shipments of commodities can be authorized at short notice from WFP's reserves: special appeals are made for larger quantities.

To speed deliveries, initial quantities may be borrowed from government or other donors' stocks against replacement when the WFP commodities arrive. (In exceptional circumstances, shipments already en route destined for other programmes in the same or other countries can sometimes be diverted.)

UNICEF and WFP are often able to complement one another in joint/collaborative programmes. WFP may also provide animal feed.

FAO

... may provide technical assistance, by the temporary reassignment of staff, and material inputs: seeds—fertilizers—crop protection chemicals—small tools and equipment for crop production and protection—veterinary and animal feed supplies—transport and storage facilities.

... also operates the Global Information and Early Warning System on Food and Agriculture which endeavours to foresee crop failures.

UNHCR

... assures protection, provides and co-ordinates assistance to "refugees." "Externally displaced persons" *may* also be included, and assistance be given to "returnees."

... is *not* normally able to provide assistance to internally displaced persons, i.e. to population groups which have not left the territory of their own country.

... is able to make rapid, initial responses to refugee emergencies but must then launch specific appeals for continuing operations. UNHCR occasionally assumes direct responsibility for projects, but more usually operates through "operational parteners" with whom it establishes formal agreements/contracts.

Under The Statute of UNHCR, a *refugee* is:
"any person who is outside the country of his nationality or, if he has no nationality, the country of his former habitual residence, because he has or had well-founded fear of persecution by reason of his race, religion, nationality or political opinion and is unable or, because of such fear, is unwilling to avail himself of the protection of the government of the country of his nationality, or, if he has no nationality, to return to the country of his former habitual residence."

Certain regional instruments, notably the OAU Refugee Convention, widen this definition. Equally, various General Assembly resolutions have widened UNHCR's original competence to act to include certain persons not falling under the statue's definition of a refugee.

Until the refugee status of individuals or groups presenting thmselves as refugees has been determined, they are considered as *asylum seekers* and still entitled to the protection of the UNHCR.

Other UN agencies

Other specialized agencies may provide technical advice in the areas of their competence. UNESCO is sometimes also able to provide some equipment and supplies for the restoration of educational institutions and cultural monuments.

Red Cross/Crescent

The national Red Cross/Crescent Society is frequently at the forefront of national efforts to provide relief and health assistance using its volunteers (including medical personnel), transport, stockpiles of relief supplies (where held), local and international donations (latter normally channelled through LRCS).

The League of Red Cross and Red Crescent Societies (LRCS)—the international federation—assists the national society, where necessary, by mobilizing and providing funds, relief supplies, drugs and personnel.

The International Committee of the Red Cross (ICRC), the founder body of the Red Cross, is an independent, private and neutral institution which acts in time of conflict to ensure that the Geneva Conventions are observed, to provide protection, medical care and material relief to victims of the conflict, and to organize tracing services for family members who have become separated. The ICRC collaborates with but operates separately from the national society.

ESTABLISHING A NEW FIELD OUTPOST

An office/outpost for an emergency operation might comprise a simple house-cum-office for a single outposted staff member, or a substantial base for an operational team with office, warehousing and maintenance facilities, separate housing, etc. In all cases, the following must be considered and attended to:

☐ Advise NYHQ and obtain approval in principle.

☐ Obtain government approval (nationally and locally).

☐ Obtain NYHQ approval of budget.

☐ Find suitable premises—rent-free or lease; check insurance.

☐ Assure staff housing, and incorporate personnel in UN security plan.

☐ Arrange necessary office transport and control of its use.

☐ Establish the best possible communications.

☐ Borrow/purchase non-expendable equipment; establish an inventory.

☐ Assure provision of expendable supplies for the office, and personal supplies for staff.

☐ Establish office procedures, administrative and financial authorities, accountability and relationships with the country office.

☐ Establish a proper accounting system; establish bank accounts if needed and possible—get approval from Comptroller.

☐ Ensure proper documentation and filing systems.

These particular actions and considerations are elaborated in the *UNICEF Field Manual,* Book E, *Emergencies,* reference note R3.

SPECIFICATIONS FOR VEHICLES

Choice and specification of light vehicles

Carefully consider the type of use expected to be made of any vehicles and the circumstances in which they will be operated.

Four-wheel drive or not?

4x4 vehicles are often assumed to be necessary for all field operations. This is not the case. Remember that, in comparison with other vehicles, 4x4 ones are:
- —More expensive to buy and may be less readily available (thereby resulting in delays in delivery);
- —Require more specialist maintenance and spare parts; *and*
- —More expensive to operate, consuming almost double the amount of fuel used by the average medium-sized saloon or pick-up truck.

Where fuel is expensive, 4x4 vehicles will be expensive to operate. Where it is in short supply, they may be a great embarassment! In some areas, however, 4x4 is clearly essential.

Diesel or petrol?

Choose on the basis of the relative availability of diesel and petrol in the areas where the vehicles are to operate, and the familiarity of local mechanics with the different types of engines.

Except where diesel is more expensive than petrol—which is rare—diesel-engined vehicles will generally be cheaper to operate and more reliable, although also being more expensive to buy in the first instance.

Where, in remote areas, the operation's trucks are diesel-engined, it may be advantageous to standardize on diesel-engined personnel vehicles also so that only one type of fuel need be supplied.

Type of body

Long-wheelbase station wagons or minibuses are ideal if large numbers of people (e.g. medical teams) are to be transported frequently. Pick-up vehicles with canvas canopies are much more versatile for loading different kinds of supplies.

If particular vehicles will be required to carry both people and goods (at the same or different times), some sort of compromise will be necessary. Double-cab pick-ups may be appropriate in some situations, or the long-wheelbase "hard top" version of the Land Rover or similar vehicles.

Make and model

Choose makes and models depending on the types of vehicles already operating in the country—for which some spare parts should therefore be available and with which local mechanics are familiar.

Within any operation, the maximum possible standardization will also facilitate the organization of maintenance and repair—especially if spare parts have to be supplied (possibly imported) by the operation itself.

In emergency operations, however, price and speed of delivery may be of paramount importance and it *may* be necessary to simply select the best of what can be obtained quickly.

Accessories, special components and spares

In general the "basic" model should be supplied, but again with due regard to what is commonly supplied and used on the country. If local agents/suppliers have standardized on particular specifications, there are probably good reasons for having done so!

In some climates, heaters may be essential (at some times of year), but air-conditioners should be avoided—they can rarely be considered to be truly essential, add appreciably to the cost of the vehicle and its fuel consumption, often break down, and may foster unwanted attitudes of elitism and extravagance.

Special options such as reinforced suspensions and supplementary filters may be appropriate if already familiar within the country. Request vehicles "as per standard export specifications for ..(the recipient country)". Consider whether towing hooks/bars, roof racks, enlarged or supplementary fuel tanks (or racks for jerry cans) may be required.

Ensure that at least a basic tool kit is supplied with the vehicle, and a set of spare parts (for emergencies, usually 15 per cent of the vehicle value according to the manufacturer's experience).

Type of tyres

The choice of appropriate tyres can be extremely important: as with other aspects, get good advice.

Tyres designed for use in sand and not good for mud, and vice-versa. Heavy duty, cross-country tyres may be the most suitable for vehicles to be used extensively on other than hard-surface roads—except in desert or semi-desert conditions when sand tyres are essential.

In general, tube-type tyres (with an adequate supply of repair kits and spare tubes as well as tyres themselves) are to be preferred to "tubeless" tyres as they can usually be repaired more easily in local workshops and are also less affected by any dents which may be sustained by the wheel rims.

Choice and specification of trucks

Consider carefully the kind of *roads, bridges* and *ferries* over which the trucks will have to operate and the kinds of supplies to be carried, thus determine what types of truck will be most appropriate. Note that:

—The movement of trucks and supplies is sometimes more easily scheduled and controlled—and more economic—using a small number of large trucks rather than many small ones. However, large trucks require better drivers, more skilled mechanics, larger workshop facilities, good roads and sophisticated spares—and individual breakdowns have a greater effect on operating capacity.

—Quick delivery and appropriate cargo bodies may be available from local assembly plants.

—Where there is no alternative to importing complete units, compromises are usually necessary between speed of delivery and preferred specifications, including standardization. (It is rarely possible to obtain large numbers of the same type at short notice.)

495

Size of truck

For *long hauls* on hard surface roads, large (20-30 ton) trucks, possibly with trailers, are often appropriate, but check/note:

—Any axle weight restrictions on routes concerned.
—Any legal constraints on the use of trailers and articulated units ("semi-trailers").
—Trailers and semi-trailers can be dangerous (particularly when empty) on bad, pot-holed roads and ferries, especially if drivers are not accustomed to them.
—Twin rear axles (although expensive) are advisable for any unit of capacity greater than 10 tons.

For *local distribution* operations:

—7-8 ton capacity trucks are often appropriate.
—Four-wheel drive may be necessary in some areas.

Other practical considerations

Restrict the number of different makes and models as much as possible to make maintenance and driver training easier and minimize the variety of spare parts which will need to be available.

Prefer trucks which are already familiar locally. Drivers and mechanics will already be accustomed to them and some spare parts hopefully be available.

Standardize on diesel-engined trucks unless there are major problems of availability of diesel in some areas.

High-side cargo bodies are best for the kinds of goods to be carried in most emergency operations, but international manufacturers rarely produce trucks with this kind of body, except to special order which takes time. (Even with standard, low sides, delivery time ex factory is normally at least 3 months.) Local/regional purchase may be possible.

Short or medium length chassis are generally best, especially on bad roads. (Some long platform trucks may however be needed if construction beams are to be carried.)

Tarpaulins should normally be provided for all trucks, and spare parts be ordered and delivered with each one.

Consult UNIPAC for further advice on specifications and delivery possibilities.

COLOUR-CODING OF PACKAGES

The Red Cross, UNHCR and some NGOs all use a common system:

Red   —foodstuffs;
Green   —medical supplies;
Blue   —clothing, tents and other relief materials.

While wishing to remain generally compatible, UNICEF's needs in *major* operations may be different, being related to a broad range of relief and rehabilitation activities in conjunction with different departments/organizations.

The following system is suggested and, if colour-coding is required, should be adopted unless a Representative feels there are compelling reasons for a different system in a particular operation:

Red   —Weaning and other children's foods.

Green   —Supplies for health services/programmes.

Blue   —Household supplies—shelter materials, clothing, cooking utensils, etc.

Black   —Supplies for water supply and sanitation programmes.

Brown   —Supplies for schools/education programmes.

Yellow   —General transport/logistics supplies.

(none)   —Administrative and other supplies.

CRITERIA FOR LOCAL PROCUREMENT

A need and the ability to deliver and use items immediately for life-saving purposes naturally overrides considerations of cost, etc., but otherwise the appropriateness of local procurement must be carefully considered in terms of the:

—Expected timing/rate of use or distribution;

—Speed of delivery possible from local and other sources;

—Appropriateness of the items available and quality thereof;

—Costs from different sources taking account of freight on imports; *and*

—Likely effects on the local market.

The particular factors which, in any programme operation, may justify local procurement (when supplies of adequate quality are available locally) are:

—The locally available items are more suited to programme needs than any that could be purchased elsewhere (e.g. indigenous seeds, utensils, garden tools, etc.).

—Servicing facilities are available only for the locally manufactured products, not for any which UNIPAC might provide from elsewhere.

—The supplies concerned are difficult or expensive to ship from outside the country (e.g. cement, PVC pipes, dangerous chemicals).

—It is desirable to stimulate the regeneration/growth of local production, and avoid undermining markets for local producers: specific objectives, criteria and assumptions in this regard are included in programme documentation.

Local procurement is also indicated for small-value orders when the administrative and shipping costs of international procurement would offset any small price benefits—hence the blanket authorization to place orders up to $5,000 on one SLN, see p. 149.

During the initial relief phase of an emergency operation, urgency of delivery may be an additional and overriding consideration. If needed items are available for *immediate* delivery locally *and* will be put to use before any supplies could be delivered from outside, local procurement may be authorized even for items not corresponding to the above criteria. The urgency and immediate availability should be documented.

If equivalent items are available in the UNIPAC inventory, local procurement will not normally be approved—especially low bulk high value items which can be airfreighted within 48 hours if necessary.

In all cases in which you believe local procurement to be justified, telex Chief Procurement (repeated Chief EOU and Director Supply Division) requesting authorization. Provide all relevant details: see Annex 41.

Take care to avoid unduly disrupting the local market—by pushing prices up or cleaning out stocks—and thus further adversely affecting the local population:

—Co-ordinate with any other interested agencies to avoid needless competition;

—If adverse effects on the market are possible, purchase and bring supplies in from outside the immediately affected area.

SIMPLE ACCOUNTING SYSTEM

FOR A SPECIAL PETTY CASH OR SPECIAL IMPREST BANK ACCOUNT IN A FIELD OUTPOST

When a bank account is possible

Where the Comptroller authorizes a *Special Imprest Bank Account* (based on a recommendation from the Representative), an appropriate, sole-signatory account is opened in the name of UNICEF.

Where a *Special Petty Cash* is to be operated, the holder opens an account at a convenient location in his/her own name (separate and distinct from any personal accounts).

Description of system of transactions

The majority of the funds on hand at any time should be held in the bank; a separate, smaller amount should be held in cash as a *cash float.*

The cash float is drawn from the account at the start and replenished to the same amount at intervals by drawing from the bank an amount equal to what had been spent (in cash) in the mean time.

Ceilings are established—by the Representative with the approval of the Comptroller—for (a) the overall account and (b) the cash float:

—Assuming accounts are to be prepared and the account replenished on a monthly basis, the account level might be equivalent to one-and-a-half times (or twice) the expected average monthly expenditure.

—The cash float level should be sufficient to meet incidental cash payments for several days at a time, avoiding keeping too much cash around at any time.

The country office makes transfers directly into the bank account.

Any large payments are made by the account holder by cheque, not in cash.

Monthly accounts are sent to the UNICEF country office showing—and substantiating with original receipts/certified *petty cash disbursement vouchers*/slips—the amounts drawn from the bank account during the month. The country office, if satisfied with the accounts, replenishes the bank account by transferring an amount equal to that drawn on the bank account in the previous month.

Accounting records

The operation of such a system requires only a cash book, a bank book and a stock of standard UNICEF payment vouchers—plus petty cash disbursement vouchers/slips to record individual, small payments to suppliers/workers not able to provide an invoice or official receipt.

The cash and bank books should preferably have hard covers, although simple exercise books may also suffice. A single book can be used, writing in the cash account entries starting at the front of the book and turning it over to write bank account entries starting from the back!

Ensure that all payments are recorded promptly. Much time—and worry—will be saved in the long run if petty cash expenditures are entered in the cash book every day, and if payment vouchers are completed (and entries made in the bank book) at the same time that any cheque is written.

The cash book

The book should have columns as shown in Figure 51/a.

Each individual expenditure entered should be covered by an appropriate receipt or disbursement voucher/slip counter-signed by the staff member, see Figure 51/b. Keep these receipts together with the cash book until a replenishment is drawn from the bank account. **501**

Figure 51/a **Cash Book**

Date	Nature of expenditure	Amount received	Amount paid out	Balance on hand

The entries and the cash balance on hand should be checked at intervals and every time a replenishment is made. The staff member should place his/her initials beside the balance figure whenever this is done as a record/reminder that the check has been made.

Figure 51/b **Petty Cash Disbursement Voucher**

UNICEF Petty Cash Disbursement Voucher   No.   ....

Office: ....   Date: ....

Paid to: ....   Currency: ....

Expenditure as incurred below:

Account to be debited: ....   Amount: ....

Signature: ....   Approved: ....

The payment voucher

Make out an appropriate payment voucher for each and every cheque which is written, whether for direct payments (e.g. to a contractor or workshop) or for replenishing the petty cash. Type them if feasible so as to have clear copies for yourself, but hand-written vouchers are acceptable:

— In the case of direct payments, the name of the individual or company to which the payment is made should be shown together with a note recording what the payment was for, and the number of the cheque. The relevant invoice must be attached, also the receipt when obtained.

— In the case of replenishments of the cash float: show "cash payments" as the payee—summarize the expenditures which make up the total under a few, appropriate major category headings—attach the original receipts and/or disbursement vouchers/slips to the payment voucher.

At some point the payment vouchers must be coded: i.e. the BAL, CCF, and project codes be entered. Agree at the beginning whether outposted staff are expected to do this or, more normally, it will be done by staff in the country office when accounts are received there.

The bank book

Make an entry in the bank book—see Figure 51/c—for each cheque written (corresponding to an individual payment voucher).

Make an entry (in the "paid-in" column) for each deposit into the account. In most situations the only deposits will be the arrival of funds transferred from the country office.

Also record—in the paid-out/cheque column—any charges levied by the bank on the operation of the account as soon as notification of a charge is received from the bank. (It will be convenient to also record these as expenditures on payment vouchers.)

Figure 51/c **Bank Book**

Date	Voucher number	Cheque number	Paid to ..... for	Amount paid in	Amount of cheque	Balance in bank

Whenever a bank statement is received, check the balance in the bank book against the balance shown by the bank as remaining in the account. Send copies of the bank statements to the country office: these will, *inter alia,* substantiate any bank charges.

Monthly submission of accounts

Prepare and submit accounts to the country office on a regular basis. This will normally be monthly; the Representative may stipulate a different schedule if necessary.

Show the balance in the bank at the start of the month, list all deposits made during the month and all payment vouchers raised (amounts withdrawn and bank charges), and the final balance. If photocopying facilities are available, a simple copy of the relevant page(s) in the bank book will suffice.

Attach the originals of all the corresponding payment vouchers (including, the attached individual receipts) to the statement sent to the country office. **503**

Additional reporting for a Special Imprest Bank Account

When preparing summary accounts at the end of the month, or whenever requesting replenishment of the account, the following must be done (either by the account holder or by the country office on his/her behalf):

— Issue a single receipt voucher to cover all funds deposited into the account during the month/accounting period; *and*

— Prepare a single payment voucher to cover the total of all expenditures incurred during the month/period including bank charges but *deducting* the cash float balance.

Where no bank account is possible

If no banking facilities are available in the area, petty cash funds will be received from the nearest UN/UNICEF office in cash and all transactions be cash. In such cases—hopefully rare—only a cash book will be needed.

When preparing the monthly accounts it may, however, be useful to group receipts/payment slips corresponding to distinct categories of activity/expenditure together attached to payment vouchers marked with that category and the total amount covered by the receipts concerned.

GUIDELINES FOR CONTACTS WITH JOURNALISTS

The following general guidelines are provided for non-information staff who may, from time-to-time find themselves being approached by journalists in the field. They may be superseded by other specific instructions issued by the responsible UNICEF Representative in any particular situation.

Establish identity and credentials

- Always ask to see the credentials of any journalist you don't know—just as you would normally ask any stranger who comes asking questions to identify him/herself.

Make a note of their newspaper, magazine or radio/TV station and a local address. Inform the Representative—or any assigned information officer—of the contact.

Understand the nature of their interest

- Try to understand the journalist's perspective and the type of story/article he/she needs.

- Answer their questions as honestly as you can—see below. Where appropriate, also try to show them another perspective.

Remember that journalists are usually seeking up-to-the-minute stories and that their interests and those of UNICEF may not always coincide. Some visiting from outside the region may, initially, have rather limited background knowledge of the situation and appreciate your help in gaining a fuller understanding.

Speaking "on" and "off the record"

Anything said "on the record" may be quoted, with attribution to the source. It must therefore be able to be officially endorsed and substantiated.

You can say that particular pieces of information you are giving are "off the record" and request that they therefore be used only for background and not be attributed to a named source.

Anything said before a live microphone or camera is automatically on-the-record. Except in an organized news conference, you may ask for a microphone or camera to be turned off if you wish.

If you are not comfortable about making on-the-record statements—or if the Representative has advised you not to give any recorded interviews without prior clearance and guidance from him/herself or an information officer—say so. You might then offer to talk off the record and to put the journalist in contact with others for further information.

Stick to facts. Avoid giving opinions, speculating or criticizing others

- Be willing to provide frankly, objectively and on-the-record any factual information you have, but use figures only when you are *sure* they are accurate.

- Keep your personal opinions to yourself. Avoid making any unnecessary comments about issues not directly related to UNICEF's concerns, particularly when dealing with of "man-made" emergency situations.

- Avoid criticizing the policies or actions of government or other agencies. If necessary explain, off-the-record, why it may not be appropriate for you—as an international civil servant—to comment. Emphasize UNICEF's strictly humanitarian mandate.

In general, emphasize that UNICEF's activities are a part of the co-ordinated, overall international assistance effort in collaboration with other agencies.

If you don't know the answer, say so

Be ready to say you don't know the answer to any particular question. Realize that a refusal to answer may be considered to be on-the-record and may itself become the story!

If possible, direct the journalist to other more authoritative sources for the replies/information sought.

N.B. These hints and guidelines apply to *all* contacts with journalists, both business and social. A journalist is a journalist twenty-four hours a day.

ANNEX 53
CONVERSION TABLES

To convert from units in the first column to the equivalent number of units in the second column, multiply by the figure shown. For example:

8 kilometres	= 8 × 0.6214 miles	= 4.97 mi
5 acres	= 5 × 0.405 hectacres	= 2.025 ha

Length

1 kilometre (km) . .	=	0.6214	miles (mi)	*1 km = 1,000 m*
1 metre (m)	=	1.0936	yards (yd)	*1 m = 100 cm*
	=	3.28	feet (ft)	
1 centimetre (cm) .	=	0.394	inches (in.)	*1 cm = 10 mm*
1 mile (mi)	=	1.609	kilometres (km)	*1 mi = 1760 yd*
1 yard (yd)	=	0.914	metres (m)	*1 yd = 3 ft*
1 foot (ft)	=	0.305	metre (m)	*1 ft = 12 in.*
	=	30.48	centimetres (cm)	
1 inch (in.)	=	2.54	centimetres (cm)	

Area

1 square km (km²) .	=	0.386	square miles (sq mi)	*1 km² = 100 ha*
1 hectare (ha)	=	2.471	acres	*1 ha = 10,000 m²*
1 square metre (m²)	=	1.196	square yards (sq yd)	*1 m² = 10,000 cm²*
	=	10.76	square feet (sq ft)	
1 square cm (cm²) .	=	0.155	square inches (sq in.)	

1 square mile (sq mi)	=	2.59	square km (km²)	*1 sq mi = 640 acres*
	=	259.0	hectares (ha)	
1 acre	=	0.405	hectares (ha)	*1 acre = 4,840 sq yd*
1 square yard (sq yd)	=	0.836	square metres (m²)	*1 sq yd = 9 sq ft*
1 square foot (sq ft)	=	0.093	square metres (m²)	*1 sq ft = 144 sq in.*
	=	930.0	square cm (cm²)	
1 square inch (sq in.)	=	6.54	square cm (cm²)	

Volume

1 cubic metre (m³) .	=	1.307	cubic yards (cu yd)	*1 m³ = 1,000 litres*
	=	35.32	cubic feet (cu ft)	
1 cubic cm (cc) . . .	=	0.061	cubic inches (cu in.)	
1 cubic yard (cu yd)	=	0.765	cubic metres (m³)	*1 cu yd = 27 cu ft*
1 cubic foot (cu ft) .	=	28.32	litres	*1 cu ft = 1728 cu in.*
1 cubic inch (cu in.)	=	16.39	millilitres (ml)	

Liquid capacity

1 litre	=	0.22	UK gallons (UK gal)	*1 litre = 1000 ml*
	=	1.76	UK pints (UK pt)	*= 1000 cc*
	=	0.26	US gallons (US gal)	
	=	2.11	US pints (US pt)	
1 millilitre (ml) . . .	=	0.0675	fluid ounces (fl oz)	*(1 ml = 1 cc)*
1 UK gallon	=	4.55	litres (l)	*1 UK gal = 8 UK pt*
	=	1.20	US gallons (US gal)	
1 US gallon	=	3.79	litres (l)	*1 US gal = 8 US pt*
	=	0.83	US gallons (UK gal)	
1 UK pint	=	0.568	litres (l)	*1 UK pt = 20 fl oz*
1 US pint	=	0.473	litres (l)	*1 US pt = 16 fl oz*
1 fluid ounce (fl oz)	=	28.41	millilitres (ml)	

Weight

1 metric ton (MT) .	=	0.984	long (UK) tons	*1 MT = 1000 kg*
	=	1.102	short (US) tons	*1 kg = 1000 g*
	=	2204.0	pounds (lb)	
1 kilogram (kg) . . .	=	2.205	pounds (lb)	
	=	35.27	ounces (oz)	
1 gram (g)	=	0.035	ounces (oz)	

1 long (UK) ton ..	=	1016.0	kilograms (kg)	*1 UK ton = 2240 lb*
1 short (US) ton ..	=	907.1	kilograms (kg)	*1 US ton = 2000 lb*
1 long (UK) ton ..	=	1.12	short (US) tons	
1 pound (lb)	=	0.45	kilograms (kg)	*1 lb = 16 oz*
	=	453.6	grams (g)	
1 ounce (oz)	=	28.35	grams (g)	

Weight of water: (at 16.7°C, 62°F)
1 litre = 1 kg; 1 UK gal = 10 lb; 1 US gal = 8.33 lb; 1 cu ft = 62.31 lb

Temperature

0°F	*=*	*−17.8°C*

From Centigrade (°C) to Fahrenheit (°F):
  subtract 32 and then multiply by 1.8 (or 9/5).

From Fahrenheit (°F) to Centigrade (°C):
  multiply by 0.555 (or 5/9) and then add 32.

0°F	*=*	*−17.8°C*
32°F	*=*	*0°C*
50°F	*=*	*10°C*
68°F	*=*	*20°C*
98.4°F	*=*	*36.9°C*
104°F	*=*	*40°C*
212°F	*=*	*100°C*

The UNIPAC catalogue (page XXXIII) provides approximate equivalents for many common metric and British/American measures.

Index

The page numbers which appear in *italics* refer to tables or figures on the pages indicated.

511

525